HUMAN HEREDITY IN THE TWENTIETH CENTURY

Studies for the Society for the Social History of Medicine

Series Editors: *David Cantor*
Keir Waddington

Titles in this Series

1 Meat, Medicine and Human Health in the Twentieth Century
David Cantor, Christian Bonah and Matthias Dörries (eds)

2 Locating Health: Historical and Anthropological Investigations of Place and Health
Erika Dyck and Christopher Fletcher (eds)

3 Medicine in the Remote and Rural North, 1800–2000
J. T. H. Connor and Stephan Curtis (eds)

4 A Modern History of the Stomach: Gastric Illness, Medicine and British Society, 1800–1950
Ian Miller

5 War and the Militarization of British Army Medicine, 1793–1830
Catherine Kelly

6 Nervous Disease in Late Eighteenth-Century Britain: The Reality of a Fashionable Disorder
Heather R. Beatty

7 Desperate Housewives, Neuroses and the Domestic Environment, 1945–1970
Ali Haggett

8 Disabled Children: Contested Caring, 1850–1979
Anne Borsay and Pamela Dale (eds)

9 Toxicants, Health and Regulation since 1945
Soraya Boudia and Nathalie Jas (eds)

10 A Medical History of Skin: Scratching the Surface
Jonathan Reinarz and Kevin Siena (eds)

11 The Care of Older People: England and Japan, A Comparative Study
Mayumi Hayashi

12 Child Guidance in Britain, 1918–1955: The Dangerous Age of Childhood
John Stewart

13 Modern German Midwifery, 1885–1960
Lynne Fallwell

14 Western Maternity and Medicine, 1880–1990
Janet Greenlees and Linda Bryder (eds)

Forthcoming Titles

Biologics, A History of Agents Made From Living Organisms in the Twentieth Century
Alexander von Schwerin, Heiko Stoff and Bettina Wahrig (eds)

Bacteria in Britain, 1880–1939
Rosemary Wall

Health and Citizenship: Political Cultures of Health in Modern Europe
Frank Huisman and Harry Oosterhuis (eds)

Institutionalizing the Insane in Nineteenth-Century England
Anna Shepherd

The Politics of Hospital Provision in Early Twentieth-Century Britain
Barry M. Doyle

Psychiatry and Chinese History
Howard Chiang (ed.)

Stress in Post-War Britain
Mark Jackson (ed.)

HUMAN HEREDITY IN THE TWENTIETH CENTURY

EDITED BY

Bernd Gausemeier, Staffan Müller-Wille and Edmund Ramsden

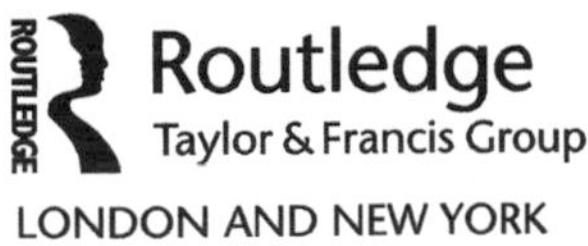

LONDON AND NEW YORK

First published 2013 by Pickering & Chatto (Publishers) Limited

Published 2016 by Routledge
2 Park Square, Milton Park, Abingdon, Oxfordshire OX14 4RN
711 Third Avenue, New York, NY 10017, USA

First issued in paperback 2015

Routledge is an imprint of the Taylor & Francis Group, an informa business

BRITISH LIBRARY CATALOGUING IN PUBLICATION DATA

Human heredity in the twentieth century. – (Studies for the Society for the Social History of Medicine)
1. Human genetics – Study and teaching – History – 20th century. 2. Human genetics – Social aspects. 3. Human genetics – Political aspects.
I. Series II. Gausemeier, Bernd editor of compilation. III. Muller-Wille, Staffan, 1964– editor of compilation. IV. Ramsden, Edmund editor of compilation.
599.9'35-dc23

ISBN-13: 978-1-138-66229-2 (pbk)
ISBN-13: 978-1-8489-3426-9 (hbk)

Typeset by Pickering & Chatto (Publishers) Limited

CONTENTS

Acknowledgements ix
List of Contributors xi
List of Figures and Tables xvii

Introduction: Human Heredity in the Twentieth Century – *Bernd Gausemeier, Staffan Müller-Wille and Edmund Ramsden* 1
Part I: Constructing Surveys of Heredity
1 Borderlands of Heredity: The Debate about Hereditary Susceptibility to Tuberculosis, 1882–1945 – *Bernd Gausemeier* 13
2 Championing a US Clinic for Human Heredity: Pre-War Concepts and Post-War Constructs – *Philip K. Wilson* 27
3 Remodelling the Boundaries of Normality: Lionel S. Penrose and Population Surveys of Mental Ability – *Edmund Ramsden* 39
Part II: Blood and Populations
4 From 'Races' to 'Isolates' and 'Endogamous Communities': Human Genetics and the Notion of Human Diversity in the 1950s – *Veronika Lipphardt* 55
5 Between the Transfusion Services and Blood Group Research: Human Genetics in Britain during World War II – *Jenny Bangham* 69
6 The Abandonment of Race: Researching Human Diversity in Switzerland, 1944–56 – *Pascal Germann* 85
7 Post-War and Post-Revolution: Medical Genetics and Social Anthropology in Mexico, 1945–70 – *Edna Suárez-Diaz and Ana Barahona* 101
Part III: Human Heredity in the Laboratory
8 From Agriculture to Genomics: The Animal Side of Human Genetics and the Organization of Model Organisms in the Longue Durée – *Alexander von Schwerin* 113
9 Cereals, Chromosomes and Colchicine: Crop Varieties at the Estación Experimental Aula Dei and Human Cytogenetics, 1948–58 – *María Jesús Santesmases* 127

10 Putting Human Genetics on a Solid Basis: Human Chromosome Research, 1950s–1970s – *Soraya de Chadarevian* 141
Part IV: Understanding and Managing Disease
11 The Disappearance of the Concept of Anticipation in the Post-War World – *Judith E. Friedman* 153
12 'The Most Hereditary of All Diseases': Haemophilia and the Utility of Genetics for Haematology, 1930–70 – *Stephen Pemberton* 165
13 How PKU Became a Genetic Disease – *Diane B. Paul* 179
Part V: Reconstructing Discipline(s)
14 The Emergence of Genetic Counselling in the Federal Republic of Germany: Continuity and Change in the Narratives of Human Geneticists, *c.* 1968–80 – *Anne Cottebrune* 193
15 Performing Anger: H. J. Muller, James V. Neel and Radiation Risk – *Susan Lindee* 205
16 The Struggle for Authority over Italian Genetics: The Ninth International Congress of Genetics in Bellagio, 1948–53 – *Francesco Cassata* 217

Notes 229
Index 291

ACKNOWLEDGEMENTS

The contributions to this volume go back to a conference organized at the University of Exeter in September 2010. The conference was kindly supported by the Max Planck Institute for the History of Science, Berlin, and through a Conference Grant by the Wellcome Trust (Grant WT092323). The event was the last in a series of workshops that were organized within the context of a long-term, interdisciplinary project dedicated to the Cultural History of Heredity, which received continuous funding in the years 2001–9 from the Karl Schaedler Foundation, Liechtenstein. For documentation of the workshops, and the project as a whole, see http://www.mpiwg-berlin.mpg.de/en/research/projects/DeptIII_Cultural_History_Heredity/index_html [accessed 29 August 2012].

We are especially grateful to Hans-Jörg Rheinberger for his indefatigable personal support, and to Claire Keyte, Birgitta von Mallinckrodt and Antje Radeck for their stellar administrative advice and help. We would like to thank Luc Berlivet, Peter Harper, Brad Hume, Djatou Medard, Hans-Jörg Rheinberger, Miguel Garcia Sanchez, Helga Satzinger, Nathaniel Comfort, Paul Weindling and Jan Witkowski, who all helped to develop the arguments presented in this book with their comments and contributions. Our thanks also extend to Ruth Ireland, Mark Pollard and David Cantor for their careful editorial supervision.

LIST OF CONTRIBUTORS

Jenny Bangham is a research scholar at the Max Planck Institute for the History of Science, Berlin. She was formerly a geneticist at University College London and the University of Edinburgh, where she published several papers on evolutionary genetics. She then moved to the University of Cambridge to complete an MPhil and PhD in the Department of History and Philosophy of Science. Her current work is about the history of mid-twentieth-century human genetics, anthropology and geography.

Ana Barahona completed her training in biology and her graduate studies at the Universidad Nacional Autónoma de México (UNAM). This was followed by a year at Harvard University with Professor Everett Mendelshon, and postdoctoral studies at the University of California, Irvine with Francisco J. Ayala. She is a full-time professor in the Department of Evolutionary Biology of the School of Sciences at UNAM. Having pioneered the historical and philosophical study of science in Mexico from 1980, at UNAM she founded the Social Studies of Science and Technology in the School of Sciences. Her interests focus on the history and philosophy of biology, and the relation between epistemology and science education. Among her published works are more than fifty specialized articles, several books, and textbooks for elementary, middle-school and college education in biology, history and the philosophy of science. She is a member of the Mexican Academy of Sciences and of the National System of Investigators, CONACyT, Mexico. She has been a member of the board of directors (2001–5), president elect (2007–9) and president (2009–11) of the International Society for the History, Philosophy and Social Studies of Biology, and a member of the International Committee of Sigma Xi, the Scientific Research Society. She is currently a member of the editorial boards of the *Journal of the History of Biology*, *Biological Theory*, *Almagest* and *Science & Education*, a council member of the Division of History of Science and Technology of the International Union for the History and Philosophy of Science (DHST/IUHPS), and vice-president of the Iberoamerican Association of Philosophy of Biology. She has been recently acknowledged as a Corresponding Member of the International Academy for the History of Science.

Francesco Cassata is Assistant Professor of Contemporary History at the University of Genoa. His main areas of interest include the history of eugenics, the history of genetics and molecular biology, the history of Lysenkoism and the history of scientific racism. His current research focuses on the history of EMBO-EMBC-EMBL and on the radiogenetic and mutagenesis programme of durum wheat at the Casaccia Nuclear Energy Research Centre in Rome from the 1950s to 1980s. His publications include *Building the New Man: Eugenics, Racial Science and Genetics in Twentieth-Century Italy* (Budapest: CEU Press, 2011), 'The Italian Communist Party and the "Lysenko Affair"', *Journal of the History of Biology*, 45:3 (2012), pp. 469–98, and *L'Italia intelligente. Adriano Buzzati-Traverso e il Laboratorio internazionale di genetica e biofisica (1962–1969)* (Rome: Donzelli, 2013).

Anne Cottebrune is a research scholar in the Institute of Medical History at the University of Giessen. She received her PhD in 2001 from École des Hautes Études en Sciences Sociales in Paris, followed by research projects at the universities of Heidelberg and Giessen supported by the German Research Foundation. Her research activities are devoted to the history of human genetics and eugenics in Germany in the twentieth century. Her publications include *Der planbare Mensch. Die Deutsche Forschungsgemeinschaft und die menschliche Vererbungswissenschaft, 1920–1970* (Stuttgart: Steiner, 2008) and 'Eugenische Konzepte in der westdeutschen Humangenetik, 1945–1980', *Journal of Modern European History*, 10:4 (2012), pp. 500–18. She is currently pursuing a research project on the history of genetic counselling in the Federal Republic of Germany.

Soraya de Chadarevian is Professor of History of Science, Medicine and Technology at the Department of History and the Institute for Society and Genetics of the University of California, Los Angeles. Her publications include *Designs for Life: Molecular Biology after World War II* (Cambridge: Cambridge University Press, 2002; paperback 2011) and the co-edited (with Nick Hopwood) volume *Models: The Third Dimension of Science* (Stanford, CA: Stanford University Press, 2004), as well as numerous other publications on the history of molecular biology and the modern life sciences more generally. She is currently working on a book on chromosomes and human heredity in the post-war era.

Judith E. Friedman completed her PhD at the University of Victoria, Canada, and has since worked as a Postdoctoral Fellow at the Max Planck Institute for the History of Science, Berlin, and as a DeWitt Stetten Postdoctoral Fellow at the National Institutes of Health, Bethesda, Maryland. She has been publishing on the history of research into non-Mendelian inheritance patterns, and editing the Genetics and Medicine Historical Network Newsletter.

Bernd Gausemeier is a research scholar at the Max Planck Institute for the History of Science in Berlin. His research focuses on the interplay of the life sciences, politics and economy in the twentieth century. He is the author of *Natürliche Ordnungen und politische Allianzen. Biologische und biochemische Forschung in Kaiser-Wilhelm-Instituten 1933–1945* (Göttingen: Wallstein, 2005), which examines biological research in Nazi Germany. He has also worked and published on the methodological foundations of the study of human heredity in the nineteenth and early twentieth centuries. His current project concerns the history of the biomedical research campus in Berlin-Buch.

Pascal Germann is a PhD candidate in the doctoral programme 'History of Knowledge' at the History of Knowledge Centre of Competence at the ETH Zurich and the University of Zurich, where he is working on a project about the history of racial research and human genetics in Switzerland. He was a pre-doctoral research fellow in the ESRC Centre for Genomics in Society at the University of Exeter and at the Max Planck Institute for the History of Science in Berlin. He is currently working as a scientific assistant at the Research Unit for Social and Economic History at the University of Zurich. His research focuses on the history of physical anthropology, blood group research, medical genetics and eugenics.

Susan Lindee is a historian at the University of Pennsylvania, where she studies historical and contemporary questions raised by human and medical genetics and genomic medicine. She is now the Associate Dean of the Social Sciences and the Janice and Julian Bers Professor of the History of Science at the University of Pennsylvania. Her books include *Suffering Made Real: American Science and the Survivors at Hiroshima* (Chicago, IL: University of Chicago Press, 1994), *The DNA Mystique: The Gene as a Cultural Icon* (New York: Freeman, 1995) with the late sociologist Dorothy Nelkin, and *Moments of Truth in Genetic Medicine* (Baltimore, MD: Johns Hopkins University Press, 2005). Lindee has also been involved in collaborations with anthropologists, including her work with Alan Goodman and Deborah Heath on the edited volume *Genetic Nature/Culture: Anthropology and Science Beyond the Two-Culture Divide* (Berkeley, CA: University of California Press, 2003) and her co-edited special issue of *Current Anthropology*, 'The Biological Anthropology of Living Human Populations: World Histories, National Styles and International Networks' (April 2012). Lindee is a Guggenheim Fellow, a Weiler Fellow and winner of a Burroughs Wellcome Fund Fortieth Anniversary Award and the Schuman Prize of the History of Science Society.

Veronika Lipphardt is a Professor at the Free University Berlin and the Research Group Director at the Max Planck Institute for the History of Science, Berlin. She has published on the history of human genetics and physical anthropology, the history of concepts of human variation (including race), and German-Jewish and European history. She is currently working on a book about human population genetics in the post-war period. Her first book, *Biologie der Juden: Jüdische Wissenschaftler über 'Rasse' und Vererbung 1900–1935* (Göttingen: Vandenhoeck and Ruprecht, 2008), dealt with German-Jewish scientists before 1935 and how they conceived of race and heredity.

Staffan Müller-Wille is a Senior Lecturer at the University of Exeter, where he is associated with the ESRC Centre for Genomics in Society and the Centre for Medical History. He has published extensively on the history of natural history, heredity and genetics. Together with Hans-Jörg Rheinberger, he co-authored *A Cultural History of Heredity* (Chicago, IL: University of Chicago Press, 2012) and co-edited *Heredity Produced: At the Crossroads of Biology, Politics, and Culture 1500–1870* (Cambridge, MA: MIT Press, 2007).

Diane B. Paul is Professor Emerita of Political Science at the University of Massachusetts Boston and an Associate in Zoology at the Museum of Comparative Zoology, Harvard University. Her work principally focuses on the histories of evolution and genetics, especially in respect to eugenics and to population and medical genetics. She is the author of *Controlling Human Heredity: 1865 to the Present* (Amherst, NY: Humanity Books, 1995), *The Politics of Heredity: Essays on Eugenics, Biomedicine, and the Nature-Nurture Debate* (Albany, NY: SUNY Press, 1998), 'Darwin, Social Darwinism, and Eugenics', in J. Hodge and G. Radick (eds), *The Cambridge Companion to Darwin*, 2nd edn (Cambridge: Cambridge University Press, 2009), pp. 219–45, and, with Jeffrey Brosco, *The PKU Paradox: A Short History of a Genetic Disease* (Baltimore, MD: Johns Hopkins University Press, 2013). Among her current projects are studies of Robert FitzRoy, captain of the HMS *Beagle*, and of how we think and should think about rare disorders.

Stephen Pemberton is an Associate Professor in the Federated Department of History of the New Jersey Institute of Technology and Rutgers University, Newark, New Jersey. His research focuses on the interwoven histories of chronic disease management and hereditary disease. He is the author of *The Bleeding Disease: Hemophilia and the Unintended Consequences of Medical Progress* (Baltimore, MD: Johns Hopkins University Press, 2011), and together with Keith Wailoo, he co-authored *The Troubled Dream of Genetic Medicine: Ethnicity and Innovation in Tay-Sachs, Cystic Fibrosis and Sickle Cell Disease* (Baltimore, MD: Johns Hopkins University Press, 2006).

Edmund Ramsden is a research assistant working on a Wellcome Trust-funded project on the history of the dog in science and medicine at the Centre for the History of Science, Technology and Medicine, University of Manchester. His present research is focused on the history of experimental psychiatry and psychobiology in the United States, and the use of experimental animals in the physiological, behavioural and biomedical sciences more broadly. He has also worked on the history of the social and biological sciences and their relations, with a particular focus on eugenics, demography and population genetics, and the history of population surveys of growth, development and intellectual ability.

María Jesús Santesmases is a Senior Researcher at the Centro de Ciencias Humanas y Sociales of the Consejo Superior de Investigaciones Científicas in Madrid. She has published on the history of biochemistry, molecular biology and antibiotics. Her current research project is on the history of cytogenetics and cell biology. She co-edited, with Angela Creager, the special issue on 'Radioisotopes in the Atomic Age' of the *Journal of the History of Biology* (2006); with Christoph Gradmann, *Circulation of Antibiotics: Journeys of Drug Standards* for the journal *Dynamis* (2011); and, with Teresa Ortiz, *Gendered Drugs and Medicine: Historical and Socio-Cultural Perspectives* (Farnham: Ashgate, forthcoming).

Edna Suárez-Díaz is a historian and philosopher of science who specializes in the twentieth-century life sciences. She is a Full Professor at the School of Sciences at the Universidad Nacional Autónoma de México (UNAM). She has published on the history of molecular evolution and the construction of objectivity in molecular phylogenetics in journals such as *Science in Context*, *Studies in the History and Philosophy of Biological and Biomedical Sciences* and *History and Philosophy of the Life Sciences*, among others. She is the editor of *Ciencia y Representación* (Mexico City: UNAM, 2007) and co-author, with Sergio Martínez, of *Ciencia e Tecnología en Sociedad* (Mexico City: UNAM, 2009). Currently she in charge of two research projects: 'Internationalization and Standardization of the Life Sciences after World War II' and 'Genes and Atoms in Mexico during the Cold War Era'. Together with Gisela Mateos, she is presently writing a book on Cold War science in Mexico.

Alexander von Schwerin is a research scholar in the Department for the History of Pharmacy and Science at the Technical University of Braunschweig. His research focuses on the history of genetics and biomedicine, historical and political epistemology, and the history of things and regulation. He is the author of *Experimentalisierung des Menschen. Der Genetiker Hans Nachtsheim und die vergleichende Erbpathologie, 1920–1945* (Göttingen: Wallstein, 2004). He has co-edited, with Luis Campos, *Making Mutations: Objects, Practices, Contexts* (Berlin: Max Planck Institute for the History of Science, Preprint 393, 2010) and, with Heiko Stoff and Bettina Wahrig, *Biologics, A History of Agents Made from Living Organisms in the Twentieth Century* (London: Pickering & Chatto, 2013).

Philip K. Wilson is Professor and Chair of History at East Tennessee State University, having previously served as Professor of Medical Humanities and Science, Technology and Society as well as Director of the Doctors Kienle Center for

Humanistic Medicine at Penn State University, and as the biomedical and health editor for *Encyclopaedia Britannica*. Following PhD studies at University College London, he has pursued research into the history of disease, human reproduction, eugenics and medical genetics, chocolate and health, geohistory, and the intersections of spirituality and medicine. His publications include the five-volume edited series *Childbirth: Changing Ideas and Practices in Britain and America 1600 to the Present* (New York: Garland, 1996), the co-authored (with W. Jeffrey Hurst) *Chocolate as Medicine: A Quest over the Centuries* (Cambridge: RSC Publishing, 2012), and book-length biographies on the English proponent of cold bathing, Sir John Floyer, the Enlightenment London surgical reformer, Daniel Turner, and Charles Darwin's illustrious grandfather, the polymath, Dr Erasmus Darwin.

LIST OF FIGURES AND TABLES

Figure 3.1: 'Stable genetical equilibrium in a population with fully assortive mating and strongly negative correlation between intelligence and family size', from L. S. Penrose, *Outline of Human Genetics* (1959) 48
Figure 5.1: Stills from two wartime public information films, *Blood Transfusion Service* (1941) and *Blood Grouping* (1955) 72
Figure 5.2: The paperwork of the depots, captured from stills from a wartime public information film, *Blood Transfusion Service* (1941) 74
Figure 5.3: Schematic showing the Rhesus locus in terms of the new Fisher-Race scheme, from 'Medical Research Council Memorandum no. 19: The Rh Blood Groups and their Clinical Effects' (1948) 81
Figure 6.1: Blood group map of Switzerland: the distribution of ABO-genes according to 'municipalities of origin', from S. Rosin, 'Die Verteilung der AB0-Blutgruppen in der Schweiz', *Archiv der Julius Klaus-Stiftung für Vererbungsforschung, Sozialanthropologie und Rassenhygiene* (1956) 88
Figure 6.2: Detail from blood group map of Switzerland 89
Figure 9.1: Joe Hin Tjio and Enrique Sánchez-Monge in Svalöf, 1947 128
Figure 9.2: Metaphase chromosomes of speltoid wheat, from E. Sánchez-Monge and J. MacKey, 'On the Origin of Subcompactoids in Triticum Vulgare', *Anales de la Estación Experimental Aula Dei* (1949) 131
Figure 9.3: Polyploidy and colchicine mitosis, from J. H. Tjio and A. Levan, 'The Use of Oxyquinoline in Chromosome Analysis', *Anales de la Estación Experimental Aula Dei* (1950) 133
Figure 11.1: Age of onset in dystrophia myotonica, from L. Penrose, 'The Problem of Anticipation in Pedigrees of Dystrophia Myotonica', *Annals of Eugenics* (1948) 155
Figure 11.2: Age of onset correlation table showing relationship of dates of onset, from L. Penrose, 'The Problem of Anticipation in Pedigrees of Dystrophia Myotonica', *Annals of Eugenics* (1948) 156

Table 6.1: Distribution of racial types in the Swiss population, from O. Schlaginhaufen, *Anthropologia Helvetica. Die Anthropologie der Eidgenossenschaft*, Vol. 1 (1946) 87
Table 11.1: Human or medical genetics textbooks, 1949–70 160

INTRODUCTION: HUMAN HEREDITY IN THE TWENTIETH CENTURY

Bernd Gausemeier, Staffan Müller-Wille and Edmund Ramsden

Ideas and knowledge about the inheritance of physical and mental characters in humans, whether normal or pathological, form one of the most important elements of intellectual and scientific life of the twentieth century. From the heyday of explicitly eugenic projects and programmes in the early decades of the century, to the reconstitution of concerns with human heredity as 'medical' and 'human' genetics in the wake of World War II, to the campaign to 'decode' the human genome at the close of the century: the definition and control of hereditary traits have been a major concern, if not a metaphysical centrepiece, of biomedicine and public health.[1] From our present-day perspective, we identify the scientific – as opposed to medical or political – endeavours in this field with the discipline of human genetics, that is, with scientific practices aiming at the determination of genetic factors affecting human characters. In this spirit, the twentieth century has been referred to, in critical retrospection, as the 'century of the gene'.[2] Yet not all projects and practices concerned with phenomena of human heredity in the twentieth century were focused on, or even concerned with, 'genes'. Anthropological concepts of race and ethnicity, for example, continued to have a legacy in human genetics, as did medical ideas about susceptibility or constitutional disposition, and sociological and psychological ideas regarding class, inheritance and ability. Moreover, many of the technologies and procedures that have been employed to detect hereditary differences – for example, serological test methods, chromosome analysis, tests of mental ability or anthropometric measurements – were imported from disciplinary contexts in which they often served a very different function to that of identifying genes. Thus the field of research about human heredity comprises a wide range of practices and ideas that transcend disciplinary borders.

This is hardly surprising. In fact, until the advent in the early 1970s of molecular tool kits of biotechnology that allowed for the sequencing and manipulation of DNA, and the development of reproductive technologies such as in vitro fertilization and cloning, humans were problematic subjects for genetic analysis.

Unlike the domesticated plants and animals that early Mendelians worked with, and unlike the highly standardized model organisms of classical and molecular genetics (such as *Drosophila melanogaster*, *Escherichia coli* or bacteriophages), humans can hardly be forced into the folds of genealogical constructs, such as 'pure lines', 'reciprocal crosses' or 'back-crosses'; nor is it easy to control confounding factors, such as nutrition, class or lifestyle, through careful experimental design.[3] Instead, researchers had to seek out highly contingent and – more often than not – idiosyncratic situations that more or less 'spontaneously' produced or enhanced phenomena of human heredity. The many problems that confront the student of heredity, as population geneticist Leslie Clarence Dunn put it so concisely in the 1950s, are 'the price [the investigator] pays for dealing with animals over which he has no control'.[4]

This is why we focus in this volume on the history of human heredity, rather than human genetics, in the twentieth century. We seek to widen the perspective from human genetics to all the concepts, practices and institutional frameworks that were involved in the production of knowledge about aspects of human nature that have been, and sometimes continue to be, considered as 'hereditary'. By focusing on a time frame from the end of World War I, when genetics had consolidated itself as an academic discipline, to the early 1970s, when the advent of molecular biotechnologies once more changed the scene, we hope to point out continuities and breaks in this broad field. By combining essays dealing with similar developments in different contexts, this volume allows for a comparative view on national, local and professional conditions. And finally, by featuring case studies from anthropology, psychology, experimental biology and various medical fields, we confront the mainstream narrative of genetics with its complement, that is to say the professional contexts that not only received methods and concepts from the science of genetics but also produced theoretical and technical approaches that became important for the whole field of human heredity. Medicine takes pride of place in the latter respect, and yet it is no coincidence that Ilana Löwy and Jean-Paul Gaudillière – the two editors of the only volume thus far which covers substantial aspects of the stories we tell in this volume – chose the more general phenomenon of disease transmission, rather than heredity, as their focus. Medicine, although a crucial context for the production of knowledge about human heredity, was not by itself a genetic science, nor was it even uniquely receptive to the tools and concepts that this discipline offered. Rather, questions of heredity, infection and immunization remained inextricably entangled for clinicians and epidemiologists.[5]

Although historical studies, especially in the history of medicine, have occasionally touched upon many of the topics outlined above,[6] there is as yet no comprehensive overview of the history of human heredity in the twentieth century. Its beginning is usually identified with the rise of Mendelian genetics, and the historiography of human genetics is still widely dominated by a 'Whiggish' perspective that prioritizes discoveries that fed into what is today accepted as truthful.[7] The notable historical introduction to Friedrich Vogel and Arno Motulsky's textbook of human genetics may serve as an example of this mainstream narrative. After giving a short overview of nineteenth-century ideas of heredity, the authors quickly focus in on two historical actors that provided the 'paradigms' with which 'the field as a science' began: Galton, the pioneer of a statistical approach to human heredity, and Mendel, the originator of the concept of particulate inheritance that was to transform a field of 'pre-scientific' speculations into a theory-driven discipline.[8] The beginnings of human genetics proper, however, are identified with the work of one man, Archibald Garrod, who first suggested the Mendelian inheritance of alkaptonuria in 1902.[9]

The attention that is often devoted to the case of Garrod in this, and other accounts, is a telling historiographical construct. Garrod was, in fact, not the only student of human heredity in his time to claim Mendelian inheritance for a human character. One only needs to remind oneself of the propensity of Charles Davenport, the founder of the Eugenics Record Office on the grounds of Cold Spring Harbour, and one of the earliest proponents of Mendelism, to claim that 'properties' like alcoholism, pauperism or 'wanderlust' were inherited according to the rules laid down by Mendel.[10] Nor had other physicians failed to notice that a number of diseases seemed to follow Mendelian patterns in their transmission across generations.[11] Like these other 'pioneers' of medical genetics, Garrod had simply observed the occurrence of a rare anomaly in one or several families and found that the transmission pattern corresponded to the one which should be expected on the basis of Mendel's laws.

What made Garrod's contribution distinctive, perhaps – especially from a late twentieth-century perspective – was that the trait he described could be detected by a biochemical test. His contribution thus embodied not only the accuracy of Mendelian statistics but also the precise definition of a trait through laboratory techniques. Tellingly, the only other example of pre-1945 progress cited by Vogel and Motulsky is also an example of a monogenic trait defined by test techniques: the demonstration by Felix Bernstein in 1924 that the blood groups are determined by alleles in one genetic locus.[12] It is understandable that human geneticists identify such cases as breakthroughs, as they have provided results that have stood the test of time. Nevertheless, this selection conveys a problematic picture of the history of human heredity and of scientific progress more generally. The 'Garrod tale', first brought up by Nobel laureate George Beadle, is obviously a revised version of the story of Mendel's long neglect.[13] It implies that in the first half of the twentieth century, the true meaning of the Mendelian gospel – and therefore the essence of genetic science and its application to medicine – was grasped by only a few outsiders in the realm of human heredity, and that, consequently and regrettably, progress in the science of medical genetics was severely obstructed.

This interpretation omits the fact that many phenomena that confronted students of human heredity defied clear-cut explanations in Mendelian terms and yet generated methodological advances that were important not only for contemporary discussions but also for the further development of human genetics. The 'long neglect' narrative also downplays the enormous impact that the eugenics movement has had on the development of the science of human heredity. As a matter of fact, most methodological innovations in the early twentieth century were produced by convinced eugenicists or triggered by eugenic concerns. Though Vogel and Motulsky underscore the close links between eugenics and genetics and their ethical implications, they only cite Galton's early work as an example of eugenically motivated research. In the end, they subscribe to the widespread view that human genetics only became a truly scientific discipline after the demise of eugenics in the wake of World War II.[14]

It should be admitted, however, that historians of science have not entirely been successful in providing a coherent alternative to this narrative of professional geneticists. There has long been a tendency to retain the broad historiographical framework adopted by Kenneth Ludmerer, in which the rise and fall of eugenics is measured against the development of genetics as a discipline.[15] According to Ludmerer, there was an early period of interaction between science and eugenics; followed by a disillusion with the scientific basis of eugenics, which, coupled with the political fallout of Nazi racial hygiene, led to a temporary inhibition of human heredity research; and, finally, a re-constitution of human genetics in the post-war era, focused on the study of blood groups and genetic problems associated with radiation, and on individuals and populations, rather than on 'races'. For Philip Pauly, like Ludmerer, eugenics ultimately failed because it was incompatible with the demands of scientific 'practice'. It was too interdisciplinary, incoherent and diffuse. It did not lend itself easily to experimental research, human generations being so far apart, their traits defying exact measurement and their behaviour precluding direct experimental control.[16] Yet Pauly's eugenics is very much 'biology' and 'genetics' based, and he focuses on individuals with very specific eugenic research programmes, such as Charles Davenport and his supporters at the Carnegie Institution of Washington. While Pauly recognizes that other disciplines were involved in the development of eugenics, in his analysis the movement seems to have depended on the input from academic biology – read genetics – for its success. Broadening our perspective to address different individuals, institutions, disciplines and national contexts provides a very different perspective on the relationship between eugenics and the study of human heredity more generally.

In their studies of British eugenics, Donald Mackenzie, Theodore Porter and Pauline Mazumdar have identified how eugenics was central to the emergence of statistical methods and to resolving the impasse between biometry and Mendelian genetics. Furthermore, they have demonstrated how direct opposition to eugenic ideas also generated considerable statistical innovations and theoretical advances.[17] The study of eugenic ideas in France, in contrast, has shown how it retained a family health orientation due to apparent transmission of disease along family lines, contributing to a social medicine in which environment and heredity were closely intertwined.[18] Daniel Kevles introduced the concept of 'reform eugenics' to try to capture the sophistication and breadth of ideas and methods used by those scientists who, though critical of mainstream eugenics, still wanted to understand and control human heredity.[19] He has recognized eugenics as a field through which numerous disciplines and movements concerned with human heredity touched and connected, knowledge was circulated, and disciplinary boundaries established and altered through time. Paul Weindling describes a similar constellation in his account of the history of German eugenics.[20] Recent work on this topic has provided a more detailed picture of the relation between the growing political acceptance of racial hygiene and the contents of medical and biological research. It has been shown that even in the context of the Nazi regime, the racial hygiene boom not only generated pseudoscientific affirmations of racialist politics, but rather boosted a further methodological differentiation of human genetics.[21]

This volume thus continues more recent concerted efforts to place the history of genetics more generally into the context of a wider history of hereditarian ideas and practices. Heredity, in a strict biological or genetic sense, was not an age-old concern of humanity. The concept itself only acquired a biological (as opposed to legal) meaning in the mid-nineteenth century through the confluence of independent traditions within medicine, animal and plant breeding, natural history and anthropology.[22] The work of John Waller and Charles Rosenberg has also helped correct the simplistic association of eugenics with Galton by examining how notions of heredity, particularly regarding marriage and disease, pre-existed and would influence later medical and statistical developments.[23] In turn, Chris Renwick has argued that Galton's vision of eugenics was shaped by, and more naturally aligned to, the social than the biological sciences.[24] Within this *longue durée* perspective, the formation of classical genetics, and later, molecular genetics, as distinct disciplines appears as a transitory moment only. Both disciplines were firmly rooted in a diversity of concepts and methodologies that had their own historical trajectories behind them, often quite independent of a properly genetic interest in transmission, and both had tools to offer in turn that quickly diffused into other research areas such as embryology, evolutionary biology or cancer aetiology.[25] To even provide an outline of the story of genetics is too complex a task for the purposes of this Introduction.[26] But the message it entails for the history of human heredity in the twentieth century is clear. It would be naive to expect a Kuhnian succession of genetic paradigms applied to the study of humans. Rather, what one should expect is a complex and ever-changing web of translations between disciplinary contexts, more akin to Ludwik Fleck's model of a 'circulation of ideas'.[27]

The contributions to this volume take up these insights from the historiography on eugenics and genetics, as well as on medicine, molecular biology and statistics. Although, as we saw above, recent studies have provided a broader and more detailed picture of the research practices and political contexts that formed the science of human heredity, important fields such as the social and behavioural sciences, epidemiology and clinical genetics, as well as crucial methods like twin research and medical statistics, have received little attention so far. Moreover, a transnational overview of the approaches to and theories of human heredity is still a desideratum. We intend to fill these lacunae by representing the diversity of approaches that were directed at or connected to questions of human heredity in the twentieth century, and by including case studies from various national settings that can highlight different scientific and political constellations shaping the perception of human heredity. Our primary interest in this is to discuss what it meant to study heredity in *humans*, that is to say, to highlight the specific methodological and social implications that arose from attempts to produce evidence regarding the inheritance of diseases, physical features or behaviour in human beings. By delimiting our time frame to what roughly coincides with Hobsbawm's 'short' twentieth century, we seek to concentrate on the period after the consolidation of Mendelian genetics and before biotechnology and sequencing techniques began to transform the field.[28] This makes sense not only for pragmatic reasons but also because for many scientists and historians, World War II is a watershed in the history of heredity research when medical genetics began to privilege the individual over the collective, and population approaches replaced racial typologies. The contributions of this volume allow us to reconsider this narrative, which has recently been challenged by Nathaniel Comfort.[29]

The essays differ widely with respect to the time span covered, the materials used and the approaches employed. Some offer micro-historical analyses based on archival sources, while others discuss long-term developments and debates. In terms of thematic focus, we can broadly distinguish between contributions dealing with questions of conceptual change, institutions, and experimental systems or objects. In view of the fact that essays often share certain thematic and temporal focal points, however, we have chosen to group contributions according to a more detailed structure that also reflects the thematic cross-relations between the texts. These are as follows: the opportunities and challenges medical and human geneticists faced in constructing statistical surveys of human heredity and interpreting their results (Part I); the pervasive importance of blood group sampling for early human population genetic studies (Part II); the conjunctions, especially with agricultural biology and medicine, produced through the import of human heredity into the laboratory (Part III); the intersection of interests in human heredity with the more general problem of understanding and managing disease (Part IV); and finally, the disciplinary reconstitution of human heredity during and after World War II (Part V). This range of topics does not, of course, reflect all of the issues a comprehensive history of human heredity in the twentieth century would have to consider. Yet it is possible to point out some general aspects that deserve attention.

Generally, the contributions show that 'heredity' assumed very different meanings in different contexts. Clinicians, medical statisticians, anthropologists and experimental geneticists took quite divergent perspectives on matters of heredity, not only because they employed different research practices, but also because their findings had different practical consequences. This may not be a profound insight, but it forces us to reconsider the supposed unity of the scientific field we know as 'human genetics'. Subsuming all scientific efforts concerning human heredity under this heading implies that all findings in this field can be established through similar methods and explained by the same conceptual framework. Apart from the fact that a coherent causal explanation for 'hereditary' phenomena is mostly an ideal rather than a reality, it also has to be noted that the study of human heredity is never about heredity alone. It always involves the consideration of those biological factors that are not hereditary. Further, the isolation and definition of traits regarded as hereditary is widely, if not always, dependent on social interests and conventions about what is normal or pathological. Finally, matters of human heredity inevitably touch upon human values. There is no absolute genetic truth independent from the social conditions constituting the framework of research. Thus what is true for *Drosophila* is not necessarily true for *Homo sapiens*.

Many essays highlight specific implications of the simple fact that human heredity is about dealing with human beings. Humans are – as all geneticists would agree, and as pointed out above – very problematic objects for genetic research. Their reproduction cannot be controlled and analysed as it is the case for most animals and plants; their individual development is seldom fully controllable; and human characters are difficult to define, especially those that tend to attract most attention from biomedical scientists, like common diseases or mental illnesses. In other words, a science of human heredity requires complex means for observing people, charting their family relations and tracking their life histories. It is essentially a matter of control and power. It is therefore no wonder that several contributions in this volume address the role of institutions that have shaped the field: record offices, hospitals, health authorities and the military.

Although several pioneering insights of human genetics, including Garrod's work on alkaptonuria, were produced on a small scale and through the observation of single families, the study of human heredity is essentially based on large administrative structures. Large-scale studies about the varying frequencies of common human traits and diseases emerged primarily where record offices, military agencies, medical services, schools and insurance companies provided consistent data, as the essays by Bernd Gausemeier, Jenny Bangham and Pascal Germann demonstrate. All of these cases, however, also show us that in spite of the growing sophistication of statistical population control in the twentieth century, it was anything but a simple task to open up data suitable for the purposes of genetic research. Large-scale statistics requires parameters that are easy to access, count and analyse. It is therefore no coincidence that matters of blood grouping feature prominently in this volume. As serological testing and blood transfusion services began to form comprehensive medical and administrative structures by the mid-twentieth century, largely due to the war efforts in different nations, blood allowed for representative surveys of populations on a scale that was soon to become global.

However, surveys did not necessarily cover large populations. In order to be useful for specific anthropological or medical needs, populations had to be selected and defined in a way that was amenable to analysis. One way was to collect random samples through national networks consisting of medical or research institutions, as Edna Suárez-Diaz and Ana Barahona demonstrate for the Mexican case. Another, followed primarily by anthropologists, was to concentrate on 'isolate' populations perceived as genealogically secluded and genetically homogeneous, as discussed by Veronika Lipphardt. In order to deal with the often heterogeneous data derived from such sources, surveying techniques had to be modified and rearranged, and new statistical techniques had to be developed to master the complexities that appeared with the growing quantity of materials. This also held true for hospitals and clinics, the oldest and most important sites for the study of human heredity. Medical institutions, especially those specializing in certain groups of diseases, were able to generate large numbers of comparable clinical histories. Yet, as Philip K. Wilson's contribution shows, available clinical data rarely conformed to the demands of students of human heredity, primarily because they usually did not comprise sufficient material about the patients' next kin. Clinical structures thus had to be remodelled profoundly in order to make them amenable to the study of genetics. Tellingly, such 'heredity clinics' did not come into being thanks to the initiatives of eugenicists who strove to form completely new structures allowing for a better surveillance of the 'hereditary ill', but instead in clinical institutions that could rely on established techniques for compiling and processing aetiological data.

Several contributions point to the rise of another institutional framework that began to affect the whole field of human heredity by the mid-twentieth century: the 'big science' structures evolving with nuclear projects. Although a significant concern about radiation damage already emerged by the 1930s, the interplay between nuclear research and genetics expanded after World War II, when wartime structures were developed into large-scale research programmes. Not only in the USA but also in all major industrialized countries, there was a concentration of radiation genetics in nuclear research centres and support by national agencies administrating the new field of big science, as evidenced by the contributions of Soraya de Chadarevian, Alexander von Schwerin and Susan Lindee. The influence of nuclear research pertained not only to the vast support provided by these agencies but also to the use of research tools and objects. Similar incentives came from agricultural research, another field increasingly characterized by global institutional networks. It was through the prior use of colchicine to produce 'bigger and better' agricultural crops that researchers were able to identify the correct number of human chromosomes, as Maria Santesmases tells us in her fascinating story of this substance. This example, along with von Schwerin's account of the role of rabbits as model organisms, provides a particularly good demonstration of the degree to which knowledge of human heredity depended on the circulation of materials, methods and people within a variety of disciplinary contexts. Such transfers not only mediated interdisciplinary relations, they were also able to induce concurrent transformations in previously separated fields. The introduction of karyotyping techniques, as de Chadarevian demonstrates, entailed considerable changes in such different disciplinary contexts as preventive medicine, criminology and sex biology.

Karyotyping is perhaps the most prominent example of a process which can be described as a 'materialization' or 'molecularization' of human heredity. Although the use of serological and biochemical blood analysis, as noted above, already generated considerable change in the pre-war era, the development and diffusion of practicable test methods in the medical realm and the use of improved animal models after World War II gave rise to a fundamentally novel perspective on human heredity. Owing to the spread of laboratory-based methods that allowed for the detection of genetic markers and chromosomal aberrations, heredity was no longer a hidden quality accessible only through statistical inference, but instead a physiological function that could be determined directly in the individual. It has to be noted, however, that this methodological transformation initially concerned only a small group of hereditary traits.

With respect to the development of concepts, the essays of this volume indicate that the Mendelian concept of particulate heredity was by no means the dominant theoretical approach to human heredity. It was undoubtedly a crucial incentive that allowed the field to become a theory-based science. The Mendelian idea of the unit character was attractive for medical scientists and anthropologists alike because it corresponded with a functional definition of physical characters and with a trend towards more precise nosological definitions. Especially in medicine, it seemed to open up new avenues for a causal understanding of diseases and, therefore, a more effective control of their distribution and development. But the Mendelian drive towards statistical precision also raised problems. It demanded highly standardized and comprehensive data. Moreover, the project of identifying Mendelian traits turned out to be more complex than expected. By the 1920s even convinced eugenicists realized that major physical characters, as well as the most common diseases, did not fit easily into the Mendelian mould. For this reason, statistical empiricism remained a dominant method in the field of human heredity. For many traits, as Gausemeier shows, determining heritability appeared a more achievable aim than establishing Mendelian ratios. The most prominent object of the new population genetics – the ABO blood group system – did not primarily attract researchers because it corresponded perfectly with the Mendelian laws, as becomes clear with Germann's and Jenny Bangham's analyses, but rather because it was a most practicable marker to study the genetic composition and the migration of groups.

Moreover, Mendelian mainstream genetics was not able to explain many phenomena that had had a long-standing place in physicians' view on heredity. The case of 'anticipation' discussed by Judith Friedman is a good example for a pre-Mendelian concept that continued to influence medical discussion. That some genetic diseases occurred earlier, and with greater severity, when passed from one generation to the next seemed a well-established and obvious fact for those who relied on pedigrees as their tools of analysis. However, anticipation was then 'explained away' by those theoretically committed to a population genetics perspective, only to be rediscovered decades later. Ideas about physical 'constitutions' as indicators of inborn dispositions to certain diseases, which are addressed by Gausemeier and Wilson, were for a long time an integral part of medical practice. While they were hardly compatible with a particulate understanding of heredity, they corresponded with physicians' need for practicable diagnostic methods.

Race was an even more persistent 'pre-genetic' concept. There is no doubt that after the experience of Nazi racial policy, the rejection of racialist thinking became an important incentive for the development of human genetics. A new generation of human geneticists, as discussed by Lipphardt and Francesco Cassata, distanced themselves not only from the concept of races as homogenous groups with a largely identical genetic make-up, but also from the research practices employed by the generation of eugenics-oriented medical scientists. And yet there are striking reminiscences of older discursive figures, even where human geneticists adopted the latest techniques in order to put their discipline 'on a solid basis' – as de Chadarevian quotes them in the title of her essay. In the new, deviant 'types' of people that were distinguished on the basis of chromosome analysis in the 1960s, one is reminded of the 'feeble-minded' and 'criminals' that had been the preferred target of the 'old' eugenics. Here typology even survived in the very name given to the new practice – 'karyotyping'.

Even while claims about absolute 'racial' differences with respect to physical and mental qualities lost credibility, the interest in 'racial' differences as an important indicator for heredity did not disappear completely. This was partly due to the fact that human geneticists continued to use populations that were selected either for their supposed homogenous genetic composition (as in the case of Lipphardt's isolates) or for their supposed diversity (as in the Swiss and Mexican cases examined by Germann, and Suárez-Diaz and Barahona, respectively). Genetic traits are often sought out in populations where they appear as 'typical'; and even where group differences are not interpreted in a discriminatory way, administrative practices may point out diversity. Thereby the interpretation of difference depended strongly on respective political contexts. It also depended on categories imported from a variety of different fields – anthropology, sociology and linguistics – whose complex histories were often conveniently overlooked in favour of their practical benefits for providing stability and order to the study of populations.

In a similar way, the general results of the volume speak against the widespread view that after World War II, the demise of eugenics cleared the way for the development of human genetics as a new scientific discipline. As the contributions of Cassata, Diane B. Paul and Edmund Ramsden show, geneticists were certainly active in identifying what they perceived to be the flaws in eugenic thinking, and in developing the idea of a break from the past. Yet their approaches were not always as novel as they claimed. Many of the ideas and methods that shaped post-World War II human genetics had been established earlier as a result of eugenic concerns. As Ramsden points out, projects initiated to vindicate hereditarian positions could ultimately undermine their own premises. Rather than as a discontinuous history divided by a watershed between eugenic ideology and genetic science, we must regard the evolution of human genetics as a dialectical process in which both partisans and critics of eugenic ideas constantly refined their methods and reframed their arguments.

Furthermore, post-war medical genetics always continued to involve elements of eugenic aspirations because, after all, it continued to be concerned with individual decisions about reproduction. Although post-war proponents of genetic counselling advanced the ideal of expert advice not interfering with the free decision of the client, new forms of analysing the genetic constitution of individuals nevertheless had an inherent tendency to create new norms for a genetically healthy society. As Anne Cottebrune argues, the rejection of authoritarian programmes of population improvement in favour of individual choice could mask an ongoing belief in the need for, and possibility of, influencing the biological future of mankind through less controversial means. Counselling was perceived as a form of preventive medicine, with expert advice influencing the fertility of clients for the benefit of society. The same faith in the power of the biomedical sciences is also evident in the adoption of karyotyping to conduct 'genetic surveys on a world scale' by the World Health Organization in the 1960s.

In view of the various contributions pointing to a 'materialization' or 'molecularization' of human heredity after World War II, there is no doubt that the methodological revolutions of the post-war period opened up a completely new – and often more precise – perception of human heredity. The new possibilities of screening for cytological and biochemical markers did bring about a completely novel form of population surveys: the surveying of 'hereditary' traits was no longer based on the measurement of the phenotype or on nosological definitions that were often disputable. Moreover, they allowed for a detection of hereditary dispositions before they manifested, thus ostensibly opening the way to a predictive analysis of heredity. But did these developments really bring about the revolutionary transformations many of its proponents predicted?

In medical genetics, the optimism evoked by some spectacular advances in testing techniques was not always grounded by a realistic assessment of their actual potential. The biochemical or cytological identification of diseases like PKU or of chromosome aberrations, as Paul shows, opened up new possibilities for prognosis and, sometimes, therapy. Yet restricted as such progress was to specific phenomena, it did not justify confident speculations that the control of hereditary disease per se was imminent. Like eugenicists of the early twentieth century, who built their cases on the basis of rare examples, medical geneticists of the post-war era remained prone to *pars pro toto* thinking.

What, after all, did medicine gain from the advances of genetics in the post-war era? Diane Paul's and Stephen Pemberton's analyses of the paradigmatic genetic diseases PKU and haemophilia provide fascinating answers to this question. The therapeutic achievements that made both diseases manageable had nothing to do with genetics but were entirely due to biochemical and clinical advances. Heredity was nevertheless important as a principle for defining the risk group. For the booming field of genetic counselling, those disorders that could be identified by biochemical and karyological means were useful exemplary cases demonstrating the possibility and effectiveness of genetic prognosis. Yet such cases remained exceptional. The emphasis on the 'genetic' nature of diseases like PKU indicates that heredity was, first and foremost, an indispensable ideological resource. Genetics became a generic term for new medical developments that had quite diverse backgrounds and consequences. Although the new biomedical technologies and constellations of the post-war era provided new concepts of human heredity, they did not change but rather reinforced the old eugenic claim that knowing the 'genetic basis' was the only way to reach a true, causal understanding of human characters and diseases.

1 BORDERLANDS OF HEREDITY: THE DEBATE ABOUT HEREDITARY SUSCEPTIBILITY TO TUBERCULOSIS, 1882–1945

Bernd Gausemeier

In the late nineteenth and the early twentieth centuries, the hereditary susceptibility to tuberculosis (TB) was one of the most discussed topics in the field of human heredity. Remarkably, the complex and substantial debates concerning this topic have left few traces in the historiography of science and medicine.[1] The reason for this neglect probably lies in the fact that these debates generated neither unambiguous results nor a coherent methodology. Historians of human heredity have tended to focus on pioneering studies regarding definitely 'genetic' human characters, notably those demonstrating Mendelian inheritance.[2] It has to be noted, however, that almost all of these paradigmatic examples – haemophilia, Huntington's chorea or alkaptanuria – were rare, distinctive anomalies that were clearly endogenous. TB, in contrast, was omnipresent, polymorphic and hardly suited to monocausal interpretations. But precisely because the idea of hereditary susceptibility to the disease was so highly ambiguous and contested, it generated a multiplicity of approaches. And since TB was – unlike most 'classical' hereditary diseases – one of the most urgent problems of social hygiene, questions about its aetiology concerned a wide circle of specialists and institutions. For these reasons, a look at the practices that informed the TB debate opens up a wider perspective on the meanings of human heredity. In this essay, I will point out some of the major methodological developments that emerged in the German context between the late nineteenth century and World War II. This survey does not intend to give a comprehensive assessment of the role of heredity played in the discussions about TB aetiology. Rather, it reflects the plurality of approaches, institutional frameworks and notions of inheritance that characterized the field of human heredity in the period when it grew into a scientific discipline.

Pedigree Collections and Insurance Statistics

Up to the late nineteenth century, TB was widely regarded as a 'hereditary' disease. The discovery of the TB pathogen in 1882 was not able to overthrow this conventional view completely.[3] For medical practitioners, it was a matter of everyday experience that certain families were more prone to the disease than others. Since the TB germ did not strike all people living under similar hygienic conditions, its impact obviously depended on a hereditary disposition, termed 'diathesis' by nineteenth-century physicians. In view of the advances of bacteriology, however, it was hardly possible to maintain this idea without providing statistical evidence, all the more so as epidemiological surveys demonstrated that the distribution of TB clearly depended on social, professional and hygienic conditions.

For those interested in substantiating the hypothesis of a hereditary diathesis, there was no obvious method of choice. By the end of the nineteenth century, there was already a variety of approaches which were all shaped by the provenance of the data employed. One option was the collection of family histories demonstrating the familial transmission of TB over several generations. The most comprehensive studies of this kind were published by the German physician Alexander Riffel in 1890 and 1905. They excelled mainly with respect to the use of masses of genealogical data: they comprised no less than the complete population history of two villages in Baden over more than a century, including causes of death and other medical information.[4] Though Riffel's approach was basically about showing that TB appeared constantly in certain lineages, hygienic aspects were not completely absent from his analysis. Most notably, the first study – which treated his home village – provided detailed accounts of the housing conditions of various families. This enabled him to argue that some families remained TB-free under circumstances that would sicken others.

Riffel's studies represented a trend beginning to take hold in the German medical community by the end of the nineteenth century.[5] There was a widespread conviction that the systematic study of pathological heredity required systematic compilation of well-documented family histories, notably of 'deep' pedigrees covering several generations. His use of voluminous genealogical data won Riffel considerable acclaim among partisans of this view.[6] TB specialists, however, were not similarly impressed. Georg Cornet, author of an influential TB handbook, slated Riffel's work as an example of uncritical – and also inaccurate – empiricism. The mere exhibition of genealogical continuity, he pointed out, was no evidence of heredity. The assumption of a hereditary disposition to TB would remain groundless in the absence of statistical evidence that revealed morbidity rates within affected families to clearly exceed those of the average population.[7]

There had, in fact, been a number of unsuccessful attempts to meet this postulate, most notably by Francis Galton, who dealt extensively with the TB problem in his book *Natural Inheritance*. Yet while Galton held that the hereditary nature of a disease or trait could be established only by analysing its frequency in an average population, his material was no less biased than Riffel's. From the stock of genealogical records he had collected through a survey among members of the English upper classes, he selected all TB-afflicted families. The figures derived from these pedigrees were ambivalent enough: among the children and siblings of TB-affected persons, there were cases of striking accumulation as well as of singular appearance.[8] Though Galton used all his statistical inventiveness, he was ultimately unable to make sense of his results. An accurate picture, he concluded, would require much broader and more precise data about the familial distribution of TB cases. He did, however, have a clear idea where such data could be found: in the files of life insurance companies.

In the late nineteenth century, insurance companies were the most important source of data about human heredity. As they inquired not only about the individual medical record of the insurants but also about the health of their relatives, insurance companies were able to compile comprehensive records about the familial occurrence of the most frequent diseases.[9] Surveys based on such records indicated that clients whose parents had died from TB were significantly more likely to suffer the same fate than the average insurant.[10] Such data were, apparently, purely empirical and allowed for no conclusions with regards to the hereditary or environmental determination of familial TB. Insurance statisticians were not out to solve such aetiological questions. Not distinguishing systematically between 'familial' and 'hereditary' disposition, they were interested only in establishing risk figures that would help to formulate guidelines for the admission or rejection of insurants.

Late nineteenth-century studies on the heredity of TB were, therefore, constricted by the obviously selective structure of their material. While the genealogical approach employed by Riffel and Galton necessarily focused on families in which TB was endemic, insurance companies tried to keep their clientele – as much as possible – free from persons prone to chronic diseases. By the beginning of the twentieth century, advances in public statistics and the medical services opened up new sources of data. Yet the availability of better statistical material alone did not inevitably generate a more coherent approach to the problem. On the contrary, different conceptions of TB aetiology and the diversity of data sources created a plurality of often incommensurable methods and conflicting interpretations.

Hospital Populations and Average Populations

The situation is best illustrated by a comparative look at two studies published in 1907, authored by two of the most important pioneers of modern human genetics, the English statistician Karl Pearson and the German physician Wilhelm

Weinberg. The two studies differed significantly not only in their conclusions but also with respect to the provenance and the arrangement of data. Pearson's work was based on patient data from a TB sanatorium near Liverpool, and the use of this material points to the structural changes that transformed TB care around the turn of the century. Specialized TB hospitals open to all strata of society only emerged in the 1890s. Up until then, treatment – in so far as there was treatment at all – took place in general hospitals and private sanatoria.[11] In addition, communal authorities began to establish TB care stations responsible for diagnosis and post-treatment surveillance. These new structures, devoted exclusively to the control of TB patients, allowed researchers to access more precise data about the occurrence and development of TB cases.

Pearson drew on material compiled by the sanatorium's medical staff, who had inquired into the health status of the patient's nearest relatives as far as it was possible.[12] He employed the same approach as in his studies about the inheritance of physical traits – that is, he calculated parent–offspring correlations in respect to the occurrence of TB. The composition of a hospital population, however, differed markedly from that of a random population. The records featured cases of patients with TB-free children or parents, but they necessarily did not include families that were completely free from TB. Pearson therefore calculated virtual non-TB individuals into his sample. Based on statistical figures estimating that TB accounted for 10 per cent of the mortality in the British population, he added nine healthy persons for one TB sufferer.[13] In other words, he sought to correct the lack of representativeness of his first-hand data by working in second-hand public data. His interpretation was even more daring. Since the parent–offspring correlations derived from his calculation conformed perfectly to those he had established for 'normal' human traits, he concluded that TB obeyed the same laws of heredity. Pearson therefore equated the appearance of TB with the hereditary disposition for TB. He did not even consider the existence of other causative factors.

Weinberg, who was working as a physician for the urban poor in Stuttgart, was not disposed to taking such a one-sided hereditarian stance. His study was based on the assumption that TB was unquestionably a social disease. For this reason, he held that the sample for a study on TB should be socially representative. This postulate alone spoke against the use of hospital records; the population investigated by Pearson, for example, was strictly working class. Moreover, hospital populations were hopelessly selective. They always exhibited an accumulation of certain diseases, usually in their most severe forms. Even statistical manipulations like those applied by Pearson could never transform hospital records into something statistically useful.[14] Truly scientific statistics on problems of pathological heredity was possible only through the analysis of complete average populations. This research concept was not easy to realize, since it demanded not only reliable and complete population records but also a precise registration of the frequency of certain diseases in the population. While most German states stipulated obligatory coroners' inquests by the late nineteenth century, medical statisticians remained displeased with the quality of public medical records. According to the influential statistician Friedrich Prinzing, the registration of cause of death was so fragmentary that it did not even comply with the most basic requirements of epidemiology.[15]

Weinberg was confident that the preconditions for his statistical endeavours existed, if anywhere, in his native country. Since the early nineteenth century, the Kingdom of Württemberg maintained a secular system of population records that allowed the tracing of genealogical relations with ease.[16] Moreover, the major cities thoroughly recorded their inhabitants' causes of death from the eighteenth century. Acting as an honorary medical statistician for the Württemberg physicians' association, Weinberg combined these data into a survey that covered all Stuttgarters who had died from TB between 1873 and 1902.[17] From this material, Weinberg compiled all those couples – 258 altogether – in which one partner had died from TB while the other had remained unaffected. He then compared the respective relatives (parents and siblings in separate surveys) of the affected and healthy partners. In both cases, he found TB mortality to be considerably – though not strikingly – higher among the next of kin of the tubercular spouses.

By using his 'spouse' method, Weinberg sought to overcome two basic problems that plagued TB statistics: first, he examined probands living under identical circumstances (which implied that no direct infection between the spouses was involved); second, he was able to juxtapose comparable 'TB positive' and 'TB negative' groups. Weinberg also took pains to control for social selection. For example, he carefully sorted his material according to occupational groups, because certain trades were known to be extremely prone to the disease. Since most of his TB-affected probands lived under precarious economic situations, he stressed that the results still needed to be compared with those from upper-class families.[18] By relying exclusively on archival material, Weinberg sought to evade another statistical problem concerning age structure. Hospital populations were widely composed of patients in childbearing age. It was therefore highly problematic to make any statistical statements as to the health status of their offspring, as children were often too young to be classified. Pearson was aware of this problem, but he was only able to correct it by inserting estimated values for the 'unsecured' part of the filial generation.[19] The generations in Weinberg's sample, in contrast, were all 'completed'.

Weinberg did not regard his study as the definitive word in the TB debate. Rather, he saw it as a demonstration of the ways in which new statistical approaches could tackle the complex problems of human heredity. His approach marked a break with the genealogical understanding of heredity that still informed Pearson's statistics, which drew primarily on cases of multiple familial occurrence. Weinberg, in contrast, aimed at the construction of comparative samples that allowed him to assess the respective influence of heredity and other possible pathogenic factors. The methodological principles developed in the TB study were formative to his later contributions to human genetics. Although Weinberg's posthumous fame as a population geneticist rests on his theoretical work concerning the distribution of hypothetical Mendelian traits in a hypothetical, ideal population, he always regarded the sober distinction between genetic and endogenous factors as the most important problem of human heredity. He would repeatedly criticize Pearson and his biometric school for systematically mixing up both aspects.[20] His conflict with the British eugenicists was also concerned with the question of whether carriers of the TB diathesis posed a major threat to the hereditary health of coming generations. While Pearson postulated an extraordinary fecundity of TB-affected families, Weinberg's statistics suggested that their overall mortality was definitely higher than in the average population.[21] Moreover, Weinberg's ideas about population genetics – which he developed in parallel to the TB study – implied that a hereditary disposition to TB, in so far as it behaved like a Mendelian factor, would not increase in frequency as a consequence of the higher fertility of its carriers.[22] This scepticism does not imply that Weinberg rejected eugenics altogether. He was an active member of the German Society for Racial Hygiene, but he maintained that claims about the omnipotence of heredity had to pass the test of rigid statistical examination. His TB study did in fact set a new standard in the German discussion. It would not, however, become as seminal as he had hoped – mainly because the field of TB statistics was occupied by a variety of surveying practices.

Regimes of Clinical Observation

Weinberg's approach was not flawless. The criterion of death by TB – especially when derived from old death certificates – was clearly less precise than the medical information provided by hospital files. Also, TB sufferers who had died from other diseases would not enter the sample. For Weinberg, this lack of diagnostic precision was clearly outweighed by the more comprehensive and representative structure of the data. TB specialists looked at things differently. A hereditary disposition to the disease did not, after all, necessarily mean a lethal outcome. It could also become manifest in the rapid development of the disease or in reduced chances for recovery. A perspective that accounted for such aetiological specificities inevitably had to draw on different data and was bound to generate different conclusions.

An interesting counter-position to both Weinberg's and Pearson's work can be found in the studies of the Hamburg physician Franz Reiche. This is not simply because Reiche was arguably the most prolific German opponent of the hereditarian position. Working as a consultant for the state insurance association of the Hanseatic cities, Reiche had access to the clinical records of most Hamburg and Bremen citizens who received treatment for TB. By the turn of the century, he began to deploy this inexhaustible arsenal of files against the diathesis doctrine.[23] Reiche's statistical investigations departed from the assumption that a hereditary disposition would manifest itself not only in illness and hospitalization, but also in the individual response to the disease. The state insurance records – widely based on his own diagnoses – allowed him to distinguish between patients who recovered, those who repeatedly relapsed and those who succumbed to the disease. In so far as there was reliable information about the health of these patients' parents, he was able to calculate if patients with tubercular parents fared worse than those without. In a survey based on 2,600 examined patients, Reiche found almost no difference between the two groups with respect to their medical record.[24] The individual ability to resist TB infection, he concluded, was evidently not dependent on a hereditary disposition. It was, exclusively, the result of the intensity of contagion. Unsurprisingly, Weinberg dismissed Reiche's patient-based statistics as non-representative.[25] While this objection was arguably justified, it is nevertheless obvious that Reiche discussed the TB problem on a level that was not accessible to Weinberg.

Reiche's position represented the mainstream in the German TB community. In the 1920s the idea of hereditary susceptibility to TB was increasingly hard to vindicate. The dramatic rise of TB cases in the aftermath of the war was an impressive demonstration of the predominant importance of hygiene and nutrition. The influence of exogenous factors such as housing and profession was much easier to substantiate by statistical evidence than was the role of heredity. At best, heredity tended to appear as a negligible factor. The TB handbook of the hygienist Adolf Gottstein, for example, mentioned heredity only in passing; it devoted much more attention to the question of whether immunity could be acquired by infantile exposure to TB germs.[26] Even a eugenically minded author like the geneticist Valentin Haecker had to admit that the statistical results on TB inheritance were too inconsistent to allow for a clear statement.[27]

This is not to say that classical hereditarian arguments disappeared completely. Genealogical studies in the style of Riffel were still produced in the 1920s, but they made little impact on the discussion. Pedigree-based claims that the disposition to lung TB was inherited as a Mendelian recessive trait raised disapproval even among the most convinced of eugenicists.[28]

This should not imply that heredity vanished completely from the discourse of TB doctors. Physicians who regarded hereditary disposition as a significant aetiological factor did not necessarily have to take interest in their patients' familial background. In everyday clinical practice, the patients' body was a much more obvious indicator of possible susceptibilities to certain diseases. The idea of hereditary diathesis was widely associated with the concept of an inborn anatomical habitus, or 'constitution'. Constitution pathology was one of the dominant trends in early twentieth-century European medicine, especially in respect to TB.[29] Yet 'constitution' was anything but a uniform concept. It did not necessarily imply typological thinking, whereby certain forms of physique were associated with certain pathological phenomena. Nineteenth-century insurance physicians, for example, employed a pragmatic form of constitutional pathology. Basic bodily measurements served as a simple means of risk determination. TB susceptibility was believed to manifest itself in a low breast circumference or general meagreness; individuals showing these 'risk symptoms' could be refused or placed in a specific insurance group.[30] This very general assumption corresponded with the long-established idea that TB mainly affected individuals of a specific *Habitus phthisicus*, i.e. weakly 'asthenic' types. Twentieth-century theorists of constitutional pathology were not always happy with this popular but rather vague assumption. As the eugenicist Hermann W. Siemens argued in 1920, there was no clear-cut statistical evidence as to the existence of TB-prone physical types; comprehensive statistical studies, however, might reveal specific bodily features – 'stigmata' – signalling a disposition to TB.[31] Siemens advocated a non-typological version of constitutionalism, according to which correlations between specific phenotypical traits and certain susceptibilities still had to be established through systematic research. For medical practitioners, however, it was much easier to draw on theoretical concepts offering a clear-cut and viable framework for classification. In the 1920s the typological system of the psychiatrist Ernst Kretschmer became particularly popular. Although Kretschmer's tripartite classification originally concerned constitutional tendencies to mental diseases, physicians also used it to assess the relation between body shape and TB disposition.[32] One such study, conducted in tuberculosis care stations in East Prussia in the late 1920s, seemed to confirm that Kretschmer's 'leptosomic' (asthenic) type was clearly more TB-prone than the 'pyknic' and the 'muscular' types.[33] Though the numerical results of these typology-based statistics looked rather unambiguous, they did not remain unchallenged. One TB expert objected by noting that 'asthenic' patients appeared so frequently in TB care stations and sanatoria exactly because they had a tendency to resist the disease; 'muscular' individuals, in contrast, would tend to succumb to TB much more rapidly.[34] Again, seemingly clear statistical evidence was called into question with reference to a possible selection bias.

Such objections were not the only problematic aspect of the constitutional approach. Obviously, 'constitution' was more than just a hereditary quality. The TB-prone 'asthenic' type, in particular, was often considered to result from TB infection during infancy. For the physician, constitutional classification provided a pragmatic way to conceptualize disposition. For those aiming to define the nature of hereditary disposition more precisely, however, 'constitution' was a rather precarious concept.

Eugenic Model Populations

The unsettled situation of the debate may have been of little relevance to physicians working in TB care. It was, however, untenable for those professionally concerned with human heredity and committed to the aims of eugenics. Eugenicists could not afford to surrender the most important problem of social medicine without a struggle. It is therefore hardly surprising that the crucial methodological innovations which reopened the debate in the 1920s and 1930s were brought forward by committed eugenicists.

One of these contributions came as a by-product of psychiatric research. In 1926 Hans Luxenburger, a researcher at the Genealogical-Demographic Department of the German Research Institution for Psychiatry (GDA) in Munich, published a survey about the frequency of TB among psychiatric patients. By then the GDA was undoubtedly the world's biggest and methodologically most advanced research centre devoted to human genetics. Its founder and director, the Swiss-born psychiatrist Ernst Rüdin, had set a landmark in the development of medical genetics with his 1916 study on the inheritance of schizophrenia. His survey was not only exclusively based on probands who had been clinically examined; it also introduced a set of statistical tools for correcting possible artefacts arising from selection bias. Rüdin's work challenged the idea that mental diseases were inherited as simple Mendelian factors, an idea then embraced by most eugenicists.[35]

The high statistical standard of the study was mainly due to the input of an external advisor – the solitary but influential Wilhelm Weinberg. It was Weinberg who taught Rüdin and his co-workers how to construct representative samples and how to avoid statistical misinterpretations. Weinberg's ideas about the statistical analysis of human heredity, partly developed in his TB study, effectively shaped the programme and the setup of the GDA. Supported by Bavarian state authorities, psychiatric clinics and the leaders of rural municipalities, Rüdin's co-workers did not restrict themselves to screening asylum patients and their families; they also surveyed whole local populations for the occurrence of diseases and physical measures. Though primarily concerned with the genetics of mental and nervous diseases, Rüdin's institute accumulated all accessible medical information, thus compiling a eugenic micro-census that allowed them to generate and combine data on all conceivable questions of human heredity. While earlier students of human heredity had to draw on approachable public records, clinical files or family histories, the GDA had at its disposal material that had been systematically assembled for the purposes of human genetics and medical statistics.

In analysing one the GDA's model populations, Luxenburger found that the tuberculosis rate among the siblings of schizophrenia patients was about four times higher than in an average population, whereas the siblings of manic depressive patients showed no such deviation.[36] In his analysis of these results,

Luxenburger speculated about a 'constitutional' factor causing a disposition to both diseases. Such interpretations were not unusual in German human genetics in the late 1920s, when it became increasingly apparent that clear-cut cases of monogenic Mendelian inheritance were rather exceptional (although eugenic propaganda continued to suggest otherwise). Accordingly, the attention of researchers shifted towards models explaining more complex genetic mechanisms and methods allowing for the detection of genetic correlations. As Luxenburger's study demonstrates, the GDA surveys were particularly well suited for the latter aim. Yet while the psychiatrist's findings pointed towards a possible genetic correlation between TB and schizophrenia, they offered no clear-cut insight with respect to the most controversial problem in the TB debate, namely the issue of the importance of a possible genetic factor, in contrast to exogenous factors. This was probably the reason why Luxenburger's work had less impact on the debates of TB experts, than that of a study initiated by another aspiring German eugenicist.

Twin Studies

In the late 1920s the physician Otmar von Verschuer, department director at the newly founded Kaiser-Wilhelm Institute for Anthropology, Human Heredity and Eugenics (KWIA), and his friend Karl Diehl, director of a TB sanatorium near Berlin, began to prepare a survey on TB in twin pairs. It was one of the first major projects which applied a method that would soon change the whole field of human heredity. Up until then, physicians had occasionally used casuistic observations on twins.[37] Verschuer, in contrast, systematically used the comparison between comprehensive samples of monozygotic and dizygotic twins, that is to say of two groups representing identical and differing genotypes. Departing from the assumption that intrauterine and postnatal conditions were identical for all twins, the approach was primarily conceived to establish precise distinctions between hereditary and environmental factors. Twin research, therefore, was not simply a complement but an alternative to existing genealogical and statistical methods. As it seemed impossible to determine exact Mendelian ratios for most assumedly hereditary traits, it was only reasonable to concentrate on demonstrating heritability, especially in contested cases. It is therefore no coincidence that one of the first large-scale twin studies addressed the disputed question of TB susceptibility.

In 1933 Diehl and Verschuer published the fruits of their project as a lengthy monograph.[38] Since his appointment as department head at KWIA in 1927, Verschuer quickly developed the institute into the leading centre for twin studies. Until the beginning of World War II, an increasing number of twin pairs were registered for psychological and physiological tests as well as for studies about disease inheritance. In addition, all twins were subjected to physical measurements. It was the interest in twins that would eventually establish the KWIA's infamous links with the Auschwitz extermination camp, a connection that bears witness not only to the institute's racialist orientation but also to the difficulties in surveying twin pairs under normal circumstances.[39]

Although twin research was aimed at producing more precise results with fewer probands, the collection of a proper twin sample was no less time-consuming than the creation of a large population survey. Verschuer and Diehl had hoped to find enough adequate pairs by using the patient records of Diehl's sanatorium and by contacting some Berlin hospitals. The first returns, however, were poor because many of the detected twins refused to be examined. Only with the help of tuberculosis care stations all over Germany, they finally succeeded in bringing together a sample comprising 127 pairs (forty-five monozygotic, fifty-three dizygotic and twenty-nine mixed sex).[40] The observations were not just restricted to pairs affected by TB but also comprised some healthy pairs living in a TB-prone environment.

The relatively small size of the sample was compensated for by detailed clinical observations. In most cases there were lung radiographs as well as comprehensive medical records for both twins. Accordingly, Diehl and Verschuer were able to compare various aspects of pathological development: the time of outbreak, the organs affected, the exact localization of infections (especially in the lung), and, in case of identical manifestation, the intensity of the local infection. On this basis, it was possible to determine different degrees of concordance or discordance for each twin pair. The problem of hereditary disposition was therefore no longer restricted to the mere presence or absence of open TB cases, but could be tackled at the level of individual manifestations. This was not a completely new perspective. Already in the late nineteenth century, physicians argued that among persons susceptible to TB, there were wide individual differences with respect to the organs or tissues that acted as gateways for infection.[41] The observations of Diehl and Verschuer seemed to confirm that in twins the infection tended to affect the same parts of the lung. The more important aspect, however, was the overall result that the monozygotic twins showed a significantly higher degree of concordance than dizygotic ones. Diehl and Verschuer confidently claimed this as clear evidence for the existence of a hereditary disposition to TB.

Published at exactly the time when the Nazi regime was about to make eugenics a central political issue, the study did not fail to make an impact on the discussion. Nevertheless, it failed to win over the majority of the TB community.[42] While many experts generally rejected the strong emphasis of heredity, some critics pointed to methodological flaws. Bruno Lange, department director at the state-run Robert Koch Institute, questioned whether the monozygotic and the dizygotic twin pairs analysed in the study had actually been living under similar conditions.[43] This was not the only weak point. Because Diehl and Verschuer arranged their material according to different degrees of concordance, the absolute numbers in each statistical group were hardly as impressive as they claimed. Much more problematic, however, was the disturbing existence of monozygotic twins for which the clinical record was clearly discordant.

It was Diehl who took the methodological criticisms more seriously.[44] Three years after their first study, Diehl and Verschuer presented an extended survey and re-examined some of their old pairs in order to rule out ambivalent observations. Raising the total number of observed pairs to 239, they were able to provide a more solid statistical basis for their claims.[45] In addition, they put more emphasis on hygienic and social conditions in the individual cases. Still, they were not really able to integrate the phenomenon of monozygotic discordance into their interpretation. After a closer examination of these cases, they attributed them to the influence of other preceding diseases.[46] In other words, they admitted that a certain part of TB infections developed exclusively due to unfavourable external conditions, regardless of the individual disposition.

By the mid-1930s it became obvious that the twin project would not generate the results Diehl and Verschuer had hoped for. In their first study they had already in fact suggested that a definite answer to the TB question would require a comprehensive screening of complete families, including precise clinical examinations and hygienic observations.[47] However, they were not willing to wait until this eugenic vision of perfect surveillance could be realized. Diehl drew his own conclusions from the intricacies of human statistics: he resorted to animal experimentation. After several years of work, he succeeded in breeding rabbits showing different forms of susceptibility. While some of his breeds developed TB infections exclusively in the pulmonary system, others were affected only in the brain, the bones or the lymph nodes.[48] Ironically, the project of Diehl and Verschuer ended up where bacteriological TB research had started: with a simulation of pathogenic development that allowed them to pass over the imponderabilities of data about humans.

For Diehl, his experimental results provided a solid confirmation of the twin study. Yet all their efforts to improve data and methods did not significantly improve Verschuer and Diehl's position in the TB community. Even under Nazism, political conditions were not as favourable to their intentions as they may have expected. Though the regime enforced rigorous sanctions against 'antisocial' TB carriers, the disease was never about to be redefined as a hereditary disease.[49] Diehl and Verschuer never argued that it should rank among the allegedly genetic anomalies sanctioned by the sterilization law. Being aware that more radical postulations would face considerable opposition in the medical community, they did not go beyond calls for more determined 'eugenic counselling'. When Verschuer and Diehl reiterated their results in the 1941 meeting of the German Tuberculosis Society – confidently presenting their work as definite proof of a genetic TB factor[50] – their conclusions were not only questioned on scientific grounds. Several attending physicians also objected that any suggestion of TB a hereditary disease should be avoided in public. In view of well-known eugenic practices, they argued, any such statement would have catastrophic consequences for people's willingness to attend physicians or TB care stations.[51] Paradoxically, the realization of eugenic measures turned against the concept of hereditarily determined TB. But the meagre support for this concept was also due to the highly ambiguous results presented by its advocates. Assembled to provide definite evidence for a hereditary disposition to TB, Verschuer and Diehl's twins ultimately demonstrated that non-hereditary factors could not be excluded from the statistical picture.

Conclusion

Up to the present day, the question of hereditary susceptibility to TB poses an especially complex challenge to human geneticists. In the age of genomic test methods, the problem is still approached by large epidemiological surveys, pedigree analysis, the investigation of model populations and twin samples, often with inconsistent results.[52] This methodological plurality is by no means unique to TB but characteristic of the medical view of heredity, which rarely concerns diseases that are unambiguously genetic. The development discussed in this essay therefore allows for some general conclusions.

First of all, it demonstrates that all knowledge about human heredity depends on, and is shaped by, institutions and structures providing data for research: hospital and census records, insurance surveys, collections of genealogical material. The development of statistical approaches would not have been possible without the advance in structures for TB care. Yet the accessibility of large amounts of patient data alone did not secure sound results. Since neither population surveys nor medical records were kept for the benefit of studies on heredity, the material had to be adjusted to the specific needs of the statistical projects. This adoption seldom went smoothly, repeatedly revealing flaws in data composition and ambivalences in interpretation. This is why many researchers deferred a definite solution to the problem to a future in which more comprehensive and standardized systems of medical record-keeping would be realized.

The statistical study of TB susceptibility, like other problems of human heredity, was subject to a specific methodological dialectic: the greater the quantity of data, the more reduced its quality, and vice versa. Surveying the TB mortality of a larger population necessarily implied a superficial definition of the disease, while a sample comprising more detailed clinical histories required restricting the number of observations. This situation also explains the striking incongruities and even methodological incompatibilities between different studies. 'Hereditary susceptibility to TB' could mean different things to a statistician calculating entries in hospital files or on death certificates, a physician following case histories over a longer period, or a pathologist comparing the results of radiographs or post-mortems. The different statistical approaches associated with these perspectives not only highlighted different aspects of the medical problem but also involved diverging understandings of heredity.

The reason for the inconsistency in understanding 'heredity' can be explained by the difficulty in defining diseases as 'characters' or 'traits'. This is especially true for pathological phenomena that were most relevant to practitioners, medical statisticians and eugenicists – apart from TB, most notably cancer and the mental diseases. These polymorphic diseases defied an undisputed definition as primarily hereditary, let alone as Mendelian traits. For this reason, the medical study of heredity was more concerned with determining heritability than with the exact identification of genetic 'causes'. A comprehensive history of human heredity in the twentieth century should, therefore, account for cases in which the boundaries between the hereditary and the non-hereditary were especially contested, as well as for the aetiological and epidemiological concepts and practices that informed the medical perception of hereditary disease.

Acknowledgements

Research for this paper was enabled by a grant of the German Research Foundation (DFG). I thank Edmund Ramsden and Staffan Müller-Wille for their comments and editorial suggestions.

2 CHAMPIONING A US CLINIC FOR HUMAN HEREDITY: PRE-WAR CONCEPTS AND POST-WAR CONSTRUCTS

Philip K. Wilson

Early US eugenic attempts at institutionalizing human heredity resulted in the formation of the Eugenic Record Office (ERO) in 1910. For the next few decades, the ERO served as a repository of eugenical information, an 'analytical index' of the traits and diseases of American families, a training centre for field workers who gathered eugenical data, an investigatory stronghold for identifying the inheritance of specific human traits, and an advice clearinghouse regarding the 'eugenical fitness' of proposed marriages.[1] Initially, ERO work was restricted to investigating institutionalized persons and select volunteer families. Over the years its aims grew towards surveying whole populations via the networking of physicians on one hand and undertaking more specific medical studies of heredity on the other. To accomplish this last aim, a Clinic for Human Heredity was proposed. However, plans for such a clinic were not realized by World War II. Only after the war, when human genetics became more embedded in medical practice, was such a clinic established. This essay discusses two approaches towards establishing medical institutions specialized in the study of human heredity: the plans promoted by the prominent eugenicist Harry H. Laughlin in the 1930s, and the genetics clinic realized by the medical geneticist Victor A. McKusick in the 1950s. Comparing these approaches highlights the profound changes in the conceptual and institutional frameworks for such projects during the mid-twentieth century.

Laughlin's Idea for a Clinic in Human Heredity

According to ERO Superintendent Harry H. Laughlin, ScD during the late 1930s, the ERO daily received inquiries from 'intelligent members of families with specific [hereditary] problems' as well as from physicians 'not specialized in human genetics' who sought ERO researchers with whom to collaborate.[2] Though the ERO had not initially intended to handle such inquiries, they found that the demands for such 'service ... [were] forced upon the[ir] attention' in ways they could not ignore.[3]

Over the course of a year spanning 1937 and 1938, the ERO gathered thirty-three specific genetics case inquiries as a special research project. These inquiries were answered 'in as clear a fashion as was permitted by the data furnished ... and by the existing knowledge of the inheritance'.[4] In reply, specific research reports were referenced, and Laughlin offered probabilities of outcomes according to Mendelian modelling. Upon completing this study, he noted two particular ERO limitations, namely: 1) the 'scarcity and inaccuracy of pertinent data presented by the inquirer'; and 2) 'a lack of knowledge of the genetics of ... particular subject-trait[s]'.[5] To rectify these shortcomings in ways that would resurrect his own faltering reputation within the eugenics community, Laughlin proposed creating a Clinic in Human Heredity 'to compute and to supply specific probabilities' regarding hereditary disease. It was believed that a 'competent and widely used Clinic' would improve 'population-quality', particularly by diminishing the 'severer ... hereditary handicaps of ... body or psyche' within only 'a few years' by following 'clinical advice voluntarily sought' regarding eugenically desirable matings.[6]

Such a Clinic in Human Heredity would serve as a training centre for physicians, a gathering point for geneticists and public health workers interested in the best approaches for preventing disease, an outlet for providing direct patient care, and a counselling centre for patients concerned about marriageability issues. More generally, this clinic would also, Laughlin argued, provide an organized interdisciplinary network of professionals collectively working towards the betterment of humanity. Such a team approach was ideal, he noted, in order to formulate a greater understanding of the hereditary predisposition that was thought to underlie a multitude of chronic diseases. By ultimately reducing the incidence of these diseases, such a heredity clinic would, Laughlin concluded, eventually come to be recognized as a key centralized national centre for promoting the 'betterment' of society.

Laughlin's strategy for the design of a heredity clinic was largely an extension of the ERO. Since the 1910s the ERO had relied predominantly upon the pedigree chart as its most common tool of assimilating and promulgating information about the nation's reproductive stock, for the most part assembled in order to assess the 'eugenical fitness' of contemplated marriages.[7] Additionally, the ERO used pedigree charts to objectify, quantify and visualize the propagation of allegedly hereditary diseases. Utilizing sheaves of pedigree charts, Laughlin had previously convinced many states to adopt his model sterilization law as the official legislative organ to involuntarily control the reproduction of their institutionalized populations.[8] Pedigree charts were also, so he argued, the 'obvious' choice to unambiguously document and visualize the diseases that were central to the operations of a heredity clinic.[9]

Laughlin's Model Clinic

Laughlin directed his initial efforts in clinic design towards adding a heredity component to physician George Draper's highly successful Constitution Clinic at Presbyterian Hospital in New York City. Draper had gained renown for studying patients with the aim of identifying particular 'types' of constitutional make-up associated with certain chronic diseases. By focusing specifically upon variations between these constitutional typologies, Draper deemed that physicians could more accurately determine the best treatment for and ultimately the prevention of these diseases.[10] His success resulted largely from designing treatment protocols that were 'situated within a narrative of moral improvement and self-restraint'.[11]

By the mid-1930s Draper had modified his initial Hippocratic view of constitutional disease to include heredity, acknowledging that the 'hereditary unit character' contributed significantly to the holistic development of one's constitution. Thus knowing a patient's 'hereditary type', he concluded, would ultimately improve physicians' accuracy in their diagnoses.[12]

Laughlin attempted to persuade the Rockefeller Foundation to expand their funding of Draper's Constitution Clinic to cover heredity in equal measure to other constitutional components. In Laughlin's words, there was 'No more profitable tie-up' for the Rockefeller Foundation than that 'between human genetics and the work of ... [Draper's] Clinic'. From the perspective of genetics, he continued, 'knowledge would advance through the development of more definite diagnostic standards ... [which] students of genetics would use ... in collecting pedigree material for ... analysis'. In turn the Constitution Clinic 'would profit from the analysis of human pedigrees ... with a view to seeking the rules by which Nature governs the transmission of definite elements of the human constitution from one generation to the next'.[13]

The Rockefeller Foundation did not, however, see Laughlin's argument in such a favourable light. Having failed to forge his desired connections between the Draper Clinic and the ERO, Laughlin sought support on other fronts. Working with the membership of the National Research Council's (NRC) Committee on Human Heredity – which included Lewellys Barker from Johns Hopkins – Laughlin attempted to secure their support in establishing a Clinic for Human Genetics. Again, his efforts were rebuffed. At this point Laughlin divested his effort to achieve his goal through two different private ventures. With the primary support of investors Wickliffe Preston Draper, Boston lawyer Malcolm Donald, US Supreme Court Justice John Marshall Harlan, and Frederick Osborn, president of the American Eugenics Society (AES), Laughlin helped co-found a group in 1937 whose initial plans included the establishment of an Institute of American Eugenics. One component of this Institute provided for the foundation and maintenance of a 'marriage clinic', to which 'persons seriously interested in the inheritance of human racial and family-stock qualities could present their specific problems for advice and information in accordance with the known facts on human heredity'.[14] The work of this newly founded group, eventually renamed the Pioneer Fund, attained many of its initial eugenical goals under Laughlin's directorship. It failed, however, to garner the support needed to found a fully functioning eugenics-based clinic.[15]

Exemplifying his characteristic fortitude, Laughlin sought yet another pathway to gain support for his clinic. Laughlin approached James E. Eddy, a wealthy lumberman and founder of the Institute of Forest Genetics in Placerville, California, with the hope of extending Eddy's interests 'from forestry to the "human tree"'.[16] Eddy shared Laughlin's vision of enabling eugenics to conquer chronic disease by establishing a Clinic in Human Heredity. He discussed this plan with California Institute of Technology geneticist T. H. Morgan, who regarded the idea as 'excellent' and suggested that it should be 'started and carried out in connection with some established laboratory such as that at Cold Spring Harbor'. He urged Eddy to provide 'permanent [financial] support', warning that it was one thing to start a clinic of this kind but quite another to 'ensure its future support'.[17]

Eddy approached Laughlin about establishing a clinic that would work closely with the ERO, whereupon Laughlin promptly drafted an 'Outline of the Organization, Staff and Service, Proposed for "The Clinic of Human Heredity"' and presented it to John C. Merriam, president of the Carnegie Institution in Washington, DC in July 1937. In it, a 100,000 cubic foot clinic was to be situated near the ERO on Carnegie property. The building would consist of the clinic's headquarters, an office and a laboratory as well as archives and library space for pedigree analysis. Staffing would include 'one eugenicist-in-charge', one investigator 'skilled in the diagnosis and measurement of human traits', one geneticist 'skilled in the rules of inheritance of human traits', one field worker, one secretary-stenographer who would also act as archivist/librarian, and one janitorial caretaker. After an initial $70,000 investment for the building and equipment, Laughlin proposed that the clinic could be run on $20,000 per annum.[18] Creating such a well-organized and maintained clinic would, he argued, become a 'model for similar clinics, many of which would be required to serve the whole field effectively, and which ... could be established in universities, medical schools ... social centers ... [or] possibly [stand] independently' as well.[19]

According to Laughlin and Eddy's plan, the clinic would work as follows: initially, patients faced with 'a particular problem in human heredity' would 'supply ... evidence from several near-kin with a description of the presence or absence [of a trait] or the degree of development of the same ... [or 'allied'] trait[s] in each named near-kin'. After analysis of the pedigree evidence, the 'findings would be reported [back] to the inquirer'. Though such findings would 'not necessarily [need to] include advice', they should state 'as accurately as possible the behavior of Nature in reference to the inheritance of the particular subject-trait' as well as the 'probabilities of the particular trait being transmitted along certain branches of a specified family tree'. Laughlin reiterated the need for establishing the clinic in close proximity to the ERO because 'the world's stock of knowledge of rules of inheritance of a given trait are on hand and available for critical application to the specific [hereditary] problem'. This expression suggests that Laughlin envisioned the basic aspects of hereditary disease as a given fact rather than a matter to be explored by virtue of comparative observations within a clinical setting. He posited that the clinic staff offer their services to the public in exchange for completed pedigree information, noting that pedigrees were of such 'great use to the archives of human heredity' that they had cost much more when procured by ERO-trained field workers, and that they were more likely to be completed if exchanged for free clinical services.[20]

Beyond an obsessive gathering of pedigrees, it is difficult to see what specific clinical duties Laughlin envisioned. No specifics were mentioned as to the medical specialties required, the number of beds to be allocated for particular kinds of patients, or whether the clinic would operate as a polyclinic in which patients would be seen for short visits without the expectation of hospitalization. Moreover, particulars as to how this clinic would precisely expand ERO initiatives remained nebulous. This vagueness in project design was hardly suited to persuading potential backers to support such a speculative venture.

Carnegie President Merriam's support would be critical for the birth of this clinic. His response, however, was not all that Eddy and Laughlin had desired. Merriam argued that since the clinic would have 'as its normal function a broad relation to health and medical problems', it would more likely achieve its clinical aims if 'connected with a great university hospital or with some independent institution of the hospital-research laboratory type'. He acknowledged that the pedigree data assembled by the ERO was indeed 'indispensable' for such a clinic; but rather than adding the expense of building a clinic on its own somewhat remote grounds, he argued that the ERO could better establish links with an existing clinic in a big city whereby the latter could 'obtain use of [ERO] materials without serious interference with the progress of the [existing ERO] research program'. In principle, he concluded that it would be wiser to keep the ERO and the newly devised clinic 'sharply separate as to responsibilities and administration'.[21]

Prompted by Merriam's response, Laughlin reached out to establish ties with the Johns Hopkins Hospital in Baltimore, Maryland. Despite persistent efforts, the specific Clinic in Human Heredity that he envisioned never materialized. Much of this was due to matters of circumstance or timing, a lack of overall management design and Laughlin's own diminishing reputation. Upon retirement, Merriam was succeeded by Vannevar Bush in January 1939. Though Laughlin immediately apprised Bush of his plans for a clinic, Bush deferred the matter until he became more familiar with overall Carnegie-funded operations. Like other US medical science institutions that endorsed eugenics, the Carnegie Institution began to distance itself from this connection. Most strikingly, the ERO was closed in December 1939 upon the Carnegie Institution's withdrawal of further financial support. Beyond such political frameworks, Laughlin's clinic concept also failed to generate intellectual resonances in a medical world that was still grappling over whether patients who presumably carried a hereditary predisposition to disease would be better served in a general clinic or one dedicated to hereditary disease.

World War II's intercession postponed the fulfilment of many pre-war medical science plans, including the creation of a Laughlin-model Clinic in Human Heredity. Still, during the war and in the early post-war years, we find an outgrowth of facilities – some even called 'Clinics' – that regularly 'offer[ed] competent advice on all phases of human heredity'.[22] These included the Hereditary Clinic of the University of Michigan, financed through the Rackham Research Foundation beginning in 1940, and the Dight Institute for Human Genetics at the University of Minnesota, which opened the following year and later secured the ERO's family trait records.[23] Other programmes were initiated in North Carolina, Utah, Texas, Oklahoma and Ohio.[24] Though not all were fully fledged clinics, these minimally staffed entities were situated within pre-existing hospital or clinic settings and offered what Sheldon Reed of the Dight Institute referred to as 'genetic consultation' and 'genetic advice'.[25]

In response to public demand at this time, 'a number of medical schools which had pioneered in medical genetics set up hereditary clinics where ... couples [with questions] could talk with qualified people'.[26] According to Frederick Osborn's later reflections, these clinics originated 'quite independently of each other, but by the logic of their situation they ... developed similar operating procedures'. The post-war 'hereditary counselor' was not, as had been the case in the ERO, to give couples authoritative advice as to whether they should have a child. Rather, the new clinic counsellors were assigned to carefully study the family records and inform each couple of 'the statistical likelihood of their having a defective child as compared to the likelihood for couples in the general population', based on 'the best information available'. They were expected to leave the decision making entirely up to each couple.[27]

To find an institution that came near the model that Laughlin envisioned, a clinical structure that not only provided genetic consultation but also undertook research and teaching whereby the entire specialty of medical genetics could advance, we turn to the Johns Hopkins Hospital in Baltimore. Laughlin had favoured Hopkins during the pre-war era as the particular site that held all of the key ingredients from which to establish a model Clinic in Human Heredity. However, it was not until the post-war period that conceptual changes and institutional reorganizations were able to bring such a fully fledged clinic into operation.

Birth of the Hopkins Clinic in Medical Genetics

The Medical Genetics Clinic at the Johns Hopkins Hospital grew out of a long-standing clinic for treating syphilis – a disease that both sufferers and healers had long suspected was transmitted, at least in part, due to hereditary factors.[28] Hugh Young, while directing the venereal disease prevention programme for the American Expeditionary Forces during World War I, had recruited Joseph Earl Moore to work in and (beginning in 1929) to supervise Hopkins's Syphilis Clinic. Moore significantly altered the operations of this clinic, housed on the second floor of the Carnegie Dispensary Building. During the 1930s this space officially became designated as the 'Medicine 1' Clinic in order to avoid further stigmatization of syphilitic patients who were seen there as outpatients. In 1938, through Moore's innovative leadership, '[p]rovisions were made whereby an entire family ... in which at least one case of syphilis was suspected, could be handled in one clinic'.[29] Establishing this family-oriented form of health care delivery within Medicine 1 was subsequently helpful in caring for families in which genetic disease ran rampant.

By the early 1950s, following the increased availability of penicillin, Moore deemed that the Medicine 1 Clinic's work 'wasn't as exciting ... as it had been'. Remembering that his voluminous files contained 'a tremendous collection of patients' [records] with all sorts of chronic diseases', he converted this space into a 'multifaceted chronic disease clinic'.[30] With its new focus on chronic disease, Medicine 1 undertook 'life-long observation of its patients'.[31] Specific 'techniques of patient follow-up and diagnostic filing', which had long seemed 'unique and invaluable' for the study and treatment of syphilis, seemed 'admirably suited for the care and study of individuals with other chronic diseases'.[32] Furthermore, Moore envisioned that studying patients with chronic disease would prove to be of 'considerable service' in 'assuming responsibility of [the] follow-up care of individuals who are of potential interest but who are not presently ill enough to justify continued attendance to a general medical clinic'.[33] Moore advocated for several research resources, including the housing of 'a clinic and a laboratory side by side'[34] as well as providing a second-to-none cross-indexed filing system of diagnostic data.[35]

In mid-1957 A. McGehee Harvey, physician-in-chief of the Johns Hopkins Hospital, appointed Hopkins physician Victor A. McKusick to take over the operations of the Medicine 1 Clinic. According to McKusick, his 'deal' with Harvey was that he would be 'permitted to develop a division of medical genetics within the Department of Medicine on the same footing as all other divisions, having the triple role of teaching, research, and patient care'. Medicine 1, already renowned for its study of chronic disease, seemed ideal to McKusick, who considered genetic disease to be the 'ultimate in chronic disease since you have it all your life. You're born with it'.[36] On 1 July 1957 McKusick officially became chief of the newly created Division of Medical Genetics, an appointment that secured his position on the pathway by which he eventually became recognized as the 'founder of modern medical genetics'.[37]

McKusick was fortunate to have 'inherited' a long-term follow-up clinic facility, a well-funded fellowship programme and an established link with the Hopkins School of Hygiene and Public Health.[38] Such a link was essential to disseminate among physicians a mindset aimed at preventing disease in future generations. Medicine 1 had a steady volume of patients[39] and well-established facilities for social service work with the families of patients.[40] Still, much was required to functionally change the operations of a busy chronic disease clinic into one with a 'sub-clinic' dedicated to that new specialty focus, 'medical genetics'.

McKusick kept close tabs on the hereditary counselling efforts that had been established in US medical centres. In November 1957 he participated in a symposium on that topic sponsored by the AES.[41] To better assure himself of what was transpiring in such clinics across the globe, he made a whirlwind tour of Europe, visiting key sites in Berlin, Cologne, Münster, Heidelberg, Stuttgart, Munich, Milan, Rome, Bern, Geneva, Paris, London, Oxford, Birmingham and Cardiff in August and September 1958.

By the end of his first year as physician-in-charge, McKusick announced the reorganization of the newly named Joseph Earle Moore Clinic (formerly Medicine 1) into a group of sub-clinics that included Connective Tissue Clinic, Growth [i.e. Cancer] Clinic, Hypertension Clinic, Kidney Clinic, Rehabilitation Clinic, Sarcoidosis Clinic, Venereal Disease Clinic and General Chronic Disease Clinic, as well as the Medical Genetics Clinic which McKusick coordinated. Building upon the existing meticulous record-filing system, McKusick prepared a systematic entry form – including pedigree data – in his 'Log Book of Medical Genetics at the Moore Clinic'. A standard file folder was to be maintained for each kindred and filed according to pedigree number. Although McKusick acknowledged that 'the great majority of information' may exist in general hospital unit records, 'special information of confidential nature, photographs, which might become damaged in the unit history, negatives of photographs, x-rays from other institutions, etc' were to be kept in these newly created clinical files.[42] Ninety-nine different genetic diagnoses were represented among the first 200 patients seen during the Medical Genetics Clinic's first six months of operation.[43] To better manage the heavy patient load, within the first few years McKusick hired three assisting physicians: Malcolm A. Ferguson-Smith, Samuel H. (Ned) Boyer and Abraham Lilienfield.

To bolster his studies in the Medical Genetics Clinic, McKusick's investigations were not simply based upon those patients who walked through the door. Between 1925 and 1930 Raymond Pearl, director of the Hopkins Institute for Biological Research, had operated a 'constitution clinic' in which patients from some 528 families had been seen when a family member 'came to the hospital for one condition or another'. McKusick followed up Pearl's family studies, with the help of Pearl's now seventy-year-old assistant. Given the 'large number of individuals catalogued in each family', McKusick anticipated being able to 'trace more than 95 per cent' of these families.[44]

McKusick's correspondence reveals much about his inquisitive method of gaining evidence about genetic disease. 'I would appreciate very much having information on the present status of your son', he writes to one family, 'Do you have other children? ... Do you think that there have been in your family any children with a condition similar to [your son's]?' When requesting a reply, McKusick included a stamped envelope.[45]

For some, he helped pay their transportation costs to his clinic, such as the $5.00 check he sent to a Washington, DC-based patient on welfare without transportation. The ever money-conscious McKusick added, 'please come by bus because it is the least expensive way'.[46] For others, his desire to review their cases was so strong that he absorbed additional costs. Writing in October 1958 to an individual in Virginia suffering from scleroderma, cataracts and Werner Syndrome, McKusick explains,

> I have recently come upon your hospital record from the times you were here as a patient ... We have been particularly interested in the trouble from which you suffer. I gather that your sister has a similar condition for which she has been under the care of one of the physicians at the University of Virginia. We would appreciate it very much if you would come to Baltimore to have a checkup some time in the near future. We can make arrangements to have you admitted to the hospital at the expense of our study assuming it ... is necessary for you to be in the hospital for only 4 or 5 days at the very most. Furthermore, I am willing to make the same offer to your sister. If you desire, we can arrange for you to be in the same room in the hospital.

Though he did not 'guarantee' his study would turn up anything that would 'work miracles', he saw to it that his work created neither expense nor inconvenience to these patients.[47] Delving into his own research funds, McKusick invited the sister's doctor in Virginia to come, too.[48]

Beyond the plans that Laughlin had envisioned for a clinic, the Medical Genetics sub-clinic at Hopkins involved both laboratory and clinical research, as McKusick's first 'Research Summary' (18 June 1959) details. In regard to Milroy's disease (hereditary edema), the clinic had studied one family and noted that another was available for further study; they planned to analyse the familial linkages, perform plethysmography, and secure lymphangiograms from those so diagnosed. In regard to the hereditary linkages suspected regarding coronary artery disease, clinicians had completed the analysis of a retrospective 1954–8 study as well as initiated a progressive study using data from recent deaths and also from a group of patients surviving coronary disease. Regarding Marfan's syndrome, a disease that captured McKusick's special attention, upper-segment/lower-segment limb ratios were compared between 2,000 school children considered to be normal and thirty Marfan's patients. Though McKusick acknowledged that Marfan's patients had been studied quantitatively for joint mobility, his Medical Genetics Clinic pursued a statistical analysis of the prognosis, expression and overall genetics of each patient in order to formulate a 'more precise definition of various parameters' of this disease.[49]

McKusick noted a number of other concurrent clinical investigations into genetic disease, including the study of mother-daughter pairs in reference to toxemia of pregnancy, the genetic and epidemiologic study of Buerger's disease, and an upcoming corneal transplant for a patient with Hurler's syndrome. Given the proximity of the laboratory to the clinic, it is not surprising to see a number of cytogenetic studies that were undertaken. One study of 160 'mongols' at the nearby Rosewood State Training School (previously known as the Asylum and Training School for the Feeble Minded) concluded that their cytogenetic chromosome analysis showed their nuclear sex to be consistent with their phenotype. Three other 'mongols' were subjected to chromosome analysis, whereupon the basic diploid number was found to be 47 in each case, though 'considerable variation' existed in this number from cell to cell, and in one case distinct structural changes were noted which required further study. Three cases of Klinefelter's syndrome were found among 250 'male defectives' studied at Rosewood. Additional chromosomal analysis had recently been undertaken by the clinic in four cases of sex anomalies. There, they found one individual with chromatin negative gonadal aplasia to have a 2n chromosomal count of 45 and an XO sex constitution, whereas an individual with chromatic positive gonadal aplasia showed a 2n count of 46 and an XX sex constitution. A case of male pseudohermaphroditism showed a 2n count of 26, with an XY constitution, and in a true hermaphroditism case, McKusick reported the 'puzzling failure to identify Y in any of [the] 25 plates' studied.[50]

As seen by McKusick's late 1950s investigations, cytogenetic studies were becoming the standard method for comparative medical genetics. Although the pedigree had not been replaced, what appeared on pedigrees reflected newly developed typological comparisons at the chromosomal level.

Conclusion

Following World War II, physicians worked more closely with geneticists, some actually becoming specialized in medical genetics as a result of their quest to better understand the genetic factors underlying many diseases. In general, these specialists deemed that by studying human heredity more intensely, they could 'make earlier diagnoses, introduce preventive measures, perhaps even develop cures'.[51] In order to more fully achieve these clinical aims, many deemed that a new operational structure – the Medical Genetics Clinic – was essential. Subsequent advancements in this field took place within such clinics, for which McKusick's restructured Moore Clinic at Hopkins served as a model.

Although some threads of Laughlin's theoretical framework are identifiable in the fabric of McKusick's clinic, the dissimilarities between pre-war concepts and post-war constructions far outweigh the similarities. Such dissimilarity was, in part, due to the changing knowledge of genetic disease as well as the distinctions between the ERO's aims and those of Hopkins. For Laughlin, the concept for the clinic was an offshoot of the ERO's existing working structure which revolved around the production, storage and analysis of pedigree charts. His plans were laid more from the perspective of an architect's theoretical framework, focusing little attention to the organization of clinical care. McKusick, in contrast, took on more of a contractor's role, remodelling the elements of the clinical setup he had inherited. His approach to medical genetics had grown out of a setting in which a wide variety of disease aetiologies had once been investigated, including that of heredity. Patients who were either seen in the clinic or whose clinical case presentations were studied retrospectively provided the core evidence that established further research protocols. This form of data management allowed McKusick to gather all possible types of data from these patients, which were deemed to hold potential for understanding a broader scope of the genetics underlying disease. In this way, the Moore Clinic provided a practical working model in which to readily and rapidly gather information from patients, include it in a comprehensive database of files that allowed for statistical analysis, and experimentally investigate select cases at the lab bench.

Acknowledgements

The author is grateful for the exemplary assistance from the entire staff at the Alan Mason Chesney Medical Archives of the Johns Hopkins Medical Institutions, Baltimore, Maryland; Special Collections at the Pickler Memorial Library, Truman State University, Kirksville, Missouri; and the American Philosophical Society Library, Philadelphia, Pennsylvania. Additional helpful insight offered by Bernd Gausemeier, Edmund Ramsden, Jan Witkowski and Nathaniel Comfort is also warmly appreciated.

3 REMODELLING THE BOUNDARIES OF NORMALITY: LIONEL S. PENROSE AND POPULATION SURVEYS OF MENTAL ABILITY

Edmund Ramsden

Introduction

When it comes to critics of eugenics from within the biological sciences, few are as renowned and respected as the British medical geneticist Lionel Sharpless Penrose (1898–1972). It was not simply that he was severe and incisive in his criticism – this was a characteristic he shared with the left-wing biologists J. B. S. Haldane and Lancelot Hogben. Penrose is considered unique in terms of the depth and consistency of his censure. While others may have tempered their criticisms by declaring a determination to distinguish a true eugenics from false, to place it on a sure scientific footing, Penrose identifies the very idea of eugenics to be fatally flawed. He is celebrated for his critique; Deborah Thom and Mary Jennings see Penrose serving as 'almost the Galileo of genetics, establishing "true science" in the face of the religiosity of the eugenicists'.[1] In more measured terms, Diane Paul sees his position to be 'a major exception' among mid-century biologists.[2]

One of the aims of this essay is to complicate this story – but not, as has been so popular in recent years, by attempting to uncover an underlying sympathy for eugenics by another of its famed critics. The power and importance of Penrose's critique will be emphasized as it is further explored.[3] We will see how his analysis of the relationship between intelligence and fertility helped contribute a more optimistic vision of man's biological future. In this, Penrose was aided by evidence of an increase in the intellectual capacity of Western nations, as measured by a series of important post-war population surveys. While evidence of intelligence increases is seen as a recent phenomenon, perceived by many to necessitate a fundamental revaluation of the methods and applications of mental measurement,[4] it has a longer history that is rarely recognized by contemporary commentators. Historians have given little attention to this new orthodoxy of intelligence increase, preferring to focus on eugenicist fears of intellectual deterioration. They have also paid little attention to population surveys more generally, in spite of their important role in continuously generating new questions and problems, new social and scientific interests and concerns.[5]

The evidence provided by the Scottish Mental Survey of 1947 contradicted the eugenic assumptions of its creators and gave critical support to those who emphasized the decisive role of environmental factors in determining intellectual capacity.[6] Its results supported Penrose's arguments of the 1930s. Penrose had drawn upon surveys of child growth that showed how stature, which has a significant hereditary component, could be increased through improved nutrition and exercise. Yet at this precise moment, Penrose also sought a genetically determinist explanation for the survey results. He developed an equilibristic model – as improbable as it was ingenious – that he extended far beyond its original purpose as a critical device. Penrose's interest in a genetic explanation for the survey findings will be seen to have resulted from his recognition that eugenicists were able to manipulate environmental variance to explain away the significance of intelligence increases. While proponents of eugenics such as Ronald A. Fisher and Cyril Burt may have partitioned and privileged genetic factors through their statistical methods, environmental factors remained critical to the arguments of the staunchest of 'hereditarians' – it was increasingly employed as a means of preserving support for projections of hereditary degeneration in the post-war era.

We will see how the arguments of both eugenicists and their critics became increasingly sophisticated and overstated in response to one another. Indeed, while much of the voluminous scholarship on eugenics has been driven by a concern to identify the social and political interests that have shaped the scientific focus on human heredity, scholars have been far less interested in examining the ways in which anti-eugenicists have developed and manipulated methods, models and evidence to realize their aims. Following Imre Lakatos, both sides remained true to a 'hard core' set of assumptions that could not be refuted and abandoned without a complete repudiation of their alternative belief systems and research programs.[7] The consequence was a continuous and creative reinterpretation of data, aided, in the language of Lakatos, by a set of flexible 'auxiliary' and 'positive heuristic principles' that maintained a 'protective belt' around those assumptions. By providing a solution through a genetic model, we will see how Penrose was able to challenge a more sophisticated eugenic argument that emphasized the important role of environmental factors, while, at the same moment, providing an important space in which *both* social and biological scientists could interpret intelligence as a genetically determined quality.

The Inheritance and Distribution of Stature and Intelligence

Height is a variable that has been particularly important to the development of statistics and the study of heredity. Its study contributed to Galton's law of regression to mediocrity and his concept of correlation – co-relating such variables as arm span and stature.[8] Height is, of course, something that all people share; it is easily measurable, stable among adults, a natural, tangible criterion that, perhaps most significantly, follows a normal distribution. For Galton, it revealed a fundamental law of deviation that would be seen in all common traits. By a considerable sleight of hand – mapping mental ability (first represented by a scale of social achievement) onto the distribution of height – Galton promoted the idea of intelligence as a natural entity, determined by heredity.[9] He argued that the analogy of stature 'clearly shows there must be a fairly constant average mental capacity in the inhabitants of the British Isles, and that the deviations from that average – upwards towards genius, and downwards towards stupidity – must follow the law that governs deviations from all true averages'.[10] Yet for Galton, height did more than serve as a useful tool for illustrating the distribution of normal characters; he also believed it to be directly correlated to mental ability:

> There is a prevalent belief ... that men of genius are unhealthy, puny beings – all brain and no muscle – weak-sighted, and generally of poor constitutions. I think most of my readers would be surprised at the stature and physical frames of the heroes of history ... if they could be assembled together in a hall ... A collection of living magnates in various branches of intellectual achievement is always a feast to my eyes; being, as they are, such massive, vigorous, capable-looking animals.[11]

The striking similarity of the curves of distribution was no coincidence. Physical size was indicative of the physiological basis of intelligence – of 'circumference of head, size of brain, weight of grey matter, number of brain fibres, &c.; and thence ... mental capacity'.

Galton's arguments were applied to the study of children's growth by two leading figures of American physiology, Henry Pickering Bowditch and William Townsend Porter. In 1892 Porter had measured 33,500 children in the public schools of St Louis from the ages of six to fifteen, collecting data on height, weight, head and facial morphology, chest girth and grip strength. He was the first to compare these physical measurements with ability at school, measured by grade level in relation to chronological age.[12] While he accepted that his analysis was inevitably crude, after plotting his results he believed that the curves of his graph expressed a 'truth' that was 'was very plain. They declare in unmistakable lines that precocious children are heavier and dull children lighter than the mean child of the same age. They establish a physical basis of precocity and dullness'.[13]

Porter's evidence was a powerful demonstration of the biological basis of differences in intellect. Henry H. Goddard, director of research at the Vineland

Training School for Feeble-Minded Girls and Boys in New Jersey, began his influential report of 1912 on the height and weight of 'feeble-minded' children: 'It has been long been known that in man there is some connection between size of body and mentality. Even among normal people, on the average, size means efficiency, – as is shown by Porter's measurements of school children'.[14] Dividing his inmates into categories that would become standard in psychology – idiots, imbeciles and morons – he found that the greater the deviation from the normal, the lower their height and weight. Small size was indicative of low intelligence. Yet in Goddard's pedigree studies, gone was the smooth, normal distribution of intelligence. He preferred the analogy of Mendel's pea crosses – tallness (normality) being 'dominant', and dwarfness (mental deficiency) 'recessive', or the 'absence of tallness'.[15] 'Feeble-mindedness' was a true Mendelian unit character. While the 'idiot' of a low-grade intelligence was 'loathsome', he did 'not continue the race with a line of children like himself'.[16] The high-grade moron was the real danger, capable of spreading the recessive gene for feeble-mindedness throughout the normal population, breeding, of course, according to a classic ratio of three to one.

Such simplistic models of inheritance drew the ire of biometricians and contributed to their well-documented disapproval of Mendelian genetics.[17] Not only did they contradict their own studies and methods, but they also raised considerable problems for eugenics. In spite of his commitment to eugenics, R. C. Punnett concluded that as rare recessive traits would be hidden by normal carriers, selection based on the incidence of defect would prove most ineffectual.[18] The defective gene became, in the words of Johns Hopkins geneticist H. S. Jennings, 'a frightful thing; it is the embodiment, the material realization of a demon of evil; a living self-perpetuating creature, invisible, impalpable, that blasts the human being in bud or in leaf'.[19]

R. A. Fisher's famed paper of 1918 allowed for a solution.[20] Then the Galton Chair of Eugenics at University College London (UCL), Fisher demonstrated how Mendelian genetics could account for continuous variation and its inheritance in a way that was consistent with the biometric paradigm. Once again turning to stature, Fisher argued that many genetic factors were involved in the determination of quantitative characters, explaining how the discontinuity of Mendelian unit factor inheritance could be reconciled with the smooth distributions of biometrical measurement.[21] Extending this argument to the problem of mental ability, there would be numerous factors for defect. Once dominance and additive variance were taken into account, many more cases could be diagnosed by psychiatrists. Further, and consistent with the abstraction that was the Hardy-Weinberg equilibrium, Punnett had assumed mating was random. However, Fisher argued: 'In stature the resemblance of husband and wife is nearly as great as that of uncle and niece; it can scarcely be doubted that mental similarity is equally, or more, effective; those who find their "affinity" among the feeble-minded, are surely not to be taken as average citizens'.[22] The result would be the production of identifiably feeble-minded offspring, even in the case of recessive genes, and 'the concentration of the defect in a limited number of strains'.[23]

Fisher's synthesis also allowed him to deal with another challenge to eugenics – the role of the environment in determining traits and characters.[24] Fraternal resemblance for stature was approximately 0.54, leaving 46 per cent requiring some other explanation.[25] He argued that it was 'not sufficient to ascribe this last residue to the effects of environment. Numerous investigations by Galton and Pearson have shown that all measurable environment has much less effect on such measurements as stature'.[26] This residue was in fact largely genetic, consistent with Mendelian principles – 'the large variance among children of the same parents is due to the segregation of those factors in respect to which the parents are heterozygous'. Genetics not only explained the existence of traits common to families, but could also account for their differences. Using parental, fraternal and marital correlations, Fisher concluded: 'it is very unlikely that so much as 5 per cent. of the total variance is due to causes not heritable, especially as every irregularity of inheritance would, in the above analysis, appear as such a cause'.[27]

Fisher had also expressed his faith in the development of new technologies that would better identify feeble-mindedness.[28] One of the leaders in developing mental tests was the psychologist Cyril Burt. Following the Mental Deficiency Act of 1913, Burt was first employed by the London County Council (LCC) to identify feeble-minded, maladjusted and delinquent children. In the 1920s he extended his focus to assessing the performance of normal children in schools. When at the LCC, he had the opportunity of working in the laboratory of Charles Spearman, who he would later succeed as professor of psychology at UCL in 1932. Burt was committed to Spearman's notion of general intelligence – which, following the work of Galton and Pearson, posited that mental ability was hereditary and distributed normally, and that factors of mind were measurable and closely correlated, just as were the physical measures of stature, weight or forearm.[29] Burt was both a skilled biometrician and a committed Mendelian, making Fisher's resolution and analysis of variance particularly important to his quantitative estimates of heritability.[30]

Surveying Child Growth and Development

While Porter's growth studies proved extremely influential, they were subject to a critique by one of the leading figures in physical anthropology, Franz Boas.[31] Through his examination of Bowditch and Porter's data and his own studies of Toronto and Worcester schoolchildren, Boas introduced the notion of 'tempo of growth' – a child 'retarded' in height or intelligence when compared to his or her peers could catch up or even surpass them. This could be established through longitudinal surveys that traced individual growth patterns through time, unlike cross-sectional studies that created a statistical artefact by adding together individuals with different rates of acceleration and retardation. Not only did longitudinal studies undermine the predictive qualities of intelligence and growth measures, but they also questioned the degree to which intelligence was dependent upon physical factors: 'Dr. Porter has shown that mental and physical growth are correlated, or depend upon common causes; not that mental development depends upon physical growth'.[32] These common causes were further analysed in a series of studies that used biometrical methods to compare the body size and form of immigrants and those of their US-born children. The considerable increase in height revealed that while differences between genetic types existed, 'the type as we see it contains elements that are not genetic but an expression of the influence of environment'.[33] This discovery 'compelled' him to conclude that as a consequence of the environment, 'the whole bodily and mental make-up of the immigrants may change'.[34]

In the United States, Boas's studies contributed to the rapid growth of longitudinal surveys of physical and mental development in children, with the Harvard and Berkeley Growth Studies, the Fels Longitudinal Survey, the Yale Normative Study and those of the Iowa Child Welfare Station.[35] In Britain, such surveys would have to wait until the post-war era. In the meantime Boas's work provided a means of critiquing eugenic fears of physical and mental degeneration. It was employed in just such a way by Lionel Penrose.

Penrose was at this time a research medical officer at the Royal Eastern Counties Institution for mental defectives in Colchester, providing a detailed clinical and genetic study of its 1,280 patients and their relatives so as to understand the causes of mental deficiency. His conclusions were profound.[36] First, he argued that there was no sharp dividing line between mental deficiency and normality. Measurements of intelligence, the standard diagnostic tool for identifying defect, were, like stature, graded throughout the population. Second, those defined as mentally deficient were not a homogeneous group; there was no single cause, such as a Mendelian recessive for feeble-mindedness, as promoted by Henry Goddard. Mental deficiency was a sociological and legal concept or definition that covered a highly heterogeneous series of conditions. Finally, there were numerous environmental and genetic causes responsible for its occurrence.[37]

Clearly influenced by Hogben and Haldane, it was to the environment that Penrose turned when addressing the broader question of intelligence decline in the entire population. In a paper read before the National Council of Mental Hygiene in 1939, Penrose emphasized the vast array of factors, hereditary and environmental, that combined to influence mental development.[38] He argued that intelligence test scores would always be too limited to fully grasp the shape of a mind, particularly when influenced by culture. With the aid of psychologist John Raven, Penrose developed his own methods to measure educative abilities for those handicapped in verbal skills.[39] He criticized the idea that the professional and clerical classes were innately more intelligent than those of the less skilled. Social inheritance was critical: 'As there is a tendency for children to enter the same type of occupation as the parents, it can be inferred that the abilities of people in the different occupational grades will resemble those of the children in these surveys'.[40]

He transferred his discussion of the problem of intelligence to the terrain of height. Drawing from Boas's challenge to Porter, Penrose argued that the rates of growth of individuals and populations were strongly influenced by nutrition and health. Penrose noted how Boas had identified an increase in the size, weight and mental development of immigrant children, becoming more like the 'American type'. Penrose concurred, noting that the average height of British children had also increased through time. As the environment improved for the socially disadvantaged, 'Is it possible', he asked, 'that intelligence, directly measured by systematic testing at intervals, might show a similar increase?'

Penrose was using Boas's evidence to challenge eugenicist fears of intellectual deterioration through differential fertility. Degeneration seemed the logical conclusion when the fertility rates identified by demographers were combined with an understanding of intelligence as determined by heredity. Fisher had long bewailed the negative correlation between intelligence and fertility, believing that lower fertility gave individuals a distinct advantage when competing in industrial society.[41] The cost of child-bearing not only encouraged childlessness, but those with a physiological disposition for lower fertility would advance, then marry, and thus effectively sterilize, others elevated for their intellectual qualities. The result was an increased differentiation between the classes, 'uniting the highest forms of ability with relative sterility or defectiveness of the reproductive instincts, at one end of the social scale; and, at the other, the lowest grades of ability with all the genetic determinants of high fertility'.[42] Fisher lent his statistical expertise to the psychologist Raymond B. Cattell in his study of intelligence and family size of children in Leicester, and to the geneticist John A. Fraser-Roberts in his study in Bath.[43] Their conclusions were similar – predicting a significant decline in the intellectual capacity of the future British population.

The Scottish Mental Survey

Eugenicists had become increasingly reliant on demography as a means of measuring differentials in fertility between social groups. An understanding of fertility dynamics would also provide opportunities for action: by encouraging the use of birth control among the lower (and presumably less intelligent) classes while encouraging childbirth among the middle classes through family allowances, the aims of eugenics could be fulfilled through general social policy. In 1936 the Eugenics Society founded the Population Investigation Committee (PIC), which quickly became the nation's leading organization for demographic research, directed by its research secretary, the demographer and sociologist David V. Glass. The founding of the PIC followed from the 1935 Galton Lecture of the Eugenics Society by Alexander M. Carr-Saunders, Chair of Social Science at Liverpool University.[44] He argued that the 'interest in numbers' could provide for a more creative, positive and attractive form of eugenics that allowed parents to realize their ideal family size.[45]

With the Royal Commission on Population established in 1944 to address the problem of population decline, the Eugenics Society and the PIC saw an opportunity for emphasizing the importance of the study of differential fertility. The Eugenics Society decided to focus on the problems of intelligence decline. The Society chose as its star witness the respected educational psychologist at Edinburgh University and the Scottish Council for Research in Education, Godfrey Thomson, supported by a written report by Cyril Burt. Thomson had, like Burt, been engaged in the development of intelligence tests to identify children with special educational needs or abilities, irrespective of class. His work had become more prominent following the Education Act of 1944, which provided free education to all. Children would be selected for grammar, technical or secondary modern schools according to their performance on the 11-plus, a battery of intelligence and attainment tests. However, when one considered the ongoing process of differential fertility, increased social mobility could, in fact, serve to deplete the nation's reserves of intellectual ability. Thomson's memorandum suggested a decline in intelligence at the rate of one percentage point per generation: 'and this is a serious matter'.[46] He was endorsed by Burt, who also estimated the decline at 1.5 to 2.0 points.[47]

They also pushed for a survey of intelligence and family size 'on a large and systematic scale' to provide empirical support for their predictions.[48] With the blessing of the Royal Commission, and grants from Eugenics Society and Nuffield Foundation, the PIC and Scottish Council for Research in Education began a survey of the intelligence of schoolchildren in Scotland. The Scottish Mental Survey measured the IQ of all eleven-year-olds at school on the days of testing, some 70,805 children. It repeated an earlier survey of the same scale in 1932 of the 1921 birth cohort. By comparing the mean scores of both cohorts, scientists would be able to measure the effects of differential fertility on the intellectual capacities of an entire nation.

While the survey did establish an inverse relationship between intelligence and family size, when it came to assessing the effects of this differential, the results were surprising. As first reported in 1948, they revealed an increase of one to two points, the exact opposite of the original prediction.[49] The survey thus presented two pieces of evidence: that the intelligence of the population was increasing through time; and yet that the less intelligent were out-breeding the more intelligent. It seemed to many observers that the only way that these two facts were could be reconciled was through recourse to an environmental explanation for the increase in intelligence. Otis Dudley Duncan, demographer and sociologist, argued that the Scottish inquiry had given a 'final and most telling blow to the theory of intellectual deterioration'.[50] Thomson admitted: 'this strengthens the environmental side of the argument'.[51]

Many committed to an environmental interpretation of traits and abilities, who had previously questioned the benefits of a mental survey, now drew from its results. For the social epidemiologists Zena Stein and Mervyn Susser at the School of Public Health at Columbia University, the surveys provided evidence of IQ as an unstable entity that fluctuated through time.[52] Just as environmental factors had increased the heights, weights and intelligence of a generation, improved nutrition and education could lift the intelligence of the subnormal child into the range of the normal. David Glass transformed the Scottish Mental Survey from a cross-sectional into a longitudinal survey, supporting other PIC surveys such as the National Survey of Health and Development, which measured the physical and intellectual growth of national samples of children and identified how various environmental factors severely impinged upon their measured intelligence, height, health and social mobility.[53] The evidence of intellectual increase did not undermine intelligence testing as a technology, but reinforced it; now, allied with the longitudinal survey, it became a force for further social reform. As Glass took control of the PIC, it was becoming far removed from the ideals of the Eugenics Society, and more in keeping with those of Hogben and Penrose.

Penrose's Model

From 1945 Penrose's criticisms of eugenics intensified. This was the year that he accepted a new position at UCL, that of the Galton Professor of Eugenics. His title undoubtedly encouraged him, and it was not until 1963 that he succeeded in having it renamed the Galton Professorship of Human Genetics.[54] With the growing awareness of the atrocities committed through Nazi racial hygiene, eugenics had now, as the historian Daniel Kevles observed, become 'virtually a dirty word'.[55] Yet, while it is generally accepted that the 'stigma of eugenics', as Penrose described it, contributed to the power of environmental explanations for human abilities and behaviours in the post-war era, Penrose now began to promote a biological model to the forefront of his critique of eugenics. As he did so, this model assumed ever-greater degrees of generality.

Penrose drew from theories of hybrid vigour, or heterosis, used by population geneticists to explain the persistence of unfavourable traits in a population through time. As had long been established in plant and animal genetics, the crossing of pure lines encouraged vigour and fertility, as out-breeding counteracted the build-up of deleterious recessive alleles. Increasingly, over-dominance was also becoming of interest, suggested by Fisher in 1918 and soon to be established in humans in the case of sickle cell by Anthony Allison in 1954.[56] Here a gene considered undesirable could confer a selective advantage, granting heterozygous carriers immunity to malaria.

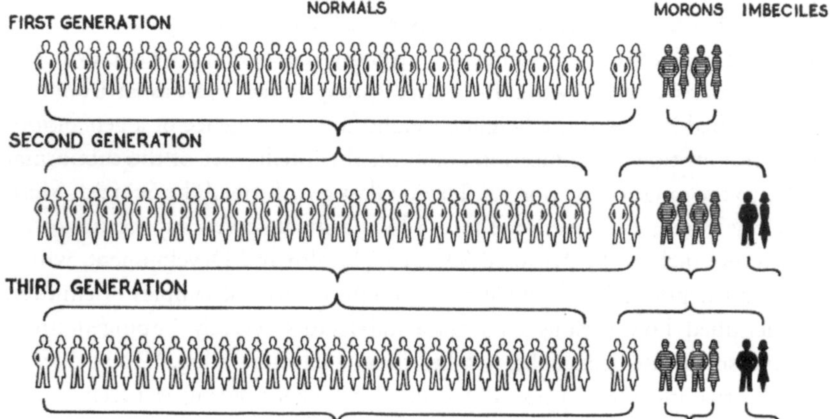

FIG. 18. Stable genetical equilibrium in a population with fully assortative mating and strongly negative correlation between intelligence and family size. Normals have genotype **AA**, morons **Aa**, and imbeciles **aa**.

Figure 3.1: 'Stable genetical equilibrium in a population with fully assortive mating and strongly negative correlation between intelligence and family size', from L. S. Penrose, *Outline of Human Genetics* (London: Heinemann, 1959), p. 117.

Penrose asked his readers to imagine a population of three main types determined by a single perfectly additive pair of allelic genes, A and a, that determined intelligence. The heterozygote, Aa, was halfway between the measurements in intelligence of the two homozygotes, AA and aa. The gene a reduced intelligence, and Penrose defined its carriers as 'morons', with reference to the ideas of Henry Goddard. This group comprised approximately one-tenth of the population, consistent with the eugenic delineation of the so-called social problem group. Those designated AA were 'normals' and made up nine-tenths of the population. Finally, a small proportion of 'imbeciles' received a double dose, aa. In terms of reproduction, the fertility of the 'normals' was below that necessary to replace their numbers, consistent with demographic studies, while the imbeciles did not reproduce at all. In contrast, and again consistent with the fears of eugenicists, carrying the gene for defect was associated with increased fertility: four per couple, over twice the national average. Assuming assortative mating, the 'moron' couple would reproduce in the next generation according to a simple Mendelian ratio: one 'normal', two 'morons' and one 'imbecile'; and thus the group as a whole: 25 per cent 'normals', 50 per cent 'moronic' and 25 per cent 'imbecilic'. Thus in each generation the 'moronic' tenth helped supplement the losses of the normal 'population'.

> The defectives are the genetical backbone of this population. If an efficient sterilization programme were instituted against this submerged fertile tenth, it would diminish the total fertility of the whole group and eventually lead to extermination of the whole race.[57]

At this point, Penrose accepted: 'The analogy between this model and human society is probably not close but it should perhaps give food for thought'.[58] A number of different alleles combined to determine intelligence. Yet he increasingly argued that this variety did not undermine his model, but strengthened it.[59] The majority of the population was heterozygous for the many factors that governed intelligence, based around the average. The greater the variation in heterozygote manifestation, the larger the number of children they would have. Once again, this highly fertile band of heterozygotes would compensate for the low fertility of the homozygotes at the extremes of distribution, of either very high or very low intelligence. Penrose believed that the model gave 'reason for rejecting eugenical theories', as, contrary to the elitism of eugenicists, 'the infertile intellectuals are found to be peripheral to a nucleus of fertile labourers'.[60] The population, therefore, existed in a state of stable equilibrium, with the 'slight' fluctuations due to fertility and environmental factors. What Penrose had done was to make the intelligence test results of the Scottish Mental Survey consistent with a genetic explanation by challenging its evidence of differential fertility. He pointed out that the method of measuring family size through a child's siblings missed a critical element of the population: those who did not have any children.[61]

Penrose continued to emphasize the role of environmental factors in the determination of traits such as intelligence. However, the genetic explanation of intelligence trends had an increasingly prominent place in his publications. This is most evident in Penrose's later treatment of his favourite analogy – height. While previously he had turned to the work of Boas, he now often referred to the work of Karl Pearson to argue that just as those at the extremes of distribution in stature, the very tall and the very short, were selected against, so to with intelligence.[62] Genetic factors were now, therefore, determining fertility. Similarly, when promoting an environmentalist argument in earlier years, Penrose had argued, contrary to Fisher, that the causes of differential fertility were more commonly 'psychological' rather than a result of 'the inherited nature of fertility'.[63] With the reduction in family size that followed increased use of contraception, intelligence would increase – large families having had restricted resources for effective child rearing. Now, however, he questioned social scientists' arguments that the use of birth control was based purely on a combination between culture and individual choice. Drawing from Galton and Fisher, Penrose increasingly argued that fertility rates in relation to intelligence were also genetically determined.[64]

Explaining the Attraction of Genetic Equilibrium

Penrose's model enjoyed a mixed response from the biological community. The population geneticist Kenneth Mather asked, 'can anyone take the model seriously? Does Professor Penrose really believe that it fairly, or even usefully, represents, albeit at a simplified level, the situation with respect to intelligence and fertility?'[65] John Fraser-Roberts described his model as 'ingenious', but then noted that it was a 'little surprising' that he should advance a hypothesis based 'simply on the analogy of single genes making for idiocy', as it 'seems out of harmony with present-day knowledge of genetic principles'.[66] It was also out of harmony with the social scientific understanding of fertility dynamics, Cyril Burt commenting that the chief 'defect' in Penrose's model was his assumption that the 'differential birth-rate is due mainly to physiological factors, whereas in my view it is mainly the effect of voluntary methods'.[67] As Penrose expanded his model, it seemed to function less as a clever parody or critical tool and more as a universal biological law.[68] So how do we explain Penrose's promotion of this model to such a degree, not only in relation to the determination of intelligence, but also to fertility dynamics? A number of events conspired to make it more attractive in the post-war era.

Firstly, under the guidance of Frederick Osborn in the USA and the psychiatrist C. P. Blacker in Britain, the eugenics movement had adapted to criticism, particularly of its programmes of sterilization focused on the mentally deficient. It shifted its focus to the promotion of voluntary family planning among the lower classes. The targeting of these populations was justified first by their high levels of unwanted fertility, and second with reference not to biological but to social heritage. Dull parents had dull children, particularly if they were undesired, and even if one assumed a sociological rather than a biological perspective. The leaders of the eugenics movement were seeking to make their aims more consistent with general social interests. The perception of fertility dynamics as socially determined and socially determining made attempts to improve directly the quality of a population more realistic. Penrose was well aware of this shift, which undoubtedly made environmentalist explanations less attractive: 'To assume that most mental variation is non-genetical in origin is, to my way of thinking, a poor defence'.[69] In presenting fertility differentials as a natural biological process, tied to innate intellectual capacity, the possibilities for eugenic improvement were more effectively denied.

Yet eugenicists had also begun using environmental factors in an even more innovative way – as a source of 'masking' an underlying process of declining genetic ability. Thomson, Burt and Cattell declared that the survey results simply did not add up. Throughout the late 1940s and the 1950s, they provided a battery of arguments to defend their original prognosis. Most controversially, they now argued that environmental factors as education and nutrition may have improved the test results while masking the process of degeneration. As Thomson explained, 'newspapers, children's journals, school reading books and the BBC' had been using the same type of item that appeared in a group test. Thomson argued that the question was still open. The claim that there was no decline was 'naive'. There had been a 'false' rise, which could 'hide a fall due to selection, which might win in the long run ... we must beware of being lulled into a sense of security by an improvement which may be apparent only'.[70]

This was an argument that they had prepared beforehand, thanks to Penrose. In a Eugenic Society symposium held on 21 January 1947, structured around Thomson's predictions, Penrose had referred to the increasing heights of Toronto schoolchildren.[71] Thomson responded by claiming that better nutrition would 'mask the selective effect'.

> We can hardly expect improved nutrition to win in the long run against persistent selection even if it scores a short-term striking success. Improved educational nutrition may similarly mask a decline in inborn intelligence, but only for a time. A race between education and selection would, I fear, end in ultimate catastrophe.[72]

Penrose was also aware of growing evidence that suggested that while the measured height of children may have increased, this did not necessarily mean that adults were getting taller, but that children were merely maturing earlier.[73] Penrose introduced his model the following year.[74] When presenting his theory to the Eugenics Society in 1949, he not only claimed victory in the debate over intelligence and fertility, but also quipped that even if the survey had revealed a decline, he would 'willingly have attributed it to environmental agencies or inaccuracies of measurement'.[75] The environmental argument had been cheapened – a means of denying the survey results by the very proponents of IQ testing and eugenics. In order to face up to the question of degeneration directly, at its core, that is, through genetics, Penrose *needed* a simple model based on single factors. As Laurence Snyder noted with regards to the problems of dealing with cumulatively acting genes, in a polygenic series the effect of an individual gene approached a limit at which it could not be distinguished from an environment increment.[76] Defenders of the argument of degeneration could always use this increment as a masking agent. Through Penrose's simplified model, any *underlying* process of selection for intelligence could be tackled in a way that challenged eugenic assumptions. Expressing his support for Penrose, Haldane argued that even if intelligence were inherited, as was blood group or eye colour, the conclusion of decline in intelligence would be 'equally false'.[77] Yet as Penrose extended this model to encompass the multifactorial structure of intelligence, it was not only necessary to demand that heterosis was a common feature in the determination of normal traits, but also, as in the single gene model, that fertility was governed by the genetic factors that determined intellectual ability, not only for idiots and imbeciles but for the entire population. Thus Penrose had not only built upon the problems for eugenic selection raised by Punnett, Hardy and Weinberg, but had also built in a solution to Fisher's response to those objections, ending up with a stable frequency of genes for intelligence within a population through time. As he argued: 'Mean adult stature has remained the same for centuries and so also, probably, has intelligence level'.[78]

Finally, on a more general level, Penrose seems to have been less than impressed with the growing tendency towards environmental explanation in the psychological sciences, stripping genetics of explanatory power. While environmental factors influenced test scores, 'the problem remains', argued Penrose, 'because, if we knew the real factors of the mind, we would find them to be manifestations of genes'.[79] For Penrose, it was genetics that provided humanity with the diversity essential to its survival. Those crippled by these genes were the unfortunate victims of the need for variability within a species. They were to be celebrated rather than despised. Indeed, the zoologist G. Evelyn Hutchinson compared the polymorphism of intelligence to the sickling gene case, arguing: 'If we introduced social mechanisms to encourage the production of more intellectuals, possibly society might perish from a dearth of stupidity'.[80] Penrose's model was proving popular among geneticists critical of traditional eugenic philosophy, who were determined to show how their own scientific advances discredited gloomy predictions of degeneration and were consistent with the ideals of a diverse and democratic society.

It was also proving popular among social scientists, particularly among sociologists concerned with educational reform and social mobility, such as David Glass and his one-time colleague A. H. Halsey.[81] Penrose's model allowed them to retain a genetic conception of IQ as the basis for social reform. Genetic ability was continuously generated and dispersed throughout the entire population. What was now required was to ensure greater social justice and efficiency through increased social mobility. Penrose's model helped sidestep the ongoing controversy over intellectual deterioration that plagued population study, costing it both social and financial capital. As Glass wrote to Penrose, 'the idea is not to have any more discussion about the correlation between intelligence and fertility', making 'it possible to obtain funds for new and really useful research, in a field which in the past has been so much the subject of prejudice'.[82]

Conclusion

At the very start of his renowned publication *The Biology of Mental Defect*, Penrose used the analogy of stature. The immense variation of height within the human species was clearly visible, just as it was also present with regards to 'intellectual stature'. However, it was the 'intellectual dwarf' that had suffered some of the harshest treatment in history.[83] He took time to document historical attitudes towards mental defect. The notion of 'stigma' was critical to his discussion. In Sparta, Rome and Protestant Europe, they were seen to be marked or sullied by evil. Yet he also observed how many saw the mentally diseased and defective as 'evidence of divine inspiration' and 'as especially innocent and holy', the term 'crétin' coming, after all, from the word 'chrétien'.[84] The belief that they were touched by God, and had necessary place in a divinely ordained natural order, encouraged the first philanthropic attempts at care and treatment in the nineteenth century. Penrose, in turn, can be seen to be giving carriers of genetic 'defect' a necessary place in a natural biological order – their destruction would engender our own, not in the sense of eternal damnation but in terms of biological suicide.

In her insightful treatment of Penrose, P. M. H. Mazumdar identifies his antipathy for eugenics as based upon the 'spiritual grounds of sympathy for the individual'.[85] Yet Penrose was equally concerned with the negative effects of the association made between eugenics and the study of human heredity. The eugenicists had, through stigmatizing individuals and groups as unworthy of posterity, stigmatized the study of medical genetics. He ridiculed eugenicists by cleverly using their arguments and evidence against them, reinventing the despised tenth as the genetic backbone of society, which carried, and suffered, the burden of biological variation. Throughout his career, Penrose used the subject of intelligence to drive a wedge between eugenics and genetics, and it joined sickle cell anaemia and phenylketonuria to become what Diane Paul describes as a 'potent symbol' of eugenicist folly.[86] However, while heterosis served as a useful means of criticizing eugenic typologies, it also provided a genetic explanation for the prevalence of human traits and diseases that would have otherwise proved difficult – carrying genes for schizophrenia, autism and even homosexuality was seen to confer some kind of selective advantage.[87]

As eugenicists shifted their perspective – from degeneracy and sterilization towards population quality and family planning – Penrose moved with them. He continuously developed his critique to take account of their use of demographic measures and social factors. While his model of genetic equilibrium seemed to be contradicted by evidence of massive generational increases in measured intelligence from the 1980s, particularly in the non-verbal (and thus supposedly more culture-free) Raven's Matrices that he had helped design, he recognized that the identification of environmental influences on test scores and the positive correlation between stature and intelligence would not spell the end of arguments of degeneration or the stigmatization of certain individuals and groups. Explaining the apparent increase in IQ is presently one of the leading topics in psychology. While some celebrate the evidence for revealing the absurdity of arguments of degeneration, others continue to argue that the increase in phenotypic intelligence (mirrored by the secular increase in height) masks an underlying genotypic decline.[88]

4 FROM 'RACES' TO 'ISOLATES' AND 'ENDOGAMOUS COMMUNITIES': HUMAN GENETICS AND THE NOTION OF HUMAN DIVERSITY IN THE 1950s

Veronika Lipphardt

For good reason, research into the history of human genetics has concentrated on medical genetics, eugenics and radiation genetics. The entanglement of research into heritable pathologies with discriminatory political and social practices has rendered human genetics a deeply problematic scientific field. Thus, when addressing the post-war era, historians have focused on the repercussions and continuities of human geneticists' interest in pathological conditions.[1] By the same token, however, human geneticists' interest in the inheritance and variation of normal traits has largely been neglected.

To be sure, the community of human geneticists cannot easily be divided up into medical geneticists on the one hand and population geneticists on the other. Often, one and the same research team investigated both pathological conditions and normal traits within a population (however defined). From one field site, it was possible to contribute to both medical genetics and population genetics. For those more interested in population genetics, it was necessary to draw on the help of already established health care systems, primarily to secure access to their test subjects.[2]

Yet for some, the primary aim was to assess human genetic variation in general – what would become known as 'human diversity'[3] – to make it epistemologically productive for the investigation of genetic characters and to establish the evolutionary history of mankind. Medical expeditions to remote places provided data for answering questions of inheritance, biological anthropology and human evolutionary history. Especially in the latter field, systematic empirical field studies in population genetics were rare before 1950, while theoretical discussions often lacking in any empirical basis prevailed.

The new approach entailed the search for normal traits that were inherited in a stable, easily assessable way and could be documented for hundreds of thousands of test subjects around the globe. Of course this interest in population genetics did not come out of the blue: it echoed earlier contributions of geneticists to the field of human racial variation. However, researchers felt that this field urgently needed to be reframed in a new terminological and conceptual vein.

In order to shine some light onto this historical episode of human genetics, this essay aims to map some of the institutional, personal and epistemic developments surrounding this new vein of research into human variation in the post-war era. In spite of substantial interdependencies and overlaps with medical genetics, I contend that those biological-anthropological studies of human populations in the immediate post-war period, seeking to provide insights into 'human racial variation', constituted the early beginnings of human population genetics as a distinct field of study.[4] Hence, in contrast to the suggestions of many historians, human population genetics did not bring about a clear break with the race paradigm.[5] As others have pointed out, largely on the basis of theoretical publications and political pamphlets by post-war geneticists, this new research vein proposed a 'populational race concept' rather than leaving race behind.[6] To take this point further, and to highlight some significant practical, conceptual and methodological continuities from the pre-war period, I concentrate on post-war studies in human genetics at the population level, providing insights into biological-anthropological aspects and into genetic mechanisms. As I will demonstrate, the concept of the 'genetic isolate' – a group of humans thought to have been reproductively isolated for a period of several hundreds or thousands of years – became critically important to this field of inquiry; and, at the same time, it was significant in its ties to older studies of race.

The Genetic Isolate: A Concept from the New Evolutionary Synthesis

In the 1950s a considerable number of empirical studies in human genetics drew on endogamous groups, or 'isolates'. Most of these groups constituted social minorities in politically tense situations, often in colonial contexts. Many geneticists considered 'endogamous groups' to be the unit that best represented a genetic and evolutionary population, that is, an 'isolate', and hence provided a sound empirical basis for population genetic investigations. 'The ultimate racial units of importance', geneticists L. D. Sanghvi and V. R. Khanolkar claimed, 'are the endogamous groups'. Indeed, endogamous groups seemed to them to provide the 'invariable and necessary framework ... for a study of genetic characters'.[7]

The conceptual turn to isolates – and the concomitant empirical turn to endogamous groups – mirrors a convergence of four developments in the life sciences: the so-called new evolutionary synthesis, the rise of population genetics, the increasing importance of serology, and last but not least (so as not to avoid the elephant in the room) the continuing legacy of the study of race. Advocates of the new approach, such as Leslie C. Dunn and Theodosius Dobzhansky, sought to transfer population genetics to the fields of physical anthropology and human genetics, two disciplines that were competing for hegemony and had to struggle with the legacies of eugenics and racial science.[8] Only population genetics, they claimed, could overcome the errors associated with the race science of the pre-war period. Discredited politically, a number of biologists considered 'race' inadequate for understanding human evolution and variation. Scientists claimed that the 'natural groupings' of mankind were to be perceived not as strictly divided, fixed and stable races, but as the product of the dynamic process of evolution. They were driven by such forces as migrations, separations, isolation, environments, mutations, variation and random drift. This was not an entirely new approach; most scientists, including German anthropologists during the Nazi regime, were not ignorant of this dynamic perspective.[9] Yet in order to distance themselves from the discredited 'old' race science, post-war geneticists emphasized the historical divide between 'fixist' and 'dynamic' notions of 'race'. Accordingly, the post-war era saw a considerable number of prominent biologists participating in anti-racist activities, such as the UNESCO initiatives in the early 1950s.[10]

Human geneticists, then, had to struggle not only with the legacy of eugenics but also with racial science. In the 1930s some human geneticists had already started to challenge the competence of racial anthropologists. The relationship between the two disciplines remained a conflicted one until late in the 1960s, with physical anthropologists often being singled out and derogated as the notorious race scientists of the pre-war period.[11] However, both scientific communities contributed to the study of human variation in the 1930s and 1940s, and by the early 1930s both physical anthropology and human genetics (especially blood group analysis) constituted the core of thinking surrounding the issue of 'racial variation'. The medical and demographical sciences were seen as providers of data to those in the centre of this collective. As a consequence, there was much cross-community membership and collaboration. Scientists of both fields (and of medical and demographical disciplines) were busy with taking measurements *and* blood samples from 'unique populations' all over the world from the 1920s until the 1960s. But whereas physical anthropology gradually lost its traditional authority over these questions, human genetics, equipped with serological tools, was increasingly entrusted as the most objective discipline for investigating human diversity and evolution.[12]

A crucial step for human geneticists in reasserting their authority was to adopt the term 'population' as the principal unit of analysis. Humans were no longer divided into races with typical traits, but instead into populations that differed in allelic frequencies.[13] This allowed for flexibility – a 'population' included groups of all sizes, such as islanders or religious communities, or even larger congregations, identical with the races of the pre-war period. 'Population' was the new buzzword in academia and international politics.[14] In genetics, the innovative substitution of 'race' with 'population' necessitated many further innovations, but also involved recourses to older 'racial' knowledge.

Historians of science have noted that experimental biology emerged in opposition to natural history, or field biology, which was mainly devoted to collection and description. In studies of genetic variation, however, geneticists turned the logic of the experiment, or the laboratory gaze, back onto the messy reality of the field.[15] In the eyes of geneticists, evolution was an experiment, and the test unit submitted to evolutionary forces was 'the breeding unit', 'the isolate', 'the Mendelian population', 'a reproductive community of sexual and cross-fertilizing individuals which share in a common gene pool'.[16] A species would be a Mendelian population, albeit 'differentiated into complexes of subordinate Mendelian populations' of races, subspecies and local populations, separated by more or less effective reproductive barriers.[17] Reproductive barriers would, through centuries, lead to the genetic distinctness of populations. Isolation of groups within the species was only relative; but through complete and long-lasting reproductive isolation from other subpopulations, a population would, sooner or later, become a new species. The results of the evolutionary experiment were populations that differed quantitatively in the frequencies of gene alleles.

Geneticists did not hesitate to apply this theoretical frame to the human species. 'By far the most complex system of Mendelian populations', leading geneticist Theodosius Dobzhansky contended, 'exists in the human species'.[18] Different from all other animal species, they noted, humans encountered and maintained very special reproductive barriers – not geographic factors, but, so to speak, typically human self-made factors. As isolating factors, Dunn listed 'language, custom, religion, economic organization, social class'. In modern societies, Dunn specified, 'social isolation tends to replace other isolating factors of the natural environment'.[19] His colleague Herluf Strandskov elaborated this idea in his publications from the late 1940s onwards:

> The primary isolating or limiting factor separating two or more nearly but incompletely closed intrabreeding populations may be only distance. However, in some instances it may be a nonbiological barrier such as a mountain range or a body of water or it may be some biological barrier, such as a predator. Relative to the human species it may be a psychological, social or cultural factor. In the latter event two or more incompletely closed intrabreeding populations may occupy the same spatial range without interbreeding to any appreciable extent.[20]

To be sure, none of the scientists provided a clear-cut definition of, or made an attempt to precisely distinguish between, consanguinity, inbreeding, incest, reproductive isolation and endogamy. The term 'endogamy', as used in the social sciences, was meant to denote strong social rules or cultural and social preferences of individuals for marrying partners from the same group, be it a religious community, a family or any other small social group. Transferred to the realm of biology, 'endogamy' became a synonym for the effects of reproductive barriers that would effectively isolate that group from the gene pool of other groups. Hence the 'genetic isolate' could refer to all kinds of barriers. In animals, most often these would be geographical ones, but social and cultural isolation was seen to be specific to humans, and identical with what social scientists referred to as 'endogamy'.

This approach was put into practice in research designs joining human medical genetics and investigations of consanguinity. It was well represented in the proceedings of international conferences on human genetics in the 1950s.[21] The conceptual tools the scientists used, as well as the sampling techniques, were partly borrowed from experimental animal genetics. However, taking this population concept from theoretical evolutionary biology and then implementing it in empirical studies of human genetics proved quite a challenge. Geneticists constantly noted that experimentation with humans was impossible: 'The study of human genetics, as everyone knows, is severely hampered by such inevitable obstacles as the unfeasibility of experimentation, the small number of progeny, and the great length of each generation'.[22]

But researchers also struggled with many other basic questions. First of all, what markers could be considered good enough for such a study? What demands would a population have to meet for an investigation of this kind? What were good methods and practices for delineating populations? What historical sources would be informative for describing a population's history? And, most importantly, how could one rule out, account for or control other factors that were known to influence gene frequencies, namely mutation, selection, inbreeding, drift and migration? These challenges led to a dynamic interplay of genetic markers, populations and history, each an epistemic tool as well as an epistemic object. I will examine this interplay after the next section, which first provides the institutional background.

Institutions for the Study of Human Variation and Genetics

In a number of nations following World War II, geneticists (in some cases, together with physical anthropologists and demographers) founded institutions dedicated to the study of early human population genetics. The scope of their agenda differed from that of institutions concentrating on genetic diseases. This is not to say that there were no overlaps, but the actors actively tried to shape the new field, which they coined 'the study of human variation'.[23] In the work of these new institutions, the concept of endogamous groups played a significant role. The groups chosen for study were often minorities in politically tense situations, several of them in colonial contexts, and the research activities show an impressive range of transnational interaction.

Two institutions were established with Rockefeller grants: first, the Laboratory for Studies in Human Variation, hosted by the Cancer Research Centre in Bombay. It was founded in 1949 by Khanolkar and Sanghvi and received *c.* $38,000 from the Rockefeller Foundation over the course of around seven years, from 1952 to 1959.[24] Second, the US-based geneticists Theodosius Dobzhansky and Leslie Clarence Dunn founded the Institute for the Study of Human Variation at Columbia University in 1952. Its members published some sixty articles within six years, dealing with various subjects related to human evolution, genetics and variation.[25] As a visitor to this institute, Sanghvi's research was supervised by Dobzhansky and Dunn, among others.[26]

In Brazil, at the Federal University of Paraná, Newton Freire-Maia established a Laboratory of Human Genetics that pursued population studies on Brazilian populations. In other countries, similar research was carried out at already existing research institutes for serology, medical human genetics or demography, such as at the Istituto Sieroterapico Milanese, or Arthur Mourant's and R. A. Fisher's laboratories at the Lister Institute and University College London.[27] As blood typing was part of many medical services at the time, blood group research was often carried out within the framework of a medical institution. This shows the connection between human genetics oriented towards either medicine or population, even if researchers interested in human variation framed their work in terms of evolutionary biology and as a search for normal rather than pathological variations.

One shared preoccupation, on the empirical and conceptual level, was the interest in 'endogamous groups', 'isolates', 'inbreeding' and 'consanguinity'. As mentioned above, there was no consensus about their meaning among those who studied isolates at the time; they were used synonymously and ambiguously, varying from author to author.[28] William C. Boyd argued in 1950: 'In its correct sense inbreeding means mating between close relatives. Unless this occurs, a population, though it might be cut off from all contact with the outside world, is not inbred; it is merely reproductively isolated'.[29] But as interesting as the inbred population was for the medical geneticist, the population geneticist preferred populations that were 'reproductively isolated', and not too closely related to each other, because this would distort the gene frequencies sought. The perfect population for the population geneticist was isolated yet characterized by 'random mating'. As it turned out in practice, groups that were selected for population genetics for their apparent isolation did in fact show a significant percentage of marriages between very close relatives.

But in spite of this tension between various degrees of desirable isolation and undesirable relatedness, both medical and population geneticists shared an interest in mating patterns and their genetic effects. These aspects of human populations were covered and quantified in numerous publications through the 1950s. Medical geneticists were interested in the effects of inbreeding as they traced patterns of inheritance of pathological traits through family lines. They also assessed the 'genetic load' of populations and compared the accumulation of harmful mutations by inbreeding with those induced by radiation exposure. The interest in inbreeding and consanguinity can be viewed as an interface where medical, nuclear, genetic and eugenic research interests overlapped, and many famous human population geneticists (James Neel and Luigi Cavalli-Sforza, for example) studied the effects of consanguinity in the early years of their careers.[30] The genetic isolate seemed a reasonable unit to study, and if a research team made an attempt to approach such a population in a remote periphery, it was efficient to collect all information of interest in one visit. Hence, medical and biological-anthropological data were collected alongside the demographic and ethnological.

Which Populations to Study? The Historical Context

The biological and anthropological interest in reproductive isolation and in the crossing or mixing of humans dates back to the late nineteenth century (and even further back to eighteenth-century discussions among scholars such as Kant and Herder). Nineteenth-century scientific race concepts had already employed the notion of human races as reproductively isolated groups in which specific heritable traits were transferred from one generation to the next. The scientific discussion of isolation and reproductive barriers has undergone considerable change from this time, but in human genetics and physical anthropology one crucial aspect was retained: the assumed coherence of isolated groups through centuries. Whereas the expression 'pure race' was used predominantly in the late nineteenth century, and assumed to be a stable entity from prehistoric times, the term 'isolation', which became more popular in the twentieth century, evokes notions of processuality, temporality and evolution. It drew on Mendelian ideas, as Mendel had used what was later called 'pure lines' and their respective hybrids (the F1 generation), and had thereby set the standard for a controlled mixture of two pure lines.

Yet the term also drew on Darwinian ideas of evolution. Scientists turned to supposedly isolated populations in a very Darwinian fashion, namely to island inhabitants or people separated by geographic barriers such as mountains or rivers, who could be studied abroad, in remote places and in colonial contexts (their administrations providing ample networks and infrastructure for such scientific projects).[31] And in accordance with what they deemed to be particularly human – namely, social and cultural barriers to reproduction – they also turned to isolates 'at home'. Minorities were outsider communities notorious for their social separation, and thus they seemed useful resources in certain regional contexts. These were often groups that were blamed for social tensions within national or imperial contexts. For Americans, Native American populations were among the most promising isolates. For Swiss anthropologists, the most obvious isolated group were the inhabitants of the Swiss Alps.[32] For Indian scientists, isolation was to be studied in the caste system.[33] Other isolated communities were the Dunker community (1952) and other religious isolates,[34] certain African tribes (1950s),[35] Western Apache (1956),[36] Australian Aborigines (from 1928),[37] the Walser and Romansh in Switzerland (1956–7),[38] and certain Indian tribes in Brazil,[39] in Arizona[40] and elsewhere. In Europe there were also the Basques and the Sámi, as well as the Roma and the Jews, though in the eyes of geneticists, these latter two seemed to represent a different type of isolation.

This turn to isolates through the influence of population genetics began in the late 1940s.[41] But each of the isolates that were now studied had long before been subject to scientific inquiry from several disciplines, with differing methodologies and in varying epistemic frames.[42] The investigation of Australian Aborigines as an isolate had a long tradition, and even more so the investigation of the Basques. Older publications were read and cited by the authors of the new publications. All sorts of cultural narratives had become embedded in the common assumptions surrounding each group and its isolation. They were transferred from the older to the newer publications, and they easily entered the research designs and explanations of human population geneticists.

The methodologies employed in population genetic studies differed significantly from older studies that had often been based on anthropometric measurements alone. Although anthropometry remained, it was marginalized as new tools such as blood group distributions or, increasingly, other genetic markers such as phenylthiocarbamide (PTC) taste sensitivity came to the fore. Diseases or new pathological alleles were also an issue, but far more emphasis was given to 'normal', non-pathological traits, such as blood groups and PTC taste sensitivity. Furthermore, in an attempt to prove endogamy or isolation, many studies used questionnaires and collected demographical data, while others combined the natural sciences with the humanities or social sciences, assessing both social endogamy and blood type distribution.

Methodological Challenges and How They Were Met

As mentioned above, it proved difficult to find good markers, good historical sources and, particularly, good populations to study. First of all, the implementation of the new quantitative approaches required mathematical innovations in order to characterize populations and, more specifically, isolates. Geneticists could draw upon important mathematical work from an earlier period.[43] In the 1950s scientists discussed laws of selective breeding, population size, and ways of assessing the impact of drift, population growth, selection, mutation, etc. on the genetical structure of a population.[44] This general mathematization of human populations provided the tools for demarcation necessary for the study of human variation. It also played out more directly at the level of human variation studies: Sanghvi, for example, established the first genetic distance measure based on gene frequencies.[45]

Secondly, much attention was paid to the respective markers and their validity. A good marker had to fulfil a number of requirements. It had to be easily available and universal, and its distribution across populations had to differ within a reasonable, workable and productive range. On the level of the individual, yes/no answers were optimal, and the distribution of yes/no individuals in populations or in geographic spaces was of greatest interest. Also, the genes should not be subject to selection (genes for skin colour, for example, varied in a cline) if they were to display evolutionary migrations and isolations and their discontinuous effects in populations. Drawing on Boyd, physical anthropologist Jean Hiernaux explained that 'the best characteristics for the study of racial differences are normal physiological characters inherited by a known genetic mechanism, not too infrequent nor too frequent, showing stable frequencies in populations and considerable variation between populations (the blood groups being the best known example)'.

At that time, the most established genetic traits that seemed adequate for such frequency analysis were the blood group systems, taste reaction to PTC and green-red colour blindness.[46] Researchers at the Columbia Institute also assessed a number of new biochemical markers from the metabolic system or from excretion, for example beta-amino-isobutryc acid excretion rates.[47] Towards the 1960s the number of potential markers showing a polymorphism that could easily be assessed grew. To establish its usefulness, however, it was also important to calibrate a new marker. This, in turn, demanded a certain number of diverse populations, so that the frequencies of the marker's alleles could be assessed comparatively. Hence, human variation became the epistemic tool for the calibration of a new marker and for the investigation of its inheritance.

The most pressing problem, however, was the choice of populations to scrutinize for allele frequencies. Demarcating a population for any empirical investigation in population genetics proved tricky and required ever more conceptual innovations. Such a population had to fulfil a number of requirements: evolutionary cohesion, that is, long-lasting reproductive isolation; accessibility; and finally, small size. In the eyes of geneticists, such endogamous populations provided ideal, quasi 'experimental' conditions for studying evolutionary processes and their genetic consequences in humans.[48]

The studies conducted in India under the geneticist Sanghvi and his colleague Khanolkar are an early example of such a research design. Sanghvi worked with Dobzhansky at the Columbia Institute and established the Laboratory for Studies of Human Variation in Bombay, and he was one of the first geneticists who employed empirically the conceptual framework of reproductive isolation. His teacher Dobzhansky had viewed India through the lens of experimental logic: 'The Indian caste system is the grandest ... genetic experiment ever performed on human populations'.[49] Sanghvi wholeheartedly agreed with this view when he wrote in 1950:

> People of India are almost under an experimental environment, broken up into a large number of mutually exclusive groups, whose members are forbidden, by an inexorable social law, to marry outside their own group ... The people of India are not just a collection of individuals, but a mass of corporate entities, whose numbers, names, characters and functions are infinitely diverse.[50]

Together with the pathologist Khanolkar and others, Sanghvi investigated castes, including immigrant castes, as endogamous groups in India. The team saw as self-evident the fact that their test populations were endogamous, pointing to their (unwritten but orally confirmed) marriage laws. For the historical demarcation of each single isolate, they cited mythical traditions, as for example the partly mythical figure of David Rahabi, supposedly from AD 1000, in the case of the Bene Israel Jews. The criterion for sampling was, then, self-identification with the caste.

Within the six groups studied, they found significant genetic differences particularly between two groups, which fell into two distinct castes. When they compared their data with studies from the United States, they concluded that the differences between these two groups were as large as the genetic differences between whites and blacks, and yet they had always been sorted into the same racial category. Accordingly, Sanghvi and Khanolkar explicitly challenged not only older racial classifications of the people of India on the basis of measurements or facial outlook, but also serological studies that had summarized Indians as one and the same racial category. At the same time, they drew new lines between human groups along social-cultural notions that seemed more plausible to them than the racial divisions of Western scientists. On the basis of their research on endogamous groups, Sanghvi and Khanolkar heavily criticized European and US scientists for lumping Indians together in an undifferentiated mass. The following lengthy quote sums up their meticulous critique of categorizations by famous leaders of their field, which they believed had brought nothing but confusion:

> It is customary in most of the European countries as well as in the U.S.A. to refer to the inhabitants of India as 'Hindus' as different from 'Indians', a term synonymous with 'American Indians'. This connotation of the term 'Hindu' has been very unfortunate and should be discarded in all scientific publications. Hirszfeld & Hirszfeld (1919), in their study of the racial distribution of ABO blood groups, presented along with their data the distribution of 'Indians'. It is impossible to say from their paper which castes and tribes were examined by them. It is known that the Indian troops in Macedonia included Gurkhas, Garowalis, Rajputs, Jats and Kumaons. Labour Transport Corps were composed chiefly of scheduled caste persons from different parts in India. It is therefore likely that their sample of 'Indians' contained a mixture of some or all of these groups. Verzar & Weszeczky (1921), in their oft-quoted illustration, compared this distribution of blood groups in 'Indians' with the distribution of gypsies in Hungary, and contrasted them with the distribution in Hungarians. It has been shown above that the group K.B. shows significant differences from D.B., C.K.P. and M.K. as regards the

> distribution of ABO blood groups. 'Indians' of Hirszfeld & Hirszfeld probably had in their sample similarly different groups. Ottenberg (1925) has called these 'Indians' of Hirszfeld & Hirzsfeld 'Hindus', who are referred to in many publications and standard works on the subject since then. All references to this work of Hirszfeld & Hirszfeld should be assessed on the basis of the above considerations. It might be stated in a general way that any investigation on the distribution of genetical characters, where the people of India are lumped together as one group without taking into consideration the ultimate endogamous groups, would probably lead to erroneous conclusions.[51]

European and US colleagues, so to speak, did not get the categories right because they were too far away from, and thus unaware of, the real differences between Indians and various Indian groups that had been isolated from another for centuries in India. As other geneticists, Sanghvi and Khanolkar relied on the concept of the 'endogamous group', the 'isolate' or the 'inbreeding unit' for achieving the practical task of sampling a population. This involved further requirements. For example, an 'isolate' would have had to be separated from other populations by means of strict endogamous marriage rules – what Sanghvi and Khanolkar described as 'an inexorable social law'.[52] In addition, it could not be too small, and families should not be too large in order to rule out inbreeding (a factor appreciated by the medical geneticist). And as for the comparison of two isolated populations and their allelic frequencies, 'racial crossing' in both past and present had to be ruled out.[53] Notably, population geneticists did not require that these units be isolated since prehistoric times, as most proponents of race concepts would have demanded. A time span of a few thousand years of isolation, or even a few hundred, was enough to bring about the desired experimental results: differing allelic frequencies. As argued by Sanghvi and Khanolkar, only one thousand years had passed since the advent of the Bene Israel Jews. With these rules, any minority, religious group or island population could be checked for its potential as a suitable genetic isolate.

However, thus far scientists had not felt a need to provide empirical proof of reproductive isolation: it had been enough to state that a group was generally known to be isolated. By the 1950s this changed. Now, in their empirical work, not only would geneticists have to account for genetic characteristics, but a considerable part of their time also had to be spent on identifying isolates, endogamous groups and their reproductive behaviour. 'Cross-breeding' was considered a problem. Hence, before blood tests and genetic analysis could be carried out, much work was invested to stabilize the group under study as an evolutionary coherent isolate. Therefore geneticists were in need of evidence for reproductive isolation on an evolutionary scale, and invariably drew on bio-historical narratives that would narrate the supposed social – and hence reproductive – isolation of the group. For this, geneticists had to rely on other experts and even on 'non-scientific' knowledge. The new population approach thus entailed overlapping interests of population geneticists with cultural and social anthropologists, ethnologists and sociologists, particularly with regard to marriage systems and social isolation.

In this way, accounts of endogamy from all kinds of sources entered deliberations about research design, mostly by a priori classifications and bio-historical narratives that would tell the history of what made the group so isolated. The accounts of linguists, demographers, ethnographers, historians, sociologists and others, as well as 'non-scientific' knowledge from myths or claims of collective identity, turned out to be essential for studies of human genetic diversity. Population geneticists drew upon narratives of group history and identity from written or oral sources. They asked their research subjects to fill out questionnaires, evaluated church or synagogue records and marriage registers as well as communal records, and conducted interviews with community officials. 'Purely scientific' explanations of 'genetic diversity' relied heavily on other – non-genetic and non-scientific – knowledge.

Conclusion

If the 'race paradigm' gave way to the 'population paradigm' after World War II, or from 'physical anthropology' to 'population genetics', this was not a smooth and easy transition. Given that the 'isolate' attracted so much attention of human geneticists in the 1950s, I first concentrate on the shift of attention from 'races' to 'isolates'. What had changed? What remained? What were the continuities and what was left behind?

In the 1950s the oft-cited turn away from discrete units of human variation, formulated in 1962 by Frank B. Livingstone – 'There are no races, there are only clines'[54] – was yet to come (though the use of this argument also dates back to eighteenth-century discussions). However, even then discontinuities between populations would not be completely disregarded. When the World Health Organization and the International Programme for Human Biology launched their large-scale transnational research projects in the mid-1960s, focused on 'primitive groups' around the globe, both institutions took advantage of a growing interest in so-called isolated, primitive people in many academic fields.[55] The notion of the 'primitive isolate' was heavily critiqued in cultural anthropology in the 1970s, but not in population genetics and other disciplines.

In physical anthropology as well as in human population genetics, many bio-historical narratives as well as a priori classifications remained, and in many cases they remain today. As each of those narratives tells the story of one group, defining that group along traditional notions of 'isolation', and aligning the latter with scientific understandings of reproductive isolation, was a convenient way of both demarcating and narrating. Tellingly, the narratives continued to coincide with larger cultural narratives and common-sense classifications. What changed, however, was the need to account for social, cultural and reproductive isolation, and for the boundaries of bio-historically defined populations, on the basis of the empirical research design.

The search for mathematically reliable accounts of isolation, for manageable markers, and for bio-historical narrations from outside of science also points to the necessity to claim a new territory. Population genetics was distinct from other fields of human genetics through its mathematical sophistication and its focus on genetically determined non-pathological physiological mechanisms. Its members also claimed to understand human evolution better than physical anthropologists did. While the distancing from medical genetics was crucially important to the field, at the same time it was essential to have enough overlapping themes and interests with those disciplines.

The search for isolation, markers and narratives went hand in hand with a new standard of integrating the test subjects' knowledge into scientific knowledge production. To investigate human biological diversity meant to engage in a dialogue with other humans, in order to elicit information from individuals about their origins and the communities from which they came. One should not herald this dialogue as a democratic and ethically correct way of engaging with test subjects, as there were still clear hierarchies of interpretation at work. Neither was this attention to the narratives of the test subjects new; but it was of much greater importance in the post-war era. For example, a 'WHO Scientific Group on Research on Human Population Genetics' would note in 1970: 'All groups have learned individuals, e.g., experts on oral traditions and those with systematized knowledge and interpretations of natural phenomena ... Such information is pertinent to their cultural and therefore biological history'.[56]

Similarly, interdisciplinary cooperation with linguists, archaeologists, social scientists and others had happened before; but now there was an indispensable need to collaborate. 'As is always the case', the French anthropologist Jean Hiernaux wrote in 1966, the definition of the units of study 'required the cooperation of an ethno-sociologist who already had gained acquaintance with the people'.[57] Hiernaux alluded to having benefited from the aid of a linguist, a demographer and an economist for his fieldwork in Central Africa.

On the theoretical level, a significant change had occurred with regards to evolutionary temporalities that elicited such cooperations. The timescale required for the emergence of diversity was reinterpreted by the mid-twentieth century. Evolutionary change could now occur to a measurable degree within a few hundred years. With this premise, scientists now turned to historical sources of all kinds and from all periods, instead of merely acknowledging archaeological or prehistorical findings.

One might wonder whether the historical actors were unaware of how problematic working with such sources could be. Whether definite evolutionary narratives could be inferred from these sources – that is, a single narrative per group – is questionable. Data might be incomplete, ambiguous, unreliable or simply not compatible with the biologists' demands. Geneticists are not fully aware of the critical methodological discussions of historians regarding their engagement with historical sources. On another token, accounts from the humanities might, in some cases, simply have reformulated older myths of origin, migration, isolation or miscegenation. There might be different understandings of endogamy, isolation or group cohesion in each discipline. It seems that geneticists addressed such problems occasionally, but this did not lead to a rigorous critique or any profound changes. In 1927 Melville Herskovits had already noted that it might be 'hazardous' and 'jeopardizing' for anthropologists' results if their genealogies were dependent on the accounts of their test subjects. Nevertheless, he regarded the problem irrelevant in the light of his research design.[58] Jean Hiernaux, in the 1960s, drew on 'numerical taxonomy' to overcome the pitfalls of a priori classification, but this attempt to establish a better practice did not survive within the scientific community. In the 1950s L. C. Dunn stated:

> The other difficulties inherent in the genetical study of human populations do not call for special comment here. Identification of family members, of the families composing a community, determination of the mating pattern and of the continuity of endogamy are problems which each investigator must face and overcome as best he may. They are, so to speak, the price he pays for dealing with animals over which he has no control.[59]

Geneticists such as Dunn proceeded on the assumption that these difficulties *could* be overcome. Eventually, the widespread stories of migration and isolation seemed too plausible and too evident to be doubted. However, had somebody invested the same amount of energy and time into proving that difficulties could *not* be overcome, he or she might have been successful in establishing a convincing argument of a very different kind.

Acknowledgements

Many thanks to Jenny Bangham and Ricky Heinitz for inspiring discussions of an earlier version of this essay.

5 BETWEEN THE TRANSFUSION SERVICES AND BLOOD GROUP RESEARCH: HUMAN GENETICS IN BRITAIN DURING WORLD WAR II

Jenny Bangham

Shortly after the outbreak of World War II, geneticist R. A. Fisher and serologist George Taylor published an appeal to workers in the newly founded Emergency Blood Transfusion Service (EBTS). Taylor led the Galton Serum Unit, a Cambridge laboratory producing blood grouping reagents for a national network of hospitals and EBTS depots. Fisher was Taylor's former boss at University College London (UCL), who had recently relocated to the agricultural Rothamsted Experimental Station in Harpenden. The letter, entitled 'Blood Groups of Great Britain', entreated blood depot medical officers to send to Fisher or Taylor the records of transfusion volunteers. They explained that the records, which included the results of blood grouping tests, constituted valuable 'genetical and ethnological data' that could:

> not only ... throw light on points that require very large numbers for their elucidation, but will open up the field, at present wholly unexplored, of the homogeneity or heterogeneity in respect to blood groups of the population of these islands.[1]

In response, the researchers were inundated with lists of donor records and blood grouping results. It represented the start of two wartime research programmes that Fisher and his colleagues conceived during these years. The first – to study the distribution of ABO blood group allele frequencies across Britain – made use of the many thousands of blood grouping records generated by the EBTS. The second – to determine the detailed genetic structure of the Rhesus blood groups – depended upon blood samples sent in from doctors and hospitals around the country. This essay is about how Fisher mobilized the infrastructure and materials of the wartime transfusion services to carve out a new research agenda for human genetics.[2]

Blood groups were exemplary Mendelian traits; during the interwar period they had been made emblematic of an 'ethically neutral' human genetics.[3] Much has been written on how blood grouping tests concurrently became a routine part of transfusion protocols,[4] while anthropological and medical journals published hundreds of papers correlating blood group frequencies with racial and nationalist narratives.[5] We know less about how blood groups were shared between doctors and geneticists, who carried out grouping tests, and how the results of those tests were negotiated, accessed and interpreted by experts with different interests. Moreover, 'blood groups' were not things that could be directly seen and manipulated. Rather, they were constituted by the circulation of highly elaborate representations and practices – e.g. donor records, blood grouping techniques, reagents, samples and nomenclatures – between different places and disciplines. I follow how people with diverse interests negotiated techniques, samples, access to willing populations and analytical expertise. Attention to these brings into view the ways that blood groups were made into genetic objects in these wartime conditions; it also reveals some of the practices and infrastructures that shaped mid-twentieth-century human genetics.

Britain during World War II is a compelling setting for such a study. The EBTS was a formidable bureaucratic institution, dedicated to the management of large numbers of people and vast quantities of blood. The Galton Serum Unit was the wartime incarnation of a laboratory that Fisher had established in 1935 at UCL with money from the Rockefeller Foundation. Fisher, like several of his geneticist colleagues, firmly believed that blood groups – as sharply defined traits that could be collected in large numbers and handled mathematically – could put the study of human heredity on a properly genetic footing.[6] In this essay, I begin by sketching the organization and activities of the EBTS, and outlining the institutional setting of the Galton Serum Unit and its influence on wartime blood grouping practices. I then turn to how the objects and practices associated with blood groups – first donor records and grouping expertise, later blood samples and nomenclatures – were exchanged, circulated and deployed. I end by discussing how Fisher, the Medical Research Council (MRC) and the University of Cambridge sought to preserve the productive wartime networks in peacetime.

The EBTS and Galton Serum Unit

Plans for the wartime transfusion service began after the Munich Crisis in September 1938, when haematologist Janet Vaughan convened an informal 'sub-committee' of medical practitioners to discuss advances in blood transfusion.[7] Vaughan's group was particularly impressed by the many interwar improvements in transfusion technique that had consolidated in Spain during the Civil War – simplified apparatus, methods of transport and bureaucratic systems for recruiting and monitoring donors.[8] Particularly pertinent to Vaughan's colleagues were improved methods of preservation: blood could now be stored for up to two weeks in central 'depots', relieving the pressure on donors to be called up in an emergency and demanding a new administrative system for managing volunteers.

Vaughan's sub-committee decided that the service should comprise a network of 'empanelling centres' for registering and testing donors, and depots for storing blood. London and the surrounding southeast would be served by four depots, in Luton, Slough, Sutton and Maidstone, while the southwest was to be managed by the Army Transfusion Service in Bristol. Each depot was to be directed by a medical officer working with a handful of other medics and nurses to bleed donors, give transfusions, sterilize equipment and work in depot laboratories. Female assistants were to be hired as clerks or trained in blood grouping; unskilled volunteers were to help with administrative work and drive ambulances. The MRC – which took over administration of the new transfusion service in April 1939 – also expected the depots to carry out research, e.g. on blood preservation methods, so many depots also employed two or three research assistants. Research was to be coordinated centrally by an MRC committee – later known as the Blood Transfusion Research Committee – which ensured that each depot was 'kept informed of the most recent developments'.[9]

Donors were to be organized through a system of 'panels', collections of index cards with the name, address and blood group of individuals willing to donate. Many volunteers were to be registered and tested at depots and empanelling stations, while mobile teams of medical officers, nurses, secretaries and transfusion technicians were to test and extract donated blood at 'bleeding centres' in towns, villages and factories.[10] The empanelling stations opened for recruitment on 3 July 1939. The MRC organized a campaign to coordinate appeals in newspapers, on the radio, through broadcasting companies and cinemas, in pamphlets and at local institutes, as well as in more specialist journals such as the *British Medical Journal* (*BMJ*). The campaign was phenomenally successful: barely a month after recruitment began, the *Times* announced that the service had registered its first 100,000 donors.[11] Figure 5.1 shows stills from a film made by the Ministry of Health to recruit new volunteers: a nurse extracts a small amount of blood from the earlobe, and laboratory workers carry out grouping tests on porcelain tiles. Blood groups were defined by mixing two samples; when red cells clumped together – or 'agglutinated' – the samples were ascribed to different groups. Agglutination was understood to be caused by soluble antibodies in the serum of one sample binding to cell-surface antigens of the other. The ABO group of a new sample was determined by mixing it with both anti-A and anti-B 'antisera' – solutions made from blood containing antibodies of a known type.[12]

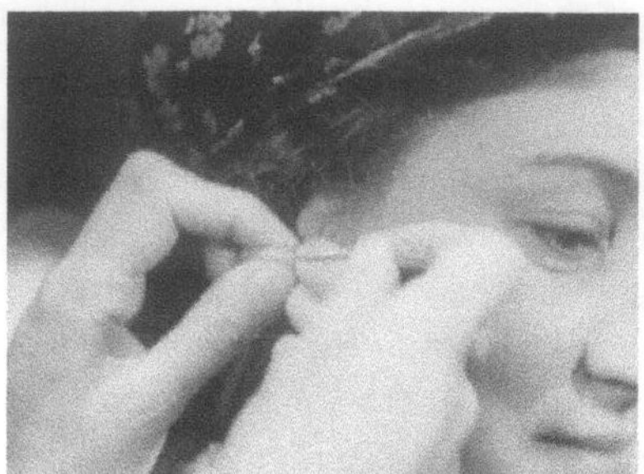

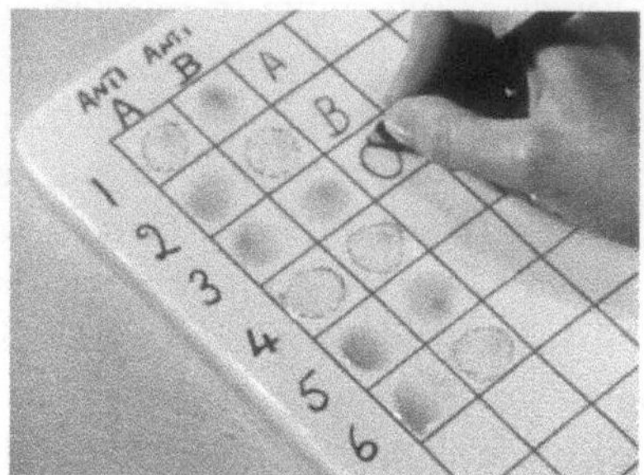

Figure 5.1: Stills from two films. The image on the left comes from the wartime public information film *Blood Transfusion Service*, directed and edited by H. M. Nieter, a Paul Rotha production (Ministry of Health in cooperation with the MRC and the Blood Transfusion Units of the Fighting Services, 1941). The image on the right is from the film *Blood Grouping*, by Cyril Jenkins Productions Ltd (Imperial Chemical Industries Limited, 1955). Images reproduced courtesy of the Wellcome Library, London, under the Creative Commons licence.

During the planning stages, Vaughan's main authority on the technical aspects of grouping tests was George Taylor. Formerly a general practitioner, Taylor had spent several years studying serology in Cambridge, before being recruited to head the UCL Galton Serological Laboratory in 1935. There, Taylor collaborated with Vaughan on researching blood groups and jaundice, and later Vaughan recruited him to the very earliest planning stages of the EBTS. Taylor was assigned responsibility to train blood grouping 'girls' to do serological tests.[13] The Galton Serological Laboratory also began producing standardized antisera for blood grouping.[14] While group O blood was to be used for transfusion, group A and B blood (containing 'anti-B' and 'anti-A' antibodies, respectively) would be used to make antisera, requiring additional tests to select those people with the highest antibody concentrations.

After the lab began producing antisera in April 1939, Taylor and Fisher agreed that if war broke out, the laboratory – comprising Taylor, research assistants Robert Race, Eileen Prior and Elizabeth Ikin, and two laboratory 'attendants', Douglas Keetch and George Tipper – would move to the Department of Pathology in Cambridge to become part of an MRC-administered Emergency Public Health Laboratory Service. As the lab's primary responsibility was to produce antisera, they needed a reliable source of A- and B-type blood. One reason for choosing Cambridge as the new home of 'the grouping serum show', as Taylor described it, was its proximity to a population of 'healthy young adults willing to be bled'.[15] Later, as demand quickly outstripped the availability of the town's student donors, the unit had to find additional regular sources, and Taylor persuaded the Air Force to allow the unit to determine the groups of men undergoing flying training.[16] As the war went on, depots gradually became self-sufficient in antiserum production, but not before its production and circulation had placed Taylor's laboratory firmly at the centre of the EBTS network.

On 29 August 1939 the Galton Serological Laboratory was ordered to move to Cambridge, where it was renamed the Galton Serum Unit. Taylor later described how the practical responsibilities of the unit established channels through which other kinds of expertise could be circulated:

> As a result of supplying serum, examining and giving opinions on troublesome samples of blood, and being consulted about blood grouping problems in general, we are in touch with very large numbers of civilian and service workers interested in blood transfusion.[17]

These 'very large numbers' were precisely what would become so precious to Fisher over the next few years. Thus the expertise claimed by the Galton Serum Unit and sanctioned by Vaughan and the MRC propelled the research laboratory into a new institutional setting. Preservation techniques meant that donations could be collected and stored at large depots, while demand for a stable population of volunteer donors was met by a new bureaucratic organization of donor panels. Embedded in this network, the unit made, tested and distributed antisera. It was this work that enabled the mobilization of donor records.

Donor Records and 'Ethnological' Data

When his laboratory moved to Cambridge, Fisher remained at UCL, although he stayed in close contact with Taylor and his other colleagues.[18] UCL soon evacuated their premises, and Fisher secured research space for himself and the 'computing and genetical sections of the Department' at the agricultural Rothamsted Experimental Station in Hertfordshire, where he had worked in the 1920s.[19] His daughter and biographer Joan Fisher Box describes the crowded wartime conditions in the plant pathology building, where Fisher's desk and calculating machine faced those of his secretary Barbara Simpson.[20] From Rothamsted, with Simpson's assistance, Fisher turned the availability of records from depots and empanelling centres around the country into an opportunity to map the geographical distribution of blood group frequencies in Britain.

Although Fisher had worked in Rothamsted for many years – on statistics and the design of experiments on crop yields and fertilizers – his greatest interest had always been problems of human heredity and eugenics. When he had arrived at UCL in 1933, he was already part of the new MRC's Human Genetics Committee, a small group of 'expert geneticists' (the MRC's words) – including J. B. S. Haldane, Lancelot Hogben and Lionel Penrose – with the responsibility to 'sketch the line of work most likely to produce definite results' in the field.[21] Early on, the committee agreed that blood groups should become central to the study of human heredity, because they could be collected in huge numbers and were amenable to statistical analysis. They could, as Fisher put it, give the study of human genetics 'a solidly objective foundation, under strict statistical control'.[22] So Fisher saw the grouping records of the wartime transfusion services as a magnificent opportunity. While the Serum Unit supplied antisera to the depots, Fisher requested donor records in return. In his letters, Fisher first reminded recipients of the 'large quantities of testing fluids' being supplied by Taylor, then asked whether they might be willing to send in their 'grouping totals'.[23] He framed the requests as an informal exchange.

Back at the depots, clerks and administrative assistants were managing hundreds of thousands of donor records, central to the depots' smooth functioning (Figure 5.2). They held donor information on enrolment cards, including name, address, telephone number, general state of health, past serious illnesses, and whether under national service obligations. Once a donor was selected, their card was marked with the date on which the blood was taken, the result of the Kahn test for syphilis and, in the relevant cases, their antibody titre. Illustrating just how central blood groups now were to transfusion, cards were often colour-coded by group. Each card was stamped with a serial number corresponding to the labels on bottles of donated blood.[24] An article in the *BMJ* reporting the day-to-day activities of the Slough depot (by then run by Vaughan) noted that within three months of opening, it had already enrolled 15,000 potential donors: 'The mere card-indexing of such a number would be regarded as a very serious business indeed for the average city office, but in this depot they seem to take it in their stride'.[25]

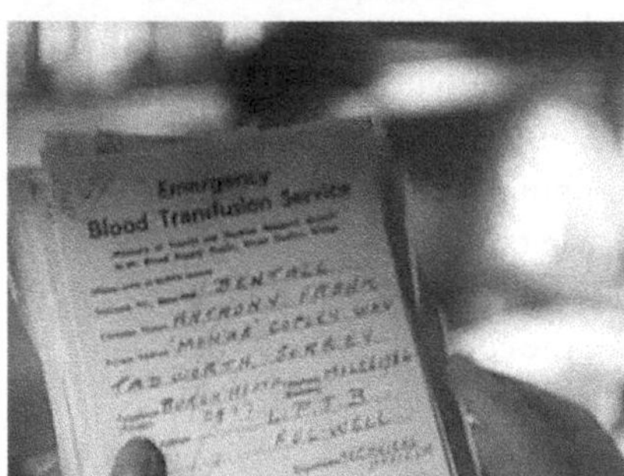

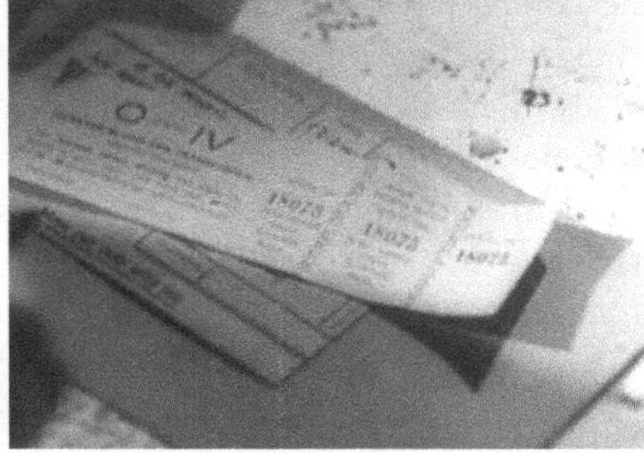

Figure 5.2: The paperwork of the depots, captured from stills from a wartime public information film, *Blood Transfusion Service*, directed and edited by H. M. Nieter, a Paul Rotha production (Ministry of Health in cooperation with the MRC and the Blood Transfusion Units of the Fighting Services, 1941). Images reproduced courtesy of the Wellcome Library, London, under the Creative Commons licence.

Fisher asked the depots for blood grouping totals: the frequencies of A, B, O and AB, summed separately for the two sexes. Many of his correspondents obliged, although whether this was part of their routine clerical work is not clear. One indication that it may not have been was that some depots did not send processed totals but instead the raw donor enrolment forms.[26] Fisher's secretary Barbara Simpson dealt with the index cards and grouping totals, as well as arranging the 'transmission by rail, car, etc. of packages of forms' and the 'avoidance of confusion between different batches'. This paperwork Fisher described as 'actual laboratory work'.[27]

Fisher and Simpson did further work on paper to make the blood group records yield genetic data, transposing the totals into allele (gene variant) frequencies. Owing to dominance between alleles, it was impossible to tell without family data whether an individual of group A had the genotype AA or AO, but at a population level a new kind of data could emerge. A basic principle of population genetics – the Hardy-Weinberg equilibrium – stated that in a large population the allele frequencies of a Mendelian gene, for example the alleles A, B and O, stand in fixed relation to each other. Using population totals, Fisher could use mathematical techniques he had developed in the 1930s to estimate the underlying allele frequencies. Work on paper – the sorting, counting and organization of cards and the manipulation of symbols – brought genetic data into view.

Fisher and his colleagues had carried out blood group surveys before. Before the war they had tested the blood of 600 individuals in London, with the express intention of testing the application of population-genetic techniques to human populations.[28] But the sample size of that survey was rapidly dwarfed by wartime data. By August 1939 Fisher and the Galton Serum Unit already had data from 58,000 people, and by February 1940 this had increased to more than 100,000.[29]

With the donor cards in hand, Fisher took the opportunity to embark on a rather different project from his interwar work. Although the Regional Blood Transfusion Service was not officially established until July 1940, provincial transfusion services were functioning well before this, and Fisher quickly began receiving results from around the country. He began to see these regional records as 'ethnographical data', rather than just materials on which to practise human population genetics.[30] He signalled his new interest in allele frequency distributions when he requested the UCL library to subscribe to the *Zeitschrift für Rassenphysiologie* [*Journal for Race Physiology*], published by the Deutsche Gesellschaft für Blutgruppenforschung [Society for Blood Group Research].[31] Despite its *völkisch* pretentions, it was one of the principal international journals for comparative work on group frequencies and race, and over half of its articles were written by international contributors.[32]

Thus the institutional structure of the wartime transfusion services, and the donor records themselves, radically shaped Fisher's research programme. A mere three months into the war, he co-wrote with Vaughan his first 'ethnographical' paper, 'Surnames and Blood Groups'. Using the Slough records, Vaughan and

Fisher reported that people with distinctively Welsh surnames had significantly different blood group frequencies from the rest of the Slough cohort. Explaining this, they alluded to 'recent industrial development associated with immigration'.[33]

In a more systematic attempt to correlate the distribution of blood group frequencies with narratives about British history, Fisher and Taylor presented a much-expanded study to the Pathology Society in Cambridge in early 1940.[34] Publishing this shortly after in the journal *Nature*, under the title 'Scandinavian Influence in Scottish Ethnology', they reported a continuous gradient in the A:O ratio from North to South Britain. Comparing these frequencies to those found in other European populations, they correlated these patterns with the standard account of British history, which put special emphasis on the Viking conquest and settlement in Shetland, Orkney and the Scottish mainland. Fisher and Taylor expected the North of England and Scotland to have had 'a greater infiltration of Scandinavian blood'.[35] So they were taken aback when they found that Scandinavian frequencies more closely resembled the ratios in the South of England, and that 'no Continental population ... comes near to the Scottish ratio'.[36] Iceland was the only European country with results comparable to those from Scotland. The authors' solution – described in the paper and more cogently in a letter by Fisher to Vaughan – was that the blood groups of the North Europeans themselves might have changed since Viking times, 'presumably', as Fisher suggested, 'by infiltration from Central and Eastern Europe'. Scotland could remain Scandinavian. Alluding to contemporary narratives about the threat to Nordic blood, Fisher commented to Vaughan: 'Almost topical, isn't it!'[37]

Almost as soon as the EBTS began its work, Fisher grasped the opportunity offered by its infrastructure and materials. At Rothamsted the donor cards were transformed from clerical tools into genetic data, quickly yielding enormous sample sizes consistent with the kind of human genetics that Fisher had envisaged in the 1930s. Using data derived from geographically dispersed depots, he and his colleagues correlated their results with historical narratives about British nationhood. Although 'ethnographic' studies were not a major or persistent theme in Fisher's career, and he soon handed over the work to two younger colleagues, it marked the inception of a two-decade 'British Blood Group Survey', which relied on data from the transfusion services.

Population Genetics and Blood Grouping Technique

Alongside research on blood group distributions, Fisher suggested using a basic tenet of population genetics to make a practical contribution to the war effort. The Hardy-Weinberg principle was described formally in the early twentieth century by the German geneticist Wilhelm Weinberg and the British mathematician George Hardy. Hardy and Weinberg independently showed that for any large population of sexually reproducing organisms, a single generation of random mating would result in stable allele frequencies that could (a simple system) be calculated using a general formula. This could be used to test hypotheses about the genetic basis of a trait (e.g. the numbers of loci involved, allelic dominance, etc.) or conversely to test basic assumptions of genetic equilibrium (e.g. random mating, large population size).

Fisher proposed to use this to evaluate the accuracy of blood grouping technique. He reasoned that any deviation from calculated population frequencies could reveal consistent technical errors by the depots.[38] Blood grouping was not always straightforward; if reagents were out of date or laboratory workers inexperienced, the group AB, for example, might be misread as B. Fisher frequently praised the careful skill deployed by his colleagues at the Galton Serum Unit, asserting that 'we are the only "professionals" in the country', but he lamented the poor results coming in from elsewhere. He suggested using the Hardy-Weinberg check as a contribution to the war effort, framing this as part of ongoing attempts to educate and discipline transfusion workers.[39]

Fisher also used the worldwide distributions of blood groups as a reference point for evaluating serological technique. Encountering a particularly obstinate set of records from Scotland, he told Taylor: 'the Glasgow series practically knocks me flat ... there are nearly 15% B's among the males, and 26% in the female list'. This, he observed wryly, could 'give rise to alarming ethnological speculation, as it probably could not be paralleled nearer than Northern India'.[40]

These protocols also became part of Fisher's exchange – mediated by the Galton Serum Unit – between genetic research and the war effort. In a letter to Taylor, he remarked that 'the detection of anomalies in grouping frequencies is one of the most useful by-products of the collections we are making'. Forced to justify Simpson's salary to the UCL authorities, who were intent on sacking anyone not contributing to the war effort, Fisher implored the MRC to plead his case, explaining that Simpson was making a 'positive contribution to the efficacy of the Blood Transfusion Service', and that through their statistical checks 'numerous anomalies and discrepancies in the frequencies of blood groups obtained have been brought to light'.[41] Unfortunately for Fisher and Simpson, his clarification came too late and UCL withdrew its funding, although in the end he pulled together money from other sources to keep her on.

For Fisher, the techniques of population genetics were universal tools that could function as effective controls in transfusion depots. This was less obvious to depot medical officers. Several issues of *Science* had mentioned the Hardy-Weinberg principle, and statistics featured regularly in more specialist biology and statistical journals, but trained physicians were unlikely to be familiar with these kinds of mathematical methods.[42] So Fisher trod carefully in his interventions over grouping technique. Wondering to Taylor how best to communicate his concerns, he suggested diplomatically disclaiming 'all technical knowledge of serological work'.[43]

Some medical officers already had misgivings about techniques advocated by the Galton Serum Unit. To group blood, most transfusion centres used the simple 'tile' or 'slide' technique, where blood samples and antisera were mixed together on sections of glass or porcelain and checked by eye for agglutination a few minutes later. The Serum Unit preferred the more reliable 'tube technique', where an antiserum was added to a series of test tubes containing serial dilutions of a blood sample, left for a few hours and then checked for agglutination using a microscope. Not only did this use more equipment and take much longer, it required an expert eye to transpose degrees of agglutination into binary data, fine for Taylor and his colleagues but unwieldy for some depots.[44]

Nevertheless, using the networks through which he circulated antisera, Taylor tried to persuade depot workers of the tube technique's virtues. Publishing his favoured protocol in the *Journal of Pathology and Bacteriology*, he suggested to the MRC that it might be a 'good plan to send [copies of the paper] to all the people who apply to us for grouping serum'.[45] And his persuasion was evidently often successful, as debates over the two methods appeared in the pages of medical journals. For example, a medical officer in Cardiff named R. Drummond read Taylor's article and wrote to the *BMJ*, declaring that although it meant 'extra work in the laboratory and more precise technique', he had 'completely discarded' grouping on slides 'in favour of tubes'. Drummond cautioned readers that he had witnessed 'two fatalities due to incompatible blood transfusion', both of which were due to 'faulty grouping by the slide technique'.[46]

Others were doubtful about being lectured by an institution clearly far removed from the front line of clinical work. In 1941 the Blood Transfusion Research Committee drew up a memorandum on blood grouping techniques in the transfusion services, which it circulated to various workers in the field before publication.[47] The ensuing correspondence hints at general impatience with the Serum Unit's techniques. Committee head Alan Drury – who, after training as a physiologist, later qualified as a doctor at St Thomas's Hospital in London – had a keen sense of what was appropriate in the transfusion context.[48] He felt that the details of the tube technique, which he tactfully reassured Taylor was 'very reliable', should nevertheless be left out of the memorandum and published elsewhere.[49] In the first draft of the memorandum, Taylor's technique got only a short mention, although his advocates had won a fuller account of it by the time the galley proofs were ready.[50]

Meanwhile, Vaughan received damning criticism of the memorandum back from the depots. Taylor had drafted the section on the problematic topic of 'cold agglutination' – whereby the external conditions of the reaction caused red cell clumping even when the two blood samples were the same – but his account was complicated, and several people thought it should be made simpler for the benefit of the clinician.[51] Brigadier Whitby, head of the Army Blood Transfusion Service, wrote scathingly that Taylor's contribution was 'simply appalling' because it 'savours of the laboratory and does not solve the bedside difficulties'.[52] The controversy over the Blood Group Memorandum was evidently severe, and Vaughan tried to smooth things over. She told Drury that she had 'written to Whitby (very sweetly)' and that she was 'supplying sedatives by telephone and letter to an almost hysterical George Taylor'.[53]

So while blood groups were frequently shared between people with different interests, the work done to make these exchanges work, and the ensuing controversies over technique, bring into view some of the diverse interests that gave different communities their identities. That Lionel Whitby could decry the Serum Unit's techniques as inappropriate for 'the bedside', while Fisher could regard the Galton Serum Unit as 'the only professionals in the country', suggests a self-conscious regard for domains of the clinic and the research laboratory. The Serum Unit occupied hybrid ground: on the one hand the central producer of grouping reagents, and on the other (as we shall see in the next section) a nationwide centre of genetic research.

Rhesus Genetics

The Galton Serum Unit's most famous wartime research programme – and one that established Britain as the leading nation in blood group genetics for at least another decade – was on the inheritance of the Rhesus blood groups. Many accounts of this are dominated by a long-standing controversy over the nomenclatures used to denote the Rhesus system, but here I use just one aspect of the story to further explore the uses of blood groups in different settings.[54]

Fisher first suggested working on the Rhesus blood groups in 1942, two years after they were first defined by Karl Landsteiner and Alexander Wiener in New York.[55] Observing that rabbit antisera immunized with blood from Rhesus monkeys agglutinated 85 per cent of human blood samples, Landsteiner and Wiener soon found a human serum that elicited the same pattern of reactions.[56] Samples that agglutinated with this serum they called Rh-positive (Rh+), and those that did not Rh-negative (Rh–). The Rhesus groups' rapid rise to clinical significance was owing to the 1941 discovery that they were responsible for a dangerous condition called 'haemolytic disease of the newborn', or *Erythroblastosis fetalis*, where an Rh– mother produced antibodies to her Rh+ foetus, causing the baby to be born seriously anaemic.

Over the next four years, the major US and British medical journals published more than eighty articles on the Rhesus groups. Early on, the genetics looked simple: Landsteiner and Wiener proposed that the Rh+ and Rh– groups were inherited via a single locus with two alleles, *Rh* and *rh*, one dominant to the other. But as they discovered new antisera, the patterns of inheritance became more complicated. The discovery of groups was a recursive process; as researchers tested larger numbers of blood samples, they defined new groups and antisera, and from family data postulated new antigens, alleles and dominance relationships.

For Fisher the Rhesus system was a compelling research topic, not least because it was the first blood group system with clear selective consequences in human populations. And the Galton Serum Unit was the ideal institutional setting to embark on this work. With Taylor and depot head Patrick Mollison, he published an appeal in the *BMJ* for doctors to send samples from mothers and babies affected by *Erythroblastosis fetalis*.[57] The unit progressed rapidly in its investigation owing to its precious links to the transfusion services and hospitals, which also sent blood samples from people suffering adverse transfusion reactions. The Serum Unit corresponded regularly with the Wiener lab, notifying them of new discoveries and incorporating their results into Wiener's scheme.[58] But researchers on both sides of the Atlantic struggled with the increasingly complex patterns of agglutination and their inheritance. By 1944 the two labs had defined the alleles Rh_1, Rh_y, Rh', Rh_2, Rh_0, Rh'' and *rh*, although they had derived their antisera independently and given them different names.

In June 1944 Taylor's colleague Robert Race described in *Nature* a proposal by Fisher for a radically new mechanism of Rhesus inheritance.[59] Instead of a single *Rh* gene with many variants, the paper proposed three tightly linked genes, each with two possible alleles. With it, Fisher and Race suggested a complete revision of the nomenclatures for the antisera, genotypes and groups, whereby each of the genes would be denoted using letters *C*, *D* and *E*, and their alleles denoted by upper- or lower-case letters, giving six alleles: *C*, *c*, *D*, *d*, *E*, *e*.[60] In this new system, the only clinically relevant alleles were *D* and *d*, with *d* corresponding to the Rh– antigen and *D* to the Rh+ antigen.

The suggestion was audacious; the idea of a tightly linked gene cluster had never been proposed for human genetics and only once in any organism.[61] Crucially, the theory made several predictions, at least one of which was soon confirmed. One was that from generation to generation the three linked loci might very rarely form new combinations (Figure 5.3). This, Fisher argued, explained why among the general population some *CDE* combinations were common, some very rare and others extremely rare. Evidence supporting the hypothesis would come in the shape of a family with blood groups indicating that recombination had taken place between two of the linked loci. To find these, large numbers of families would have to be tested, so it was an experiment well suited to a laboratory with strong links to medical services. The unit was perfectly positioned to acquire samples representing the very rare allele combinations; using these, they soon established, for example, that the order of the linked genes *C*, *D* and *E* was in fact *D*–*C*–*E*.[62]

Rh BLOOD GROUPS AND THEIR CLINICAL EFFECTS 17

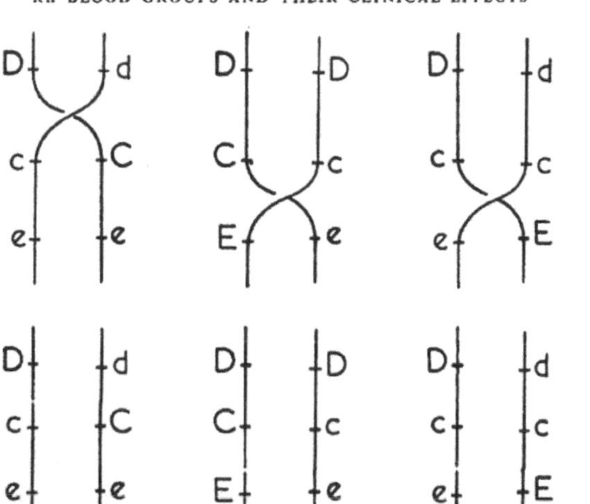

FIG. 3. Fisher's theory of crossing-over, as an explanation of the less frequent chromosomes in a population.

Figure 5.3: Schematic showing the Rhesus locus in terms of the new Fisher-Race scheme, from 'Medical Research Council Memorandum no. 19: The Rh Blood Groups and their Clinical Effects' (London: HMSO, 1948). The three genes *D*, *C* and *E* were so tightly linked that only very rarely did recombination break up the alleles. Some allele combinations were therefore common (top row), while others, which created recombination, were extremely rare (bottom row). The researchers predicted that the rare combinations would only be recovered from testing many thousands of blood samples. Image reproduced under the UK Open Government License, http://www.nationalarchives.gov.uk/doc/open-governmentlicence/.

The Rhesus groups were soon routinely tested in transfusion depots, hospitals and the surgeries of general practitioners. The journals *Lancet* and *BMJ* published their first accounts of the Rhesus groups in January 1942, and they were soon recommending that *any* transfusion recipient who had been pregnant or who had received a previous transfusion should only be given Rh– blood.[63] From 1943 depots tested donors for Rh– and Rh+ and reserved stocks of Rh– blood for pregnant women and patients needing repeat transfusions. Rh– individuals were issued with 'special group cards', a practice that, Vaughan and Panton later reported, was a 'means of educating both the public and the general practitioner in the importance of Rh tests in maternity cases'.[64]

Moreover, the medical significance of the Rhesus groups brought the principles and terminology of human genetics into the mainstream medical literature. Even the first explanation of Rhesus in the *Lancet* explained that 'about 72% of children from all Rh+ x Rh– matings should be Rh–'.[65] Before the Rhesus groups, genetic terminology had been relatively absent from medical journals; a cursory search suggests that the term 'genotype' was used only five times by the *BMJ* before 1942 (two of these were about the ABO groups and paternity testing). By contrast, between 1942 and 1950 the term was used in twenty-six articles, all but two about the Rhesus groups.[66] Rhesus incompatibility had made its genetics significant for medical prognosis. This is not to say that the Rhesus blood groups single-handedly brought genetics into medicine – after all, the early 1940s also saw the first British textbooks of human genetics for medical students – but in Britain they did help usher genetic terminology into the medical lexicon.[67]

To summarize, earlier in the war blood group 'genetic' expertise had been localized in Rothamsted and Cambridge. With the Rhesus groups, and their serious pathological consequences, genetics entered into the clinical sphere. Rhesus groups were now significant for a range of different workers – to geneticists, owing to their very complex patterns of inheritance and their selective ramifications, and to doctors because of their implications for transfusion and pregnancy – helping to explain why there was such a long-running controversy over its nomenclatures.[68] Competing nomenclatures reflected the identities and functions of the Rhesus groups – genetic and diagnostic – in different settings. Some argued that the genotype terminology should reflect the patterns of antisera reactions, which had central importance to clinicians. Many geneticists argued that the antisera should reflect the names of the antigens and their alleles. Thus while research and clinical communities successfully shared the Rhesus groups, they had commitments to different practices.

Conclusion

Blood groups were predominantly medical objects. They could only be collected in large numbers because of their significance in the clinic. But they also took on different identities in different settings. Donor records were organizational tools in the depots, but they were raw data on human inheritance at Rothamsted. Samples collected for diagnostic purposes in the hospital were transported to the Galton Serum Unit and re-appropriated for genetic research. Blood groups were serological tools in the clinic, but in Cambridge they were phenotypes made to yield examples of rare allele combinations. Blood groups were made to stand for different things, and workers in different settings prioritized different aspects of their practices. That the Galton Serum Unit was only partially successful in exerting its authority on serological techniques used in the depots signals their different interests and resources.

What does the story say about the significance of human genetics during this period? Locally, it helps to characterize the kind of human genetics Fisher stood for. He extended the jurisdiction of genetics into a new domain, as part of a longer programme to establish the authority of a new kind of human genetics. In 1942 the chairman of the Human Genetics Committee, J. B. S. Haldane, captured his colleague's aspirations for the field when he commented that 'in the study of human genetics, statistical methods replace the various technical devices, such as milk bottles and etherizers, which are familiar to the Drosophila worker'.[69] Fisher went further, regarding the Hardy-Weinberg equilibrium, and the mathematical techniques based on it, to have universal applicability, even recommending it as a routine standard for the clinical laboratory.

Yet the story also shows that the reach of human genetics was still relatively limited. When Fisher first established the Galton Serological Laboratory in 1935, he had received funding from the Rockefeller Foundation's 'Medical Sciences' programme, owing to the great promise of blood groups in establishing linkage with clinically relevant traits, an approach also endorsed by the MRC. But these aspirations were still very speculative; by the outbreak of war neither Fisher's nor any other laboratory had yet established linkage, and human genetics had certainly not yet lived up to its promise of relevance to medical practice. With Rhesus, the story changed: owing to the dangers of mother–foetus incompatibility, genetic terminology and knowledge about human inheritance began to enter into the medical literature, albeit in a carefully mediated form.

In 1943 Fisher was appointed as the new Professor of Genetics in Cambridge, and he hoped that after the war Taylor and Race would remain there and resume their original positions in his Serological Laboratory. The MRC had other ideas. They wanted to continue funding genetics but sought to bring it under the same roof as a broader range of blood transfusion research: 'a Unit of this nature is best situated in a large centre of population, such as London, where access to clinical material and records is easily obtainable'.[70] To Fisher's dismay, the MRC won out. When hostilities ended, Race was appointed head of the Lister Institute's new Blood Group Research Laboratory, specializing in blood group genetics, although the two men continued their productive collaboration for many years. The MRC chose to reinforce the laboratory's productive institutional links with medicine where the abundance of material was to be found.

Acknowledgements

Thanks to Nick Hopwood, Nick Jardine, Boris Jardine, Staffan Müller-Wille and the participants of the History Workshop in the Department of History and Philosophy of Science, Cambridge.

6 THE ABANDONMENT OF RACE: RESEARCHING HUMAN DIVERSITY IN SWITZERLAND, 1944–56

Pascal Germann

Race was a key concept in human genetic research during the first half of the twentieth century. It was especially important with regards to research on human diversity. From the Enlightenment, the biological diversity of humanity had been largely interpreted in terms of supposed racial differences. Historical research in the last decade has challenged the view that the history of racial research in the twentieth century should solely be read as the history of its decline. Rather, it revealed that the concept of race has proved astounding in its persistence in many respects.[1] However, the concept of race appears to have lost much of its significance in interpreting human differences around the middle of the twentieth century, with new concepts and interpretations of human diversity gaining ground at the expense of the old racial classifications. The concept of race lost its function as a key epistemic category. How did this change come about?

The literature in the history of science offers two main explanations. The first ascribes a decisive role to politics.[2] From this point of view, it was no longer considered appropriate after 1945 to continue using a scientific term that was so associated with the crimes of the Nazi regime. Historians of science, in contrast, especially those who take a discipline-based approach, emphasize the importance of developments within science itself.[3] They attribute the waning significance of the concept of race not to politics, but to a shift in scientific thinking that can be described as the transition from a typological view to the more dynamic models of population genetics. In a way, both of these explanations have their merits, but also their respective shortcomings. The first approach neglects the inner dynamics of science, and the second one underrates the influence of politics on science.

In her study on the human genome diversity project, Jenny Reardon offers an alternative view while using the concept of 'co-production' as a framework. This allows an examination of how scientific knowledge and political order form together.[4] In a similar way Staffan Müller-Wille suggests, in an article about the UNESCO statement on race, that the changes and challenges of the concept of race could be more plausibly delineated by taking into consideration the interaction between science and politics.[5] In this essay I will take up this interactionist standpoint. From this perspective, I do not regard science and politics as separate spheres. Rather, I hope to show that scientific research and politics are intertwined and entangled. I have loosely based this view on Volker Roelcke's plea for a historical-political epistemology, in which he states that knowledge production has an intrinsic political dimension.[6]

Moreover, I will unite this emphasis on the political dimension of science with a focus on local contexts in which research on human diversity was conducted. When examining the history of the race concept in the mid-twentieth century, historians have tended to consider debates in Britain and the USA, the popular anti-racist literature written by geneticists or cultural anthropologists, and the international debate surrounding the UNESCO statement on race.[7] In doing so, they focused on the global negotiations and circulations of knowledge, paying little attention to the actual production of knowledge on human diversity and the very different local conditions under which research practices took place. In this essay I argue that the continuity, change or marginalization of the concept of race was dependent not only on the political rejection of racialism and the global spread of new scientific concepts, but also on local contexts shaped by specific research conditions, epistemic cultures and political discourses. In the production of knowledge on the biological diversity of humanity, research practices, styles of scientific thinking, material requirements, medical contexts and political cultures interact in manifold ways. I will attempt to shed light on some of these interactions using the example of blood group research in Switzerland.

In the space of just a few years, a shift occurred in the representations and concepts of human diversity. A comparison of two particular works clearly illustrates this change. In 1946 the most comprehensive study of biological human diversity in Switzerland was published: Otto Schlaginhaufen's *Anthropologica Helvetica*.[8] In two hefty volumes, the Zurich-based anthropologist and eugenicist presented the results of a large-scale anthropological project lasting over twenty years and drawing on the anthropometric data of more than 35,000 conscripts enlisted for the Swiss Army physical examination. Schlaginhaufen's project was typical of the racial anthropological approach to population studies in the first half of the twentieth century. Human diversity was conceptualized entirely in terms of racial typologies. The research project's most important findings were summarized in a small table that shows the percentage of the Swiss population made up by each of the various races (Table 6.1).

Table 6.1: Distribution of racial types in the Swiss population, from O. Schlaginhaufen, *Anthropologia Helvetica. Die Anthropologie der Eidgenossenschaft*, Vol. 1 (Zurich: Orell Füssli, 1946), p. 686.

Nordische Rasse	1.571%
Osteuropide Rasse	0.285%
Ibero-insulare Rasse	0.615%
Alpine Rasse	1.41 %
Litorale Rasse	2.47 %
Dinarische Rasse	2.31 %
Im Ganzen	8.661%

A different picture of the biological diversity of the Swiss population was painted by Siegfried Rosin's work a mere ten years later.[9] Published in 1956, this study was based on a huge collection of blood group data. The centrepiece was a large, foldable map showing the geographical distribution of the ABO blood group in Switzerland that came to be embraced simply as 'the genetic map of Switzerland' (Figures 6.1 and 6.2). According to Rosin, two of his research findings were especially noteworthy. Firstly, the Swiss population displayed an astounding genetic heterogeneity. Regarding genetic diversity, Switzerland could be described as a mosaic made up of small areas that displayed 'sharp contrasts', particularly in the Alps.[10] Secondly, Rosin stressed that the biological boundaries in no way coincided with the religious, linguistic or political ones.[11] Racial classifications played no part in Rosin's interpretation. In fact, the word 'race' does not even appear once in the whole work. So why did Rosin abandon the old terms, classifications and interpretations?

The history of this research project shows that the shift was anything but inevitable. A close look at Swiss blood group research in the middle of the twentieth century provides evidence that there was neither an irreconcilable gap nor a smooth continuation between scientific population genetics and racial typology. I will argue that the scientific transition delineated below was not a straightforward paradigm shift. Rather, it was a complex process resulting from changes in data arrangements, practices of representation and concepts. Moreover, all of these transformations were shaped by global trends as well as by local contexts in which scientific research was interconnected with national discourses, political institutions and administrative practices in manifold ways. In the first part of this essay, I will reconstruct the development of this blood group project. The second part will deal with the political dimension of blood group research. I will then address a shift in interpretations of genetic diversity in Switzerland before returning to my initial question: why did the concept of race no longer play a role in these interpretations?

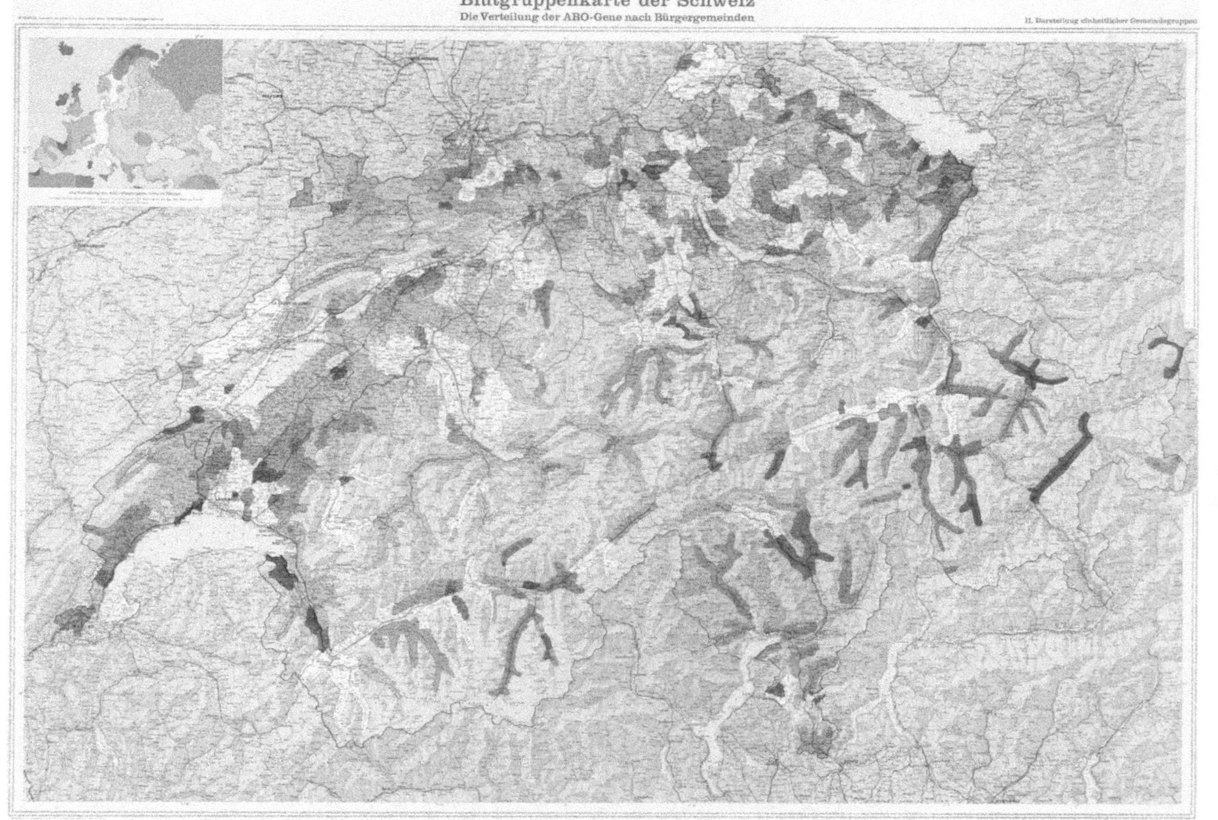

Figure 6.1: Blood group map of Switzerland: the distribution of ABO-genes according to 'municipalities of origin', from S. Rosin, 'Die Verteilung der AB0-Blutgruppen in der Schweiz', *Archiv der Julius Klaus-Stiftung für Vererbungsforschung, Sozialanthropologie und Rassenhygiene*, 31:1–2 (1956), pp. 17–127, n.p. The shadings represent the relative frequency of blood group genes, with white denoting areas with an average frequency. The tone of the shading represents the deviation from average, whereas greater intensity denotes greater deviation from the average. An intense dark grey colour, for example, shows areas where the allele predisposing for blood group O is much more frequent than the average Swiss population. Image reproduced courtesy of Zurich Central Library.

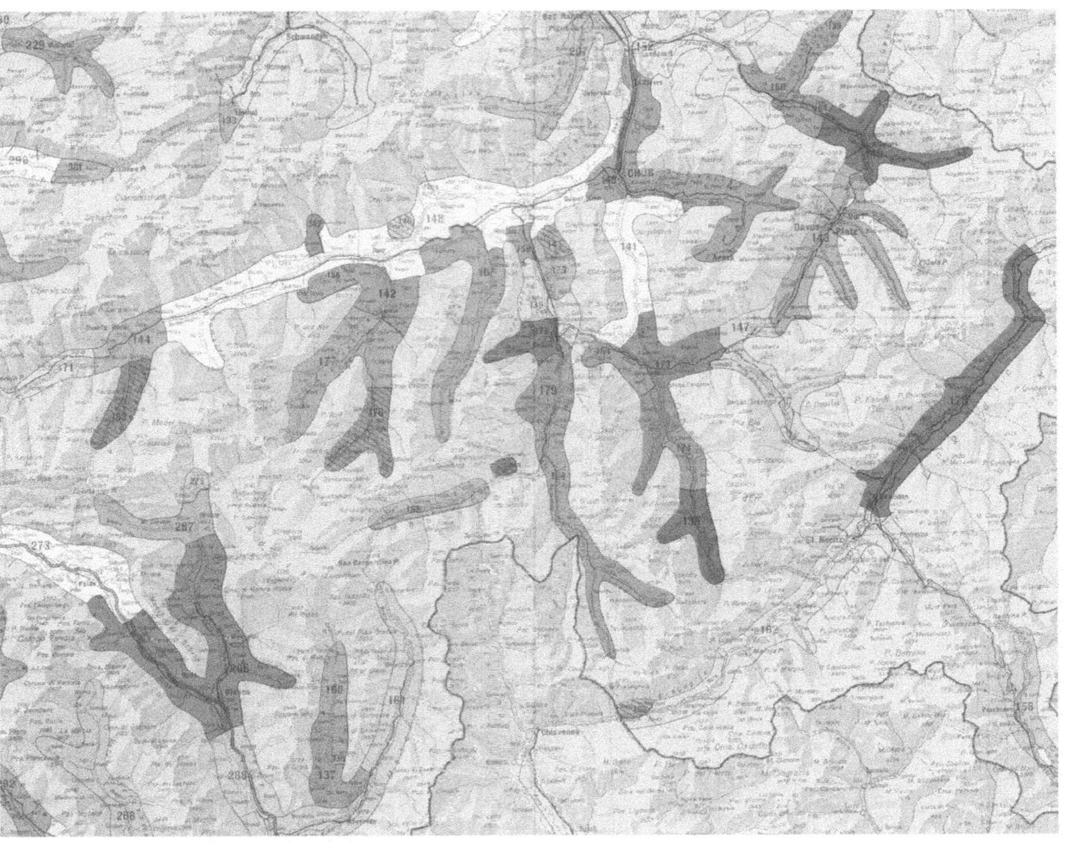

Figure 6.2: Detail from blood group map of Switzerland.

The Swiss Blood Group Project, 1944–56

The origins of Rosin's research project can be traced back to World War II.[12] The Zürcher Arbeitsgemeinschaft für Blutgruppenforschung (Zurich Society for Blood Group Research) won the support of General Henry Guisan in 1944 for a gigantic research project in the field of blood group genetics. This was particularly prestigious because Guisan was the commander-in-chief of the Swiss Army during World War II, and he was held in high esteem in Switzerland.[13] The general commissioned lists featuring the blood groups of all soldiers along with their 'municipality of origin' (this term is stated on all Swiss documents of identification, as we will see below). The result was a collection of blood group data for more than 270,000 soldiers, an amount that corresponded to approximately 7 per cent of the Swiss population. A look at the project's initiators reflects the close cooperation between genetics, medicine and racial anthropology. Originally, the *Arbeitsgemeinschaft* assembled three renowned professors from the University of Zurich: Ernst Hadorn, the most important pioneer of developmental genetics in Switzerland; the physician Hans Rudolf Schinz, an internationally known expert in radiation biology; and finally, the racial anthropologist Otto Schlaginhaufen. They were joined later by Jakob Eugster, professor for geographic medicine, and statistician Siegfried Rosin.

The project was driven by different interests. On the one hand, Swiss military officials who facilitated the project were pursuing practical goals regarding national defence. They hoped that the disclosure of blood group distribution all over the country could be helpful for building up an efficient blood donor service. This was regarded as a high military priority in Switzerland during World War II and at the beginning of Cold War.[14] On the other hand, the scientists involved anticipated that in the future the Swiss Army could regularly deliver huge amounts of blood group data, which would allow for an ongoing national research project. Not least, these prospects were also connected with eugenic visions of controlling the 'Swiss people's genetic substance', as Ernst Hadorn emphasized in a newspaper article.[15] For the purposes of eugenics and human genetics, blood group data provided a particularly favourable material, because blood groups are easily definable Mendelian traits. Moreover, the blood group project had relevance to medical science. Rosin pointed out that the examination of correlations between blood groups and diseases was a promising research field.[16] Tellingly, most of the project's initiators had medical research experience relating to epidemiological and genetic surveys. Hans Rudolf Schinz, for instance, conducted studies on the genetics of cancer, and, in cooperation with Siegfried Rosin, he carried out a statistical survey on cancer mortality.[17] Jakob Eugster also combined genetic and epidemiological research in his extensive study on goitre and cretinism in the 1930s and 1940s.[18]

At the start, however, the blood group project was most deeply connected to racial anthropology. Although it was soon revealed that there were no direct links between blood groups and racial 'types', blood group research became one of the main research strategies of racial scientists in the first half of the twentieth century. Otto Schlaginhaufen was a founding member of the Deutsche Gesellschaft für Blutgruppenforschung (German Society for Blood Group Research), which espoused a *völkisch* agenda and was committed to promoting seroanthropological race research.[19] From the 1920s seroanthropologists had been trying to reveal that there were considerable differences in blood group frequencies between peoples, races and nations.[20] Swiss blood group research initially followed this approach, aiming to provide new insights into the racial composition of the Swiss population.

The early analyses of blood group data were thus entirely motivated by racial anthropology research interests. The first work was published in 1946 by the physician Alfred Schütz, who was engaged in the Swiss Army's Blood Typing Service.[21] His research was based on only part of the corpus of army data. One of Schütz's findings was that the Romansh- and German-speaking regions of eastern Switzerland seemed to exhibit different blood group distributions. From this, he concluded that the linguistic boundary also had significance with regards to racial biology.[22] Schütz's work triggered a boom in seroanthropological research in Switzerland and was well received internationally. This led to intensive serological studies being carried out on the so-called Walser, a German-speaking minority in the eastern Alps.[23] However, criticism of Schütz's work soon mounted, and it came, among others, from the Bernese zoologist Siegfried Rosin, a pioneer of mathematical biology. But the criticism did not concern Schütz's racial interpretation. Rather, critics singled out his statistical calculations, claiming that they were methodologically inadequate.[24] It became clear that evaluating the blood group data was a complex task that required elaborate statistical and mathematical methods as well as organizational efforts.

The Zurich Society for Blood Group Research responded to this challenge by introducing a more specialized division of labour. Otto Schlaginhaufen's Anthropological Institute, which was well versed in dealing with large volumes of data, took over the job of sorting and counting the records. Furthermore, the research group recruited Rosin to conduct the statistical analysis.[25] This job was a welcome opportunity for Rosin to apply the statistical models and mathematical methods he had developed for population biology. In retrospect, Rosin judged that the main value of his work lay in providing an 'exemplary evaluation of a material which is unique to the whole world'.[26]

For several years, the funding of the project remained insecure. Otto Schlaginhaufen was Chairman of the Julius Klaus-Stiftung für Vererbungsforschung, Sozialanthropologie und Rassenhygiene (Julius Klaus Foundation for Genetic

Research, Social Anthropology and Racial Hygiene).[27] The eugenic foundation stepped in to fund the serological project. However, this commitment to such a large project was ill-timed, as during the 1940s the foundation suffered economically from inflation and decreasing interest profits. Moreover, the publication of Schlaginhaufen's *Anthropologica Helvetica* in 1946 placed further stress on the foundation's budget.[28] Thus the research group had to search for further sponsors. Two appeals, one to the Section of Medical Services of the Federal Military Department, another to the newly founded national blood donor organization of the Swiss Red Cross, were rejected. Although the Red Cross acknowledged the importance of blood group serology in the field of 'racial research',[29] its Central Committee took the view that the organization should not fund 'purely scientific' projects.[30] These financing problems became more severe once it became apparent that the statistical analysis and data calculations were more time-consuming and cost-intensive than originally projected.[31] The problems were solved when, in 1952, the Swiss National Science Foundation (SNF) was founded. As one of the first projects, the blood group project received a huge grant from this key institution of national research funding.[32]

Finally, in 1956 Rosin published his findings, together with a detailed explanation of his statistical methods, in the journal of the Julius Klaus Foundation. Another grant from the SNF also allowed for the publication of the large coloured gene map.[33] The work was very well received among both scientists and the media in Switzerland, and Rosin was presented with Switzerland's most prestigious science award, the Marcel Benoist Prize.[34] The media were especially keen on Rosin's blood group map. The popular magazine *Die Woche* published a story with the title 'Das A und O des Schweizer Blutes' (The A and O of Swiss Blood). A photo depicted Rosin sitting in front of his blood group map while a cross heading announced the 'big surprise' revealed by the celebrated study: 'Switzerland is a blood mosaic'.[35] In the newspaper *Neue Zürcher Zeitung*, Ernst Hadorn wrote an article that described the map as the first in the world to accurately show the distribution of genes within a population. The rest of the world, claimed the newspaper, would envy Switzerland's breakthrough in genetic geography.[36]

The Swiss blood group project is typical of human diversity research in the mid-twentieth century, when blood group research was booming around the globe. There was scarcely a country in Europe where no large-scale national, or at the very least a regional, blood group project was under way. Country-specific studies found their way into comprehensive surveys, and there were also international cooperations between blood group researchers. Rosin, for instance, worked with the British serologist Arthur Ernest Mourant.[37] Yet while Swiss serological research developed in line with international trends, it was distinctively shaped by its national political context.

The Political Dimension of Blood Group Research

National blood group projects have an inherently political dimension. They raise questions regarding the homogeneity or heterogeneity of the national population, the status of national minorities and relationships with neighbouring countries. Research on human genetic diversity produces images and concepts of the population that can reflect, confirm or challenge political structures. They have the potential to weaken or strengthen social, cultural and political differences.

This political dimension took different shapes in different national contexts. In Greece, for example, the discourse about the relationship between the Greek majority and the Slavic minority informed a controversy about the interpretation of blood group data during the 1950s. In 1957 the Romanian anthropologist Alexander Manuila concluded in a seroanthropological study that the Greek population was subject to a 'Dinaric influence'.[38] Subsequently his Greek colleague Ioannis Koumaris[39] accused him of being politically biased. Koumaris claimed that Manuila's results were distorted by his political intention to serologically unite the Hellenics with the Southern Slavs. Koumaris insisted on a genetic dividing line between Greeks and Slavs, which he saw as divergent races.[40] Population genetics research lent biological significance to the barriers created in the Greek Civil War between the Greek majority and the Slavic-Macedonian minority, as well as between Greece and its socialist neighbours. And genetic research had the potential both to reinforce and to undermine such barriers.

In Switzerland, meanwhile, debate centred on linguistic and religious boundaries. Swiss anthropologists saw it as one of their principal tasks to investigate whether these boundaries had any biological significance.[41] Conflicts between religious and linguistic communities had always been regarded as a threat to national stability. Indeed, until the nineteenth century, religious divides repeatedly caused civil wars. Switzerland's very development as a nation state had been based on a series of agreements aimed at building consensus and bridging these divides. During World War I, a deep divide between the French- and German-speaking parts of Switzerland opened up.[42] As a consequence, national identity discourses in Switzerland developed narratives and imagery that bridged these ethnical, linguistic and religious gaps. 'Unity in diversity' was one of the central slogans of Swiss nationalism in the middle third of the twentieth century. This was a time of growing national self-adulation, when Switzerland sought to distinguish itself from the outside world. The country's regional, religious and linguistic diversity was held up as a national asset that found its political expression in the federalist structure of the nation. Although this emphasis on diversity in Swiss national narratives also had an integrative function, it did not lead to a pluralistic attitude towards minorities in general. Rather, the discourse of Swiss diversity was accompanied by powerful discourses and practices that strove to exclude everybody who did not fit into the range of esteemed 'Swiss heterogenity': the Jews, the vagrants, the eugenically 'unwanted'. Thus 'difference' and 'diversity' were only welcome within the limits of the common notion of 'Swissness'. Tellingly, when linguistic and regional diversity was celebrated emphatically in the 1930s, eugenic ideas and practices, as well as restrictive and repelling policies towards foreigners, also reached a peak.[43]

The federalist discourse of national diversity also found resonance in Swiss science policy. At the foundation ceremony of the SNF on 1 August 1952 – significantly scheduled on Swiss National Day – the foundation's president, Joseph Kälin, affirmed that the federalist structure was the 'essence' of Switzerland and that the principle 'unity in diversity', which he referred to as Switzerland's 'Lebensgesetz' (vital law), also applied to national science.[44] Rosin's depiction of genetic diversity fitted neatly into this national self-image. Unlike earlier anthropological studies, his blood group survey downplayed the boundaries that had always been seen as problematic for national unity, namely the religious and linguistic. Accordingly, the Marcel Benoist Prize judges highlighted the study's 'surprising' finding that these boundaries had no biological basis whatsoever.[45] The picture of a heterogeneous mosaic fitted the Swiss Confederation's self-image as a nation better than racial classifications splitting the nation up into a number of groups associated with neighbouring countries and with specific languages. This may be one of the reasons why Rosin's genetic map was so positively received by the Swiss media.

However, the political dimension was not restricted to the public sphere. It was also an inherent aspect of the research practices themselves, as a closer look at Rosin's analysis reveals. Blood group research is not concerned with the characteristics of individuals, but with the frequency of a certain feature within a group. As Lisa Gannett and James Griesemer have convincingly demonstrated, a priori classifications are a prerequisite for defining groups.[46] This is where politics comes into play. In order to chart the distribution of traits in space, one has to rely on geographical or ethnic categories and administrative structures. The choice of these categories determines the way data are generated and arranged. Already in its formative stage, knowledge about genetic diversity has a fundamentally political dimension.

Rosin made a momentous decision in this regard. He based his blood group statistics on the political unit known as the *Heimatgemeinde* ('municipality of origin'). According to this peculiarly Swiss concept, every Swiss citizen is also a citizen of a municipality that is traditionally defined by his or her ancestors' origin. Naturalized persons exempted, the 'municipality of origin' is – at least in theory – identical with the residence of a male ancestor before the national state's foundation in 1848. In Switzerland the allocation of citizenship is organized according to the *ius sanguinis*. In the early Swiss federal state, at least, this principle of ancestry did not draw on an ethnical concept of nationhood. Rather, it was implemented in order to maintain the autonomy of the municipalities and the cantons in accordance with a federalist order. Even though racial ideologies never gained crucial significance in the construction of Swiss national identity, during World War I racial and ethnic concepts of Swiss nationhood emerged that influenced policies regarding foreigners and the practice of naturalization.[47] In this context, the 'municipality of origin' became increasingly associated with notions of genealogical and ethnical origin.

By building on this notion of ancestry, Rosin hoped that he could reveal the gene frequencies of bygone ages. Alfred Schütz and Otto Schlaginhaufen already emphasized the great value of the 'Heimatgemeinde' as an organizing principle for anthropological studies.[48] Schütz identified the political term 'Heimatgemeinde' with the genealogical term 'Abstammungsort' (place of ancestry), and he stressed that the category allowed them to reveal the original geographical distribution of racial groups and peoples.[49] In this regard, Rosin's classifying practices followed a tradition of racial anthropology that attributed biological meaning to political citizenship.[50] However, in contrast to Schütz and Schlaginhaufen, Rosin deliberately disregarded all known ethnic, religious and linguistic boundaries on the grounds that their significance for the distribution of gene frequencies was uncertain.[51] Choosing the municipality as the decisive entity of data organization made the analysis much more difficult. It is probable that this was the main reason why the statistical analysis of the data took so much more time and required considerably more financial means than was originally predicted. The gene frequencies of more than 3,000 municipalities had to be calculated, and due to a lack of data in less populous municipalities, there were serious problems regarding statistical significance.[52] Rosin defended his decision with the assertion that the Swiss data offered a unique opportunity to focus on the 'smallest geographical units'.[53]

This assertion signals a shift in research interests. Small, isolated populations had now come to the foreground, in the place of large racial groups.[54] In terms of research practices, this shift was favoured by specific political requirements, namely by the federalist structure of Switzerland. Trivially, the classification by municipality of origin was only possible because it is stated on all Swiss identification documents. Rosin emphasized that the huge differences within small areas revealed by his study were the most striking characteristic of Switzerland's genetic geography. But it was only by detecting blood group frequencies at the municipality level that these differences emerged. Consequently, the mosaic picture of a genetically heterogeneous Switzerland is essentially based on the choice of municipality as an underlying category. In a review of Rosin's study, the American human geneticist Richard H. Post recognized the crucial importance of this categorization. He emphasized that the 'degree of heterogeneity' throughout

Switzerland was impressive because the result would be strikingly different from other European studies. He added: 'One wonders whether a gene frequency distribution study of other countries based on units as small as these communities might give similar results'.[55] Implicitly, Post acknowledged that different research results and different genetic geographies rested upon the matrix of observation deployed to pinpoint the distribution of traits. The way population geneticists choose to collect their material is confined, enabled and shaped by the political context. In the case of Rosin, this context was determined by the political order and discourse of Swiss federalism.

Maps illustrating findings of population genetics purport to represent natural regions. There is a widespread tendency among population geneticists to reduce the Alps to natural topographical barriers standing in the way of genetic exchange. In this spirit, the Swiss human geneticist Ernst Hanhart referred to the isolated communities of the Alps as 'nature's laboratories of human genetics'.[56] Alpine populations thus appear as entities formed by nature. However, as discussed in this section, the blood group maps also represented politically defined spaces shaped by given classifications, demarcations and topographies of significance. Blood group maps are a form of palimpsest through which the underlying political coordinate systems are visible, imposing structures on genetic geographies. In Switzerland's case, the political order of federalism can be seen in the intricate structure of its genetic cartography. Federalism is often regarded as the best answer to Swiss diversity. Concerning genetic diversity, this relation is rather the reverse: federalism was not a response to diversity but the precondition for representing diversity.

From Race to Genetic Drift: Interpretations of Human Diversity in the Alps

How then did Rosin interpret the astounding diversity of Switzerland's genetic geography? As a representative of mathematical population biology, Rosin drew on new approaches developed by British and American population geneticists. He was familiar with such concepts as genetic drift and isolation, which offered explanations for genetic differences between populations. However, like other researchers dealing with the genetics of blood groups, Rosin in no way rejected the concept of race. He merely rephrased it in the language of population genetics. Races were no longer groups of individuals displaying common features, but rather defined as populations differing in the distribution of gene frequencies.[57] Within the meaning of this definition, it was impossible to assign individuals to specific races. Meanwhile, it allowed them to integrate the notion of race into the conceptual framework of population genetics.

In any case, Rosin was interested in questions of racial difference. For example, he regarded his blood group research as a way to trace migration patterns. Rosin assumed that immigrant groups would exhibit a different blood group distribution than the indigenous population. This would have pointed to racial differences.[58] However, questions of race lost their significance as the blood group project progressed. Broad racial categories were not helpful when it came to understanding the mosaic of small populations. How, for example, could it be claimed that there were racial differences between two neighbouring mountain villages with markedly different serological profiles when there was an almost total absence of linguistic and cultural differences between the two? Such an interpretation, though, would not have been completely incompatible with the thinking of population genetics, since leading theorists like Theodosius Dobzhansky and Leslie Dunn declared that even small, isolated villages could be referred to as 'races' in a biological sense.[59]

However, racial interpretations are always dependent on pre-existing classifications and narratives that make the application of the term 'race' socially relevant and plausible. Tellingly, racial interpretations in Swiss blood group research proved most persistent in regard to the ethnic minority of the Walser. In the 1950s scientists discovered that Walser populations featured a significantly higher percentage of blood group O than the surrounding populations.[60] The racial interpretation of this result was made plausible by the existence of a common 'biohistorical narrative'.[61] According to a historical narrative tinged with Darwinism, the Alemannic tribe of the Walser had migrated to the eastern Alps in the Middle Ages, where they adapted superbly to the harsh living conditions of the high mountains and increasingly supplanted the indigenous population. Thanks to a pronounced tendency to marry within the group, the story goes on, the Walser preserved their original character, race and culture.[62] Such narratives served as rhetoric strategies that made racial conceptualizations more convincing and solid. Rosin, too, by no means ruled out racial interpretations of the Walser population. However, his national blood group survey showed that high percentages of blood group O were also found in Alpine valleys with no Walser settlements. Furthermore, the project revealed significant differences between the two major, geographically separate, Walser settlements.[63] These findings were hardly compatible with a 'racial' interpretation of the blood group frequencies. Ultimately, the notion of a mosaic of small Alpine populations left little room for a racial classification in practice.

Rosin thus turned his attention to concepts that offered explanations for Switzerland's heterogeneous blood group composition. In so doing, he threw up some far-reaching questions for population genetics.[64] He believed it was possible that a hitherto unknown selection effect was at work in the Alpine valleys that led to differing blood group distributions. However, he thought it was more likely that the genetic diversity in the Alps was due to the effects of genetic drift. Genetic drift is the term used to describe random fluctuations in genetic frequency from one generation to another. The striking human genetic diversity in the Alps could thus be explained not by the presence of different races but quite simply by the effects of chance. Although Rosin regarded his interpretations to be provisional, they influenced the further course of discussion and research.[65] The Swiss blood group project, which started as a contribution to racial anthropology, finally contributed to the demise of the race concept in the field of human diversity research.

Conclusion

Which factors brought about the abandonment of race? The huge quantities of data offer little by way of an explanation. The shift cannot be attributed to a victory of empiricism over the classifications of racial anthropology. More important were changes in the representations, models and concepts that transformed data into facts. Does that mean that the abandonment of race was the consequence of a paradigm shift in favour of population genetics? The new questions, methods and concepts of population genetics did indeed alter the concept of race and diminish its importance. Racial classification was no longer the *via regia* in the investigation and interpretation of human diversity. However, portraying this as a paradigm shift would be too simplistic. The story of the Swiss blood group survey shows that this shift did not come about through a complete overthrow of concepts and research practices, but rather occurred successively within the framework of a research project. In this case, the marginalization of the race concept was primarily a consequence of developments within the research process. Rather than a clear watershed, we see a series of step-like alterations in research practice, institutional settings and scientific culture that finally resulted in a transition from racial anthropology to population genetics. These shifts were based on local conditions that restricted the plausibility and relevance of racial interpretations. The Alpine region, as represented in the genetic maps, proved to have many dimensions. It is a topographically formed, discursively described, politically governed and socially dissected space. All of these dimensions affected the anthropological and genetic geographies.

The case of Swiss blood group research points up the inherent political dimension of human diversity research. The analysis of Rosin's research practices has highlighted that the construction of ancestry and genetic geography were inextricably linked to the political order of citizenship. The publicly celebrated image of the heterogeneous 'blood mosaic' was enabled by the political order of Swiss federalism and nurtured by the national discourse of 'unity in diversity'. While it did not run counter to eugenic visions of population control, it left little room for racial conceptions and classifications. Rosin's population genetics as well as Schlaginhaufen's racial anthropology were political endeavours less in the sense that they were driven by a certain ideological agenda. Rather, their research was political in so far as it was practically shaped by specific institutional and discursive conditions, and it brought new representations and visions of national order into being. Human diversity research is political per se, as it depends on political structures, throws up questions on provenance, belonging and identity, and opens up new horizons for political actions.

Acknowledgments

I would like to thank Mitchell Ash, Bernd Gausemeier, Veronika Lipphardt, Staffan Müller-Wille, Edmund Ramsden, Helga Satzinger and the anonymous referees for their helpful comments on this essay, although, of course, all opinions are my own.

7 POST-WAR AND POST-REVOLUTION: MEDICAL GENETICS AND SOCIAL ANTHROPOLOGY IN MEXICO, 1945–70

Edna Suárez-Diaz and Ana Barahona

Introduction

The history of science focused outside of Europe and the United States has contributed to our understanding of the construction of knowledge in two ways – through the theories of diffusion and dependency. The first centres on the spread of metropolitan knowledge through nations on the periphery.[1] The second is centred on the asymmetrical relationship between centre and periphery, characterized by the latter's inability to build an autonomous system of scientific and technological innovation, and the importation of foreign knowledge by local elites.[2] Despite their obvious differences, both types of theories have produced national accounts of science and technology in peripheral countries which are restricted to local events, and which ignore the international context. In neither case is there an emphasis on global or reciprocal connections, or a focus on circuits of practices that may help explain the construction of knowledge at both the regional and global level.

The rise of postcolonial studies in the history of science has emphasized the need for interconnected histories. As Sanjay Subrahmanyam has suggested, we need 'connected histories as opposed to comparative histories'.[3] These would need to be written from a symmetrical point of view. While interconnected histories require a focus on the circulation of people, technologies and materials, symmetrical accounts demand the acknowledgement of local resistances and the recognition that the practices of more marginal partners help shape the knowledge and practices at the hegemonic centres. Perhaps nowhere in the scientific arena is there a more pressing need for interconnected symmetrical studies than in the anthropological sciences.

The serological and genetic study of indigenous populations in Mexico is a case in point. From the 1930s onwards, Mexico was internationally recognized as a leader in the study and 'management' of indigenous populations. Its leadership was a result of the social revolution that convulsed the country (1910–17) and the resulting policies and institutions that were established to deal with a largely rural (and very poor) indigenous population. John Collier, anthropologist and commissioner of the Office for Indian Affairs of the United States from 1934 to 1945, acknowledged the practical and conceptual advantages of practical anthropology in Mexico. He also recognized important allies in his Mexican counterparts. Collier, together with Mexican anthropologist Manuel Gamio (like Collier, a student of Boas; see below) and Moisés Saénz, a philosopher, diplomat and educator, organized the first Inter-American Congress of Indigenous Affairs in 1940. This took place in Pátzcuaro Michoacan, Mexico, with considerable support from both countries.[4] Ernst Gruening, from the Interior Department of the US, emphasized that the Pátzcuaro conference had a peculiar quality:

> it is a fact that in most of the interchanges of perspectives and services, the US find themselves in the position of donor: that is an unilateral relation and, in the long run, undesirable. Real friendship and understanding, if they are to be valued, must be promoted by reciprocal relations. In this context the discussions on the life and management of indigenous populations constitute a privileged area because many of the Latin American countries, notoriously Mexico ... can make definitive contributions for the matter. They can give us something.[5]

Yet what was it, exactly, that the Mexican approach to indigenous populations could give to their counterparts in the United States? From the mid-1930s Mexican anthropology had been driven by an aggressive *culturalism*: the classification of human groups needed to be based on cultural criteria such as language, while racist approaches towards large indigenous populations needed to be firmly rejected. Such views had practical implications for the indigenist policies of the post-revolutionary regimes, although they were at times interpreted as a communist threat by other Latin American countries, such as Brazil.

For Collier and his American allies during the interwar and war years, Mexico had something valuable to contribute. It was the perfect mediator for the diffusion of pan-American *indigenismo* to the rest of South American countries, one that recognized a certain amount of political autonomy (self-determination) for indigenous populations, as well as the 'link between the indigenous peoples of the United States and those of the Latin American countries, that no European nation could break'.[6] The culturalist agenda of the Mexican anthropologists contributed to a common language shared by US policymakers focused on indigenous population policies, until Collier's resignation in 1945.

Although this scenario suffered profound transformations after World War II (including the loss of interest in Latin America, with the new focus on Europe), it set the framework for health and education policies focused on Mexican indigenous populations. As economic resources flowed in the years following World War II, and health institutions were created during the 'Mexican miracle' (1950s–1970s), a new generation of medical doctors performed serological and genetic research on indigenous populations. While these doctors had studied in the United States and the UK, they used the newly created *indigenista* infrastructure, and, to varying degrees, they sought to accommodate their research within the *indigenista* rhetoric. A first account of the research of some of these scientists is the subject of this essay.

A case study focused on the connections between elite anthropologists, public functionaries and medical doctors working at national research laboratories while collaborating with US scientists allows us to understand how research practices can serve very different political interests, as well as the transnational circuits sustaining practices and knowledge. It also illustrates the great diversity of studies of human populations after the war, contradicting the narrative of a 'post-war individualism' in genetics which is implicit in European and US histories of human genetics during this period.[7] In what follows, a brief introduction to the Mexican *indigenista* policies and institutions is presented in the first section, which establishes the broader context of post-revolutionary rhetoric and health policies within which research on indigenous populations took place from the mid-1940s through to the mid-1960s. The second section offers a survey of the research of Mexican doctors on indigenous populations in the 1940s and 1950s, in particular the work of Manuel Salazar-Mallén. The third section focuses on Salazar-Mallén's student Rubén Lisker, who was in charge of extensive genetic and biochemical surveys of indigenous populations in Mexico in the 1960s. Salazar-Mallén and Lisker's research programmes illustrate the intersection and the tension between the *indigenista* rhetoric and policies, and the individual interests of medical geneticists who were part of the post-war international circuits studying the genetics of human populations.

Indigenous Policies and Health Services

The Mexican government had a vigorous agenda with regards to indigenous affairs during the decades following the revolution. The revolution that took place between 1910 and 1917 had been fuelled, to a large extent, by the demands of Mexican rural indigenous populations. The most vocal revolutionaries, such as Emiliano Zapata in the southern states, expressed agricultural demands, and more precisely, for land distribution and laws that would be fair and respectful of ancient, indigenous communities, their local traditions and social organizations. Poverty and social inequities have long afflicted indigenous populations, and Zapata's motto *Tierra y Libertad* ('Land and Freedom') illustrates this basic component of the social revolution in Mexico.

Very soon after the end of the revolution, in 1917 the Mexican government created the Department of Anthropology (Departamento de Antropología) within the Ministry of Agriculture (Secretaría de Agricultura), as well as the Department for Education and Culture for the Indigenous Race (Departamento de Educación y Cultura para la Raza Indígena) in 1921, along with many other agencies concerned with the indigenous groups. The concept of 'race' was instrumental in deciding who was indigenous in the first years following the revolution. Nevertheless, by the mid-1930s the idea of 'culture' and, specifically, linguistic difference came to the fore with the *indigenista* policies of the Mexican state. This new perspective was the result of a very sophisticated indigenous agenda, fed by research into social and cultural anthropology, archaeology and linguistics that began during Lázaro Cárdenas's presidency (1934–40).

Critical to this new perspective was the influence of German-American anthropologist Franz Boas and his students in Mexican cultural anthropology. Manuel Gamio, who is considered the founder of Mexican anthropology, studied under Boas at Columbia University between 1909 and 1911, and was considered to be one of his best students. Following his return to Mexico, Gamio developed the basic ideas of the *indigenista* doctrine, a 'modernizing nationalism' that aimed at the integration of the indigenous populations with the modern, mixed or *mestizo* nation.[8] The influence of other students of Boas, including Alfred Kroeber and Edward Sapir, who had studied the languages of Native American populations, was also profoundly influential in Mexico during the 1930s and after.[9]

It was in this context that the National Institute of Anthropology and History (Instituto Nacional de Antropología e Historia, INAH) was created in February 1939 by presidential decree. Archaeologist turned anthropologist Alfonso Caso[10] (along with other well-known anthropologists such as Pablo Martínez del Río) was a key figure in the founding of the institute, and became its first director. Two years later, in 1940, Caso was member of the group of intellectuals, including Saénz and Gamio in Mexico and Collier in the United States, who organized the first Inter-American Indigenous Congress in Pátzcuaro. During the congress, the participating countries agreed upon a set of policies and commitments, including the creation of the Inter-American Institute for Indigenous Affairs, to be directed by Saénz.

In 1948, when the Mexican National Indigenista Institute (INI) was created, with Caso as its founder and first director, it was conceived as a chapter of the Inter-American Institute for Indigenous Affairs. Throughout the following decades, the INI was considered a leading indigenous agency at the pan-American level. Caso had been rector of the National University of Mexico (UNAM) from 1945 to 1946, before directing the INI, thereby becoming a member of the political and intellectual elite. He was an actor of critical importance in the construction of policies, institutions and ideologies of post-revolutionary Mexico.[11]

The term 'indigenous affairs' does not convey the fact that the '*indigenista* perspective' has even been described as a *style of thought*: 'it comprises all the policies and politics applied by non-indigenous people to indigenous people'.[12] Such policies had a crucial role in the ideology of post-revolutionary Mexico, connected as they were with nationalistic sentiments, and they helped legitimate an independent Mexican state. In particular, during the period between the 1940s and 1970s, Mexican *indigenismo* was characterized as being: a) unilateral: that is, *from* the state; b) unidirectional: *towards* the indigenous people; and c) single-purpose: incorporating or integrating the indigenous people into the *mestizo* nation.

More specifically, access to education and health services was seen to be the most important means of integrating indigenous communities into the rest of the *mestizo* nation. The paternalistic character of the Mexican state was seen as a tool to remedy historical, social and economic inequalities. Thus, as Caso declared in the early 1960s, 'For us, the peoples of the Americas anthropology is not something that is purely theoretical, nor that serves an immediate purpose; it is a discipline entrenched in our hearts and in our lives'.[13]

As the public health and educational policies of the new Mexican governments evolved between the 1940s and the late 1960s, the INI, the Ministry of Health (Secretaría de Salud y Asistencia Pública) and the Ministry of Public Education (Secretaría de Educación Pública), provided resources and mediation between rural indigenous communities and central (federal) policies and agencies. An important factor in this mediation was the creation by Caso, in 1951, of dozens of Coordinating Centres (Centros de Coordinación Comunitaria) to help implement INI's policies. The Coordinating Centres were strategically located, allowing rural physicians, teachers, anthropologists and representatives of the indigenous assembly to gather to discuss both the contents and the modes of implementation of the federal policies designed in Mexico City. The effect of these Coordinating Centres on the development of *indigenista* policies has yet to be acknowledged by historians of Mexico. As we will see below, they also provided support for research on the medical genetics of indigenous populations in the 1960s.[14]

Studies of Indigenous Populations after World War II

The names of Caso and Pablo Martínez del Río appear continuously in the acknowledgements of papers dealing with serological and genetic studies of indigenous populations between 1945 and 1970. They are always referred to as facilitators of the blood samples taken from Mazatecan, Zapotecan, Tarahumaran, Lacandonian and many other indigenous groups in rural Mexico. Like everywhere else in the world, the main material in the scientific study of Mexican indigenous populations was blood. The cultural anthropologists acted as mediators between the urban scientists and the rural communities, obtaining the samples or facilitating the work of doctors and nurses at the Coordinating Centres. But in spite of all the similarities to research carried on in other countries, the work of Mexican geneticists was unique in several respects.[15] The context provided by the Mexican *indigenista* agenda meant that serological and genetic research was not carried out with the goal of classifying populations or delivering individual medical counselling. The study of blood was subordinated to the identification of indigenous variations that, eventually, could lead to specific strategies suitable for treating the maladies that effected indigenous Mexican populations, such as malaria, anaemia and paludism. This became more entrenched with the development of the new electrophoretic methods in the 1960s that allowed surveys of abnormal haemoglobins and enzyme deficiency (see the next section). Nevertheless, for the majority of these studies, the tension remained between the local *indigenista* agenda and international research on human population genetics.

Overlapping with the national *indigenista* agenda, the post-World War II environment of international scientific and technical collaboration helped shape Mexican health institutions and policies. Mexican scientific and health institutions were deeply intertwined with international and foreign agencies such as the International Atomic Energy Commission, the US Ministry of Health, the National Institutes of Health and the British Medical Research Council. The Mexican medical elite had studied in the United States from the mid-1920s and continued to do so well into the 1960s.[16] These doctors brought the practices of full-time careers in public medicine and scientific research back with them into Mexican medicine, even though the Mexican context was very different to that of the USA.

The revolutionary promises of social justice and health and education for every Mexican citizen created an atmosphere that permeated the post-war, post-revolutionary institutions and the new intellectual elite. It was during this period that the first national research institutes of the Ministry of Health were created, including the National Institute of Cardiology (created in 1944) and the National Institute of Nutrition (created in 1946). All of these institutes were constituted as locations for state-of-the-art research in biomedical sciences, but also as embodiments of a political project that aimed to bring social services to marginal, including indigenous, populations. This was not mere rhetoric.[17]

One of the first researchers to do research on the blood variations of indigenous populations in Mexico was Mario Salazar-Mallén, a physician who had graduated from the School of Medicine at UNAM in 1935. The following year he travelled to New York, where he pursued studies on haematology and allergy. On his return to Mexico, he settled as a full-time researcher at the General Hospital (created in 1905). Seeking to understand the inheritance and distribution of pathologies of the immune system, he became interested in the study of human populations. He published, together with his collaborators, a study on the distribution of the ABO groups in indigenous and *mestizo* populations in 1944.[18] This paper was soon followed by the seminal paper by Alexander Wiener and a Mexican colleague from Guadalajara, J. Preciado Zepeda. Published in 1945 and titled 'Individual Blood Differences in Mexican Indians, with Special Reference to the Rh Blood Types and Hr Factor', Wiener and Zepeda's data were incorporated into Arthur Mourant's survey on the distribution of human blood groups.[19] Wiener had started a world sample of serum components more than a decade before, focusing on different populations around the globe, including Afro-American, Jewish, Chinese, Australian and Mexican populations, with the goal of designing a blood-printing tool for criminal identification.

During the early 1950s, working closely with colleagues from UNAM, Salazar-Mallén published several papers on the blood agglutinogens of the Mexicans, publishing in journals such as the *Annals of Eugenics*. Between 1944 and 1952 he published different blood type surveys of *mestizo* (urban) and indigenous populations.[20] He found a high frequency of O, M and CDe blood types and some of the more recently discovered agglutinogens. The frequencies were similar to those of other Amerindian populations.[21]

Salazar-Mallén's research in this period was made possible through a British Council grant, which gave him the opportunity to visit Dr R. R. Race's laboratory in London. Race provided Salazar-Mallén not only with training and advice, but also with a generous amount of testing sera. From 1949 R. Sanger and R. R. Race had been committed to the characterization of blood groups around the world, becoming two of the leading experts in the field.[22]

But Salazar-Mallén's research in Mexico was also possible due to his connections with the cultural anthropologists, even before the INI was created in 1948. In the 1940s and early 1950s, he followed the trend set by human geneticists and serologists in studying the ancestral relations of Amerindians to Mongoloid groups (the high frequency of the S agglutinogen in Otomies and Tarascans was taken as an evidence of their Asiatic ancestry). As the *indigenista* institutions took shape in the 1950s, Salazar-Mallén frequently used the INI infrastructure. In the 1952 paper, for instance, he thanked 'Prof. Alfonso Caso, Pablo Martínez del Río and Rafael Molina Betancourt (who) gave very valuable help in the selection of our samples and in facilitating the co-operation of the Indians. Ing. Francisco Grajales and Lic. Corona del Rosal made our visit to the Chamula and the Otomi zone feasible'.[23] The help of the INI authorities in the research of medical geneticists continued well into the following decade, when Caso again intervened to provide geneticist Alfonso León de Garay, director of the Genetics and Radiobiology Programme at the National Nuclear Energy Commission (Comisión Nacional de Energía Nuclear, CNEN) with access to Lacandonian communities in order to get blood samples.[24] As we will see in the next section, the local INI authorities at the Coordinating Centres also made Lisker's surveys possible.

Moreover, from the mid-1940s and up until the mid-1950s, research on the distribution of blood components took place within a pressing political context: the need to develop a sense of *nation* in a country that only recently had been fiercely divided along class, religious and racial lines. The idea that the Mexican nation would be fully realized with the racial admixture or *mestizaje* of the European and Indian ancestors was a very powerful ideology.[25] But, as we have seen, the urgency to build a nation had a practical side too. While Salazar-Mallén's research may not have had any practical consequences, other medical geneticists started to look for relevant disease traits. Adolfo Karl, for instance, based at the National Polytechnic Institute (Instituto Politécnico Nacional), pursued research on the connection between blood components and the presence of haemolytic anaemia in the indigenous populations of Oaxaca at the end of the 1950s.[26] Karl's small survey did not succeeded in finding haemoglobin variants, but this kind of research was pursued in a more systematic way by Salazar-Mallén's student Rubén Lisker.

Rubén Lisker's Work in the 1960s

Lisker's extensive and systematic surveys of the indigenous populations of Mexico remain one of the most important contributions to the study of human populations after World War II.[27] A student of Salazar-Mallén, he had also graduated from the School of Medicine at UNAM in 1948. Lisker spent four years (1953–7) at the Michael Reese Hospital of Chicago to pursue research on haematology under Karl Singer. While at Chicago, Lisker met the young Arno Motulsky, who is considered one of the founders of today's pharmacogenomics.[28] This was the start of a long collaboration, and in 1965–6 Lisker returned to the United States with an NIH grant to continue his collaboration with Motulsky at the University of Washington, Seattle, Washington.[29]

Beginning in 1960, Lisker's research laboratory at the Hospital de Enfermedades de la Nutrición (known later as the Instituto Nacional de la Nutrición Salvador Zubirán) focused on the relations between anthropological considerations and medical applications. In Lisker's words, 'the study of human populations has a clear interest not just for anthropological studies, but for its medical uses'.[30] Following the earlier studies by Karl and Salazar-Mallén, Lisker began a long-lasting research programme on genetic haematological traits in Mexican populations.[31] However, he not only focused on the differences in frequency of blood groups. With the emerging trends and technologies of the 1960s, he also focused on enzymes and other blood components, such as the deficiency of the glucose-6-phosphate dehydrogenase (D6PD) and the presence of abnormal haemoglobins and albumins in the Mexican indigenous population.

Moreover, Lisker's surveys were designed following the linguistic classification of indigenous populations of the cultural anthropologists, and in particular the glotto-chronological system of Morris Swadesh.[32] This decision permitted him to continue his systematic research of indigenous populations in a way that was unparalleled by his predecessors. During his surveys of Mexican populations, Lisker had access to hundreds of blood samples from dozens of populations, some of them coming from unreachable groups such as the Coras and Lacandonians of the Mayan jungle. At first Lisker had the aid of the INI anthropologists, but by the mid-1960s they were able to take advantage of INI involvement in the Ministry of Health's national campaign, partly financed by the US Public Health Service, to eradicate paludism among rural populations (Campaña Nacional para la Erradicación del Paludismo).[33]

In 1962 Lisker and his group found two individuals belonging to the Mixteca linguistic group, living in Oaxaca, with red cell G6PD deficiency.[34] This finding was striking in its contrast to the rarity of this deficiency in Mexican *mestizos* (generally urban populations) and another 600 indigenous samples, some of them also from a Mixteca group but from a village in the high mountains, where malaria was not present.[35] This finding evoked the possibility that malaria was acting as a selective agent in the lower populations. But there was a second hypothesis: maybe the cause was the 'admixture with Negroes'. The presence of G6PD deficiency seemed to be correlated with distance to Cuajinicuilapa, a village where African populations had settled in Oaxaca during colonial times. Lisker decided that it was this second hypothesis that was the most probable.

By 1964 Lisker had access to a huge sample due to his connections with authorities linked to the malaria eradication campaign: 1,931 adult males who were surveyed by Mexican doctors for the enzyme anomaly and the presence of haemoglobin S (the haemoglobin variant related to sickle cell anaemia). The results again indicated that the enzyme deficiency correlated with the African settlements dating back to the sixteenth century.[36] More important for its practical consequences, however, was the connection of G6PD deficiency with haemolytic anaemia (rupture of the red blood cells) following treatment with the anti-malarial drug primaquine. In this case, Lisker could prove that his surveys of haematological traits of indigenous populations had a practical application in the context of the malaria eradication campaign.[37]

The discovery of blood enzyme and protein variants in Mexican populations, such as haemoglobin *Chiapas* and haemoglobin *Mexico*,[38] followed the close scrutiny of blood groups and other antigens thought to be characteristic of Mexican populations, such as the well-known Diego blood group. Haemoglobin *Mexico* was first found on two Zapotecan individuals (from the Oaxacan Mountains) and ten individuals from *mestizo* populations, from a sample of 281 *mestizos*, 193 Zapotecans, 20 Mazatec and 263 Mayan. The fact that it was found in *mestizo* (admixtured) populations seems connected with the name Lisker chose, reflecting the origin of the Mexican nation.

After the finding of haemoglobin *Mexico*, Lisker realized that the usual abnormal haemoglobins were infrequently found in Amerindian populations. When they were, this was 'due to mixture with other ethnic groups'.[39] He recognized, however, that the encounter of rare or 'private' haemoglobin variants was not exclusive to Mexican populations. Moreover, the study of these abnormal haemoglobins did not reveal physiological deficiencies in the carrying individuals, and the findings seemed of no relevance to medicine. Nevertheless, the samples again revealed the close relationship between the Lisker laboratory and the Mexican anthropologists, this time from the Department of History at UNAM.

Lisker's extensive research of Mexican indigenous populations not only provided a more detailed and systematic map of their genetic variation (for instance, if compared with Arthur Mourant's general observations about Amerindian populations),[40] but a new image of the genetic make-up of the Mexican nation. His continued emphasis on the role of African ancestry is now part of the 'ethnic mosaic' that characterizes Mexico. Furthermore, he provided one of the first population studies with therapeutic applications in the context of the malaria eradication campaign. It is here that the 'nationalizing modernism' of the *indigenista* agenda is best illustrated as a set of policies addressing a health problem that was almost specific to indigenous populations.

Conclusion

Mexican studies of indigenous populations relied on the technical expertise of American and British technologies and institutions, and on the fieldwork, personal connections and assumptions of the cultural anthropologists and post-revolutionary institutions directing Mexican *indigenista* policies after World War II. The personal connections between medical doctors and prestigious anthropologists and archaeologists such as Alfonso Caso and Pablo Martínez del Río, as well as the INI infrastructure (including the Coordinating Centres) after the 1950s, were crucial in the development of a social medicine focused on indigenous populations. What is peculiar to the Mexican research agenda, however, is the idea that unveiling the genetic diversity of indigenous populations would facilitate the application of health policies to target these communities specifically.

The cultural anthropologists and their institutions acted as mediators between the indigenous communities and the city labs at the new health institutions in Mexico City. The medical geneticists imported the technologies and practices of immunology, biochemistry and genetics that they had learned in London, Chicago and New York. These techniques operated within the broader context of studies of human population variation after World War II. However, the local *indigenista* agenda set the tone and the context where this research was performed. Moreover, the availability of blood samples was possible thanks to the mediation of anthropologists. In sharp contrast to the development of individualist and private health services in the post-war United States, Mexican scientists used serological and biochemical techniques to address the characterization and health problems of marginal populations, and approached them as 'groups' or 'collectives', not as individuals or families. The explicit aim was to establish federal health policies that met the needs of particular indigenous communities. Often, however, the *indigenista* agenda seemed to have served more as a means of justifying the scientists' pursuit of their own research interests in a context of increasing international collaboration after World War II. Only in a few cases, like the transnational malaria eradication campaign, were their results instrumental in bringing specific health services to rural communities.

Our account highlights the tensions between the international and the local arena, but also their overlapping character. In contrast to the prevalent nationalistic accounts, our focus is the interconnectedness and circulation of people and tools. The continuing mediation between INI anthropologists and doctors and geneticists from the research hospitals marks a first circuit in the circulation of knowledge and materials in the study of human populations in Mexico. This is a circuit that links not only rural and urban settings, but also the linguistic, cultural approach to human diversity and the biological search for characteristic traits (blood type frequencies, abnormal haemoglobins and so on). The biological research reinforced the cultural criteria: by targeting indigenous groups, medical geneticists gave new meanings to the pervasive dichotomy of the *indigenista* doctrine. Lisker's realization of the importance of African ancestry did not change the dichotomy between indigenous communities and urban *mestizos*, but it certainly enriched its character.

A second circuit links Mexican scientists and social anthropologists to the international circulation of knowledge, people and technologies. The presence of intellectual elites is crucial here to understand the mediation between foreign institutions and international agencies, and local agents and practices. Medical doctors and anthropologists had studied in the USA and the UK, and they maintained their international collaborations after their return to Mexico. This meant financial support to buy new materials and techniques (such as electrophoresis apparatus) and to travel to learn the new techniques of analysis. It was also a source of social prestige that ensured their privileged role as agents in the shaping of the national agenda. Despite the charged political context of the *indigenista* policies, one cannot rule out that the doctors had their own agenda. This more covert agenda was more in tune with the aims of international research projects, in the context of which they had been educated and continued their collaborations. The contribution of the Mexican geneticists to the study of human populations after World War II was, after all, not just a local development but part of a transnational agenda.

Epilogue

In 2004 the Mexican Congress approved the creation of the National Institute for Genomic Medicine (Instituto Nacional de Medicina Genómica, INMEGEN,). This was part of an organization within the Mexican public health system's national institutes that brought together research and clinical intervention. In parallel to their focus on the medical applications of genomic knowledge, INMEGEN scientists have directed their resources to the study of ancestry and population structure of 'the Mexicans'. Knowledge of the structure of the Mexican population, they claim, will inform the development of a Mexican genomic medicine and suitable health policies and strategies. In so doing, INMEGEN scientists have relied on notions and fieldwork from cultural anthropologists, but also on research previously done by Lisker and his group that began in the 1960s.

Acknowledgments

We want to thank Bernd Gausemeier, Staffan Müller-Wille and Edmund Ramsden, organizers of the international workshop on Human Heredity in the Twentieth Century at Exeter University in 2010, who gave us the opportunity to join forces to approach the social history of medical genetics and *indigenismo* in Mexico. We also want to thank all the participants of the workshop for their useful comments on a previous version of this work. Finally, this research was part of a research project at UNAM (PAPIIT IN303111) and CONACyt 152879. We also thank Alicia Villela for her research assistance.

8 FROM AGRICULTURE TO GENOMICS: THE ANIMAL SIDE OF HUMAN GENETICS AND THE ORGANIZATION OF MODEL ORGANISMS IN THE LONGUE DURÉE

Alexander von Schwerin

History of science and science studies have become increasingly interested in models and modelling processes in recent years. One reason for this is the awareness that the understanding of experimental science begins with the understanding of experimental practice. As scholars have long recognized, reasoning through experimental animals became the lingua franca of biologists entering the twentieth century, and the choice of organism has proven critical to scientific development.[1] From an epistemological point of view, this kind of reasoning is far more complex than it may seem at first glance. This is because animals are not the only 'ingredient' needed in modelling: 'Model organisms can be seen as a specialized subset of the more general class of model systems, where the latter usually encompassed not only the organism but also the techniques and experimental methodologies surrounding the organism'.[2]

Historically speaking, the mode and experimental arrangement of models has changed significantly since the emergence of organized experimental biology. Cheryl Logan has described how nineteenth-century rationales for the choice of test organisms in physiology were transformed after 1900. This change was driven by various developments in biological thought and theory, the requirements of the experimental method and new technologies of experimentation.[3] As a consequence of the formation of Mendelian genetics, geneticists and physicians alike sought to contribute experimentally to the understanding of human heredity with respect to medical problems. Such approaches differed from 'common' biological experiments in one crucial respect. Their aim was not, in the first instance at least, to produce knowledge of a particular biological mechanism; it was to establish, from animal experimentation, specific mechanisms in *humans*. In this respect, it was similar to Claude Bernard's pioneering endeavour to reveal human physiology through animal experiments. This procedure was by no means undisputed, and drew considerable criticism from physicians.[4] Throughout its history, the comparative approach to human genetics struggled with the challenge of applying animal models that could count as representative for *human* traits and diseases.[5]

This essay will not trace the entire history of comparative experiments. Rather, it will focus on institutions that were specialized in breeding experimental animals. Prominent examples are the Bussey Institution, the Jackson Laboratory and the facilities of the German Research Foundation. These institutions served the specific demands of medical researchers who used small mammals such as mice, rats, Guinea pigs and rabbits in their experiments.[6] From the early 1920s genetic breeding techniques were introduced within the context of systematic and commercial breeding to standardize test animals. Since these breeding facilities were also able to provide a variety of mutant strains, they became the cornerstone in the history of comparative genetics.[7] These institutions deserve special attention because they were formative for the organization of genetic research, and particularly the organization of studies of mutants.[8] This essay traces a long trajectory starting in the 1920s in the breeding facilities of the German Research Foundation, the basis for the first German research programme in comparative medical genetics. It ends with the foundation of the German Mouse Clinic in 2001. It underscores the continuity of a specific research tradition, from early agricultural genetics to today's genomics. This continuity, did not manifest itself in terms of a linear progress, but involved the many breaks and contingent configurations common to the development of new research fields.

Phase 1: The Emergence of Comparative Medical Genetics at the Intersection of Agriculture and Eugenics

In order to outline the emergence of comparative genetics, I will focus on the German geneticist Hans Nachtsheim.[9] In 1921 Nachtsheim was appointed departmental head in the Institute for Genetics at the City of Berlin's Agricultural College. Nachtsheim focused his genetic research on 'economically valuable traits' in rabbits, such as the colour and the quality of the fur. At that time, rabbits were used extensively in the fur industry. Nachtsheim insisted on the potential of Mendelian genetics for animal breeding and promised to create new 'economical and performance breeds'. He was able to obtain his material for breeding by becoming, in 1924, the chairman of the German Rabbit Breeder's Organization. There were approximately three million rabbit breeders in Germany. This meant that about sixty million rabbits inhabited the breezy gardens and dark corners of the cities – about as many as the people living in the German Reich. Nachtsheim engaged in exhaustive discussions over the right way to keep and breed rabbits. He always kept his eyes open for rare variants that might exist in a breeder's stock, or new variants that had emerged. His mission was to collect specimens of all such variants, to analyse the genotype, and to keep a list of rabbit genes and their alleles as a tool for genetically informed breeding. This was, for Nachtsheim, synonymous with 'rational breeding'.

Shipments of genetically standardized rabbits to clinics were a by-product of Nachtsheim's genetic expertise. This double use was encouraged by Erwin Baur, the director and founder of the Genetics Institute at the Agricultural College. When public spending for university facilities fell short in the aftermath of World War I, Baur found a new ally in the Emergency Foundation of German Science (which later became the German Research Foundation or DFG). From the early 1920s the DFG invested large sums in the establishment of an experimental animal-breeding infrastructure to support experimental medicine. Owing to Baur's skills in scientific management, the DFG agreed to finance the long-desired animal facilities on the grounds of the genetic institute in Berlin-Dahlem. In return, Baur's assistants supplied rabbits, rats and mice for medical research.

Nachtsheim and Baur were aggressive in their promotion of experimental biology as decisive to social progress. Breeders were not alone in encountering this missionary zeal, but were joined by many of Nachtsheim's *Volksgenossen*, whom he considered unaware of the true dangers of genetic degeneration. Interestingly, fur rabbits paved Nachtsheim's way into the field of eugenics and allowed him to become the central figure in comparative medical genetics in Germany. In 1925 a new strain of rabbits entered Germany from France. The skins of the so-called Rex rabbit seemed as precious and refined as the skin of a marten ('Edelpelztier'). Breeders were ecstatic.[10] In 1927 Nachtsheim responded by publishing a rather iconoclastic article that defined the Rex rabbit as a degenerate animal on the basis of a single trait: the unusual microscopic anatomy of the Rex's hair. The cause of the change from the smooth fur typical of other rabbits he considered to be a pathological gene.

As early as 1925, a few cases of paralyzed limb in Rex rabbits had been observed in Nachtsheim's institute. At first Nachtsheim suspected that an employee had handled the animals improperly. In the context of the pathological-agronomic experimental system, the paralysis was first interpreted as a corollary trait of the Rex gene. When, afterwards, it became clear that the paralysis was inherited separately, the paralysis was freed from the fur of the Rex and became a phenomenon in its own right. The pathologist Berthold Ostertag, with whom Nachtsheim cooperated, identified it as syringomyelia, a neuro-degenerative syndrome well known in humans. The Rex rabbit now served as model for the pathological process of syringomyelia, becoming part of the neuropathological debate regarding limb paralysis. It was at this point that Nachtsheim started to breed rabbits displaying traits similar to human diseases, as well as those with agriculturally interesting traits. Nachtsheim's interests in the inheritance of traits had emerged from his large-scale experimental animal facilities, via the artisanal practice of rabbit breeders. But they were fuelled by eugenic concerns.

After the Nazis seized power in Germany in 1933, Nachtsheim framed a research programme for transforming mammals into models for human genetics. In order to make his plans more intelligible to non-experts, Nachtsheim invented the term '*vergleichende Erbpathologie*' ('comparative genetic pathology').[11] By 1941, when he joined the prestigious Kaiser Wilhelm Institute for Anthropology, Human Heredity and Eugenics (KWI), the transformation of Nachtsheim's experimental system from agricultural genetics to modelling rabbits for human diseases was complete. There were approximately twenty different breeds of rabbits that functioned as models for human diseases, including epilepsy, degenerative disorders of the nervous system (e.g. Parkinson's disease), the blood system and the eye, and growth disturbances.

Nachtsheim cooperated with various medical specialists, such as the ophthalmologist Hellmuth Gürich from the Charité university hospital. Gürich examined Nachtsheim's rabbits ophthalmoscopically and described a clouding of the lens of the eye in terms of the typical signs of cataract, a widespread degenerative disease in humans. One of the two cataract strains descended from a buck Nachtsheim had purchased from the railroad official and fancy breeder Bernhard Wragge in the north-western city of Oldenburg in 1931.[12] The second strain derived from a mutation in one of Nachtsheims's innumerable breeds.

Comparative genetics became a field of general interest in the 1930s. While the leading German genetics journal *Zeitschrift für induktive Abstammungs- und Vererbungslehre* published only two articles on the topic during the 1920s, there were about twenty during the 1930s.[13] Most of this work focused on pathological traits. Obviously, Nazi biopolitics boosted interest in comparative genetics, but the trend was also due to inner-scientific developments. One stimulus was the growing interest in developmental genetics. The zoologist Alfred Kühn explained the instrumental value of pathologic mutants for genetic research, as they would 'multiply the targets for studies in the mode of gene action'.[14] Nachtsheim's colleagues at KWI, and his group in particular, were committed to the concept of 'Phänogenetik', that is to say, the study of the gene-controlled expression of certain traits.[15] However, the mammal-based research strategy was much more costly than using fruit flies and more dependent on large facilities. Fortunately, Nachtsheim had animal houses at his disposal at the Berlin agricultural college, which he used for agricultural research purposes. From its very beginnings, comparative genetics was characterized by a fortuitous conjunction of different interests, material cultures and institutional frameworks.

Phase 2: Animal Models for Evaluating the Dysgenic Impact of the Atomic Age

Comparative genetics fared poorly in the immediate aftermath of the war. The Red Army slaughtered most of Nachtsheim's animals when they occupied Berlin, and German politics after 1945 had more pressing concerns than the nurturing of experimental objects for genetics. However, the dawning of the Atomic Age would change this situation. Due to the spread of nuclear techniques in factories, laboratories and clinics, the health of an increasing number of technicians, physicians and patients was endangered through contact with radioactive materials. By the mid-1950s this risk stimulated the scientific interest of biophysicists, physicians, radiation biologists and geneticists. However, it took further stages of translation before the connection between comparative genetics and atomic energy bore fruit.

Step by step, Nachtsheim revitalized comparative genetics at the former KWI. His rabbit department was the only part of the KWI for Anthropology that the Max Planck Society continued – from 1953 onwards – as the Max Planck Institute for Comparative and Medical Genetics.[16] Nachtsheim was keen to rebuild the rabbit strains with the aid of new researchers. One was the student Udo Ehling, who took care of the cataract strains. The first of the two strains was extinguished by a bombing raid in 1945. However, as Nachtsheim used to systematically cross his invaluable disease models, the gene was preserved in a different rabbit strain. For his literature study on 'Hereditary and Non-Hereditary Cataracts of Humans and Mammals', Ehling received his biology degree and secured an appointment at the Max Planck Institute.[17] In 1953 he started his own investigations into the phenogenetics of hereditary cataracts.

In the mid-1950s Ehling was inspired by William L. Laurence's atomic bomb coverage 'Dawn over Zero'.[18] Ehling joined the physicist Ernst Krokowski at the radiological institute to investigate the effects of radiation on the emergence and development of cataracts.[19] Ehling and Krokowski collaborated well together and did not hesitate to seize new radiobiological tools. The state of the art in medicine or biology was to order radioisotopes freshly produced in atomic piles, packed and shipped from the United States or the United Kingdom.[20] In the summer of 1956, they decided to delve more deeply into phenogenetics with the help of radioisotopes. They studied the uptake of radiophosphorus in bones. For that purpose they turned to other rabbit model mutants, now using breeds with skeletal anomalies. Ehling visited Europe's centre for the learning of radioisotope techniques, the Atomic Energy Research Establishment (AERE) near Harwell, Oxfordshire.[21]

Radioisotope courses were part of British governmental efforts to promote atomic energy applications. There were also radiobiologists at Harwell who performed comprehensive experiments with mice in order to determine the real danger emanating from radiation. Only a state-financed institution could tackle this question, and these were the AERE and the National Laboratories in Oak Ridge (ORNL), Tennessee, that had been established to house the Manhattan Project's uranium enrichment facilities. The mouse radiation programme of the Biological Division at the Oak Ridge laboratories was, in fact, the largest in the world. Known as the 'mega-mouse project', it was one of the key projects relevant to radiation safety policy. It is also recognized to have led biology into the world of big science.[22] William (Bill) Russell headed the facility in collaboration with his wife, Liane. One single experiment that had been running since the late 1940s involved 100,000 mice.[23] 'Big Biology', an expression coined by ORNL director Alvin Weinberg, seemed to pay off, as the Russells developed a mutagenesis test – the specific locus test (SLT) – that became crucial for the determination of limit values for radioactive contamination.[24]

Nachtsheim saw an opportunity to launch a similar joint venture with the West German atomic programme. West Germany adopted an atomic energy programme soon after it regained national sovereignty in 1954. Nachtsheim argued for a considerable investment in mammal genetics in order to supplement research at Oak Ridge and Harwell. Nachtsheim's institute offered a good place to start; however, many more facilities were needed to raise an appropriate number of animals for standardized mutant screening. In 1958 the German Ministry for Atomic Affairs approved 273,000 marks to extend the breeding facilities in Berlin-Dahlem.[25] Nachtsheim also ordered Ehling to apply for a US Public Health International Fellowship to join the Biological Division in Oak Ridge. The plan was that Ehling would learn how to build big biology while working with the Russells in the famous 'Mouse House'. In 1959 Ehling and his wife left Berlin for the United States.

Ehling was ambitious, and in order to exhibit his radiobiological skills he decided to try to establish a new mutagenesis test on the basis of dominant mutations. Even the Russells had failed to realize a dominant locus test (DLoT) because dominant mutations were extremely rare. Ehling reflected in his memoirs: 'The chance to solve this difficult task was minimal. If it turned out to work, the results would be very important for the risk estimation of radiation induced damages on human genes'.[26] In Berlin the choice was rather limited; in Oak Ridge there were plenty of inbred mouse strains at their disposal.[27] How would they choose the right strain? Ehling considered his recent work together with Krokowski on skeletal anomalies in rabbits: these were suitable traits for quantitative tests because they were distinct and easy to detect. Thus Ehling searched the Mouse House for strains with skeletal anomalies. This decision changed the daily routine of the Ehlings, as the dissection, preparation and examination of 1,133 mice skeletons was time-consuming. Working all day and during the night, Udo only managed to finish the experiments with the help of his wife, Heidede.[28]

When the Ehlings returned to West Germany in late 1961, the situation had deteriorated dramatically. The hope that comparative mammalian genetics would be established on a firm and secure basis had dissipated. Nachtsheim was at the end of his career, and the Max Planck Society decided to abandon mammal genetics in favour of an institute for molecular genetics.

From a more general perspective, the linkage of eugenic concerns and atomic energy policy was rather fortunate for West German genetics. It reinstated genetic research as an urgent scientific need. Actually, genetics – including both molecular and human genetics – profited enormously in these years, thanks to the generosity of the Ministry for Atomic Affairs.[29] Comparative genetics, however, lost out. While Nachtsheim's stocks of model rabbits had managed to survive the swastika, they did not survive molecular biology. Nachtsheim was embittered. There was no future for his rabbit stocks when Nachtsheim decided to leave Berlin and retire. Yet there was still one arrow left in his quiver, courtesy of his pupil Udo Ehling.

Phase 3: From Radiobiology to Toxicogenetics of the Consumer Society

From 1961 Udo Ehling worked with the radiation biologist Otto Hug. Hug had been searching for a specialist to run the genetics laboratory at the Experimental and Education Centre for Radiation Protection (GSF), a large research centre in a suburb of Munich. Ehling had, in the meantime, moved from Oak Ridge to Munich, and he was now well acquainted with the tasks of radiation biology. Like the Oak Ridge laboratories, the GSF was a state-funded research institution within the German atomic energy programme. Thus Nachtsheim's investment finally paid off: Ehling had successfully found his way into comparative genetics. However, working in an institution like the GSF demanded that he abandon comparative medical genetics for comparative mutation genetics; and there were further new duties involved, as this section will show.

From now on Ehling's career and the development of his comparative endeavour would be connected to the GSF; yet his connection to Oak Ridge remained important. The Ehlings soon interrupted their Munich time and returned to the Biological Division for another four years. When they arrived, the global situation had changed; the good old days of big radiation biology were almost over. Soon after their arrival in late 1963, the head of the Biological Division, Alexander Hollaender, explained to Ehling that new problems had emerged for mammal geneticists. Hollaender was knowledgeable as a gifted science manager. With the Moscow Treaty that very same year, the atomic powers ceased nuclear bomb tests above ground. Scientists now shifted their attention from radioactivity to the chemotoxical problems generated by the consumer society. As the

Special Director on Research Development at the World Health Organization proclaimed: 'The action of chemical mutagens, including radiation effects, is considered one of the fundamental bio-medical problems affecting health on a global scale and relates importantly to the biological future of man'.[30] Hollaender planned a huge chemogenetical research programme for the Biological Division at ORNL and promised Ehling: 'You are now 36. In 10–15 years you can have a big program, bigger than the Russell's'.[31] As it turned out, the time was not yet ripe; Hollaender would only realize part of his vision at Oak Ridge.

Instead of remaining at Oak Ridge, Ehling accepted an offer from the German Department for Scientific Research to become the head of an enlarged Department of Genetics at the GSF. Ehling arrived at the GSF in the summer 1968, carrying with him the chemogenetical research programme he had elaborated for Hollaender. His move coincided with significant changes in research politics. The Ministry for Scientific Research was considering prospects for the future of its Big Science Facilities (*Großforschungseinrichtungen*). The GSF was about to witness a long-lasting transformation into a centre for environmental research and general medical prevention.[32] Ehling benefited from this development. When he first met the Ministry's official, Dr Georg Straimer, in the Oak Ridge's Holiday Inn to negotiate his future prospects, it seemed that Ehling was the right man to manage West Germany's fifty-five-million DM contribution to big biology.[33] In summary, when the modern buildings and facilities for biological research, the 'Biologikum', were finished, Ehling had breeding facilities for 90,000 (later extended to 140,000) mice and rats per year at his disposal – the largest facility in the world after the Mouse House at ORNL.[34]

Around this time, toxicogenetics formed as a discipline and as a form of 'scientific activism'.[35] In 1969 the Environmental Mutagen Society (EMS) was founded in the USA. A year later the European branch of the EMS was formed on the occasion of an international conference on mammalian radiation genetics held at the GSF.[36] Sixty-five members attended the meeting in July 1970. Obviously, as Hollaender noted, there was 'tremendous interest in Europe in the problem of pollution', but there was almost no toxicogenetic work done with mammals, except in Germany.[37] It is quite striking that several German mammalian geneticists were working in toxicogenetics, the most prominent being Friedrich Vogel, another pupil of Nachtsheim's.[38] However, it was Ehling whom the Ministry for Scientific Research entrusted to organize a programme to design toxicogenetic tests.[39]

The most urgent need in the nascent field was to develop standard mutagenicity tests for screening chemicals for toxicological, carcinogenic, teratogenic and mutagenic effects. Most test systems thus far developed were based on simple organisms that were easy to handle, such as the model of radiation genetics, the fruit fly *Drosophila*. But their relevance to humans was contested.[40] Ehling began to study the possible genetic risks of antineoplastic drugs.[41] At that time the common assumption was that cytotoxic drugs used in cancer therapy were mutagenic, but experts differed in their opinions over how serious these effects were. Ehling was rather ambitious in his attempt to elaborate a method for the quantification of toxin-induced genetic risks. He argued that these efforts could be modelled on the experiences gathered in research on the genetic risks from radiation: 'The attempt to explore the genetic hazards to humans through chemical mutagens should be based on the data observed in radiation genetic experiments with mammals'.[42] In practical terms, this implied transforming the established radiogenetic test systems into toxicogenetic test systems. Hence Ehling chose two tests systems he was acquainted with from Oak Ridge: the dominant lethal test (DLT) and the specific locus test (SLT). In 1973 he presented the results at the First International Conference on Environmental Mutagens at Asilomar, California.[43]

Since both DLT and SLT were expensive test systems, Ehling eventually fell back on the experimental approach he had tried in the early 1960s at ORNL, the dominant locus test (DLoT) using skeletal mutants. This test was rather difficult to design, but it was worth the effort as, once established, it would be much more effective and cheaper when used for the routine screening of chemicals.[44] Ehling managed to further elaborate the DLoT in the course of 1970s.[45] When he first presented his results, they were quite well received; however, criticism was raised by his old master, Bill Russell. Ehling, stung by this criticism, tried hard to improve the method. In the process, he drew upon his earlier scientific work with rabbits and chose cataracts as the test trait in mice.[46] The cataract gene turned out to be the perfect indicator to indicate mutagenic activity of toxins in a standard dominant locus test.[47]

Ehling's efforts paid off, and he gained the greatest recognition a toxicogeneticist could wish for: his tests were acknowledged in guidelines for radiation and chemogenetic risk assessment of various international organizations and national agencies such as the United Nations Scientific Committee on the Effects of Atomic Radiation (UNSCEAR) and the US Environmental Protection Agency (EPA). In 1982 UNSCEAR stated that Ehling's group 'validated the usefulness of the cataract system for both radiation and chemical mutagenesis studies'.[48] At that time, nobody would have assumed that 'comparative toxicology' (Ehling) was rooted in comparative medical genetics.[49] In fact, the DLoT was a hybrid of the radiogenetic test systems and experiences from comparative medical genetics. From that point, only a few more transfers were needed to convert this test system back into a model system for comparative medical genetics.

Phase 4: The Introduction of Supermutagens for Modelling Genomics

The 1980s are known as the decade when the Human Genome Project was initiated. It can also be considered as a time when mammalian genetics began to operate on a new scale. The prerequisites for this turn also emerged within the toxicogenetic site in Munich, where Ehling was still busy inventing, evaluating, improving and standardizing the mouse test system for protection against the hazards of technical civilization.

A crucial step was taken when Ehling and his group introduced a new chemical compound in the toxicogenetic experiments at the GSF animal house: ethylnitrosourea (ENU). This happened in the context of Ehling's elaboration of the DLoT. Ehling was determined to show the advantages of his test, instigating a series of experiments that involved all of his personnel at the GSF Department for Genetics. The aim of these experiments was to show that the DLoT was both reliable and even more effective than Russell's SLT.

These experiments differed from previous chemogenetic experiments in one crucial detail. As Ehling's assistant Jack Favor explained: 'such comparisons are most meaningful' – that is statistically reliable – when 'the yield of mutations in both test groups is large enough'.[50] There were two ways to realize this precondition: either to raise the number of animals used, or to apply a more potent mutagen. The latter was the obvious solution because it was more economic. Ehling was also familiar with 'supermutagens', having shared an office with the microbiologist Heinrich Malling in Oak Ridge.[51] A number of potent mutagens had by now accumulated in Ehling's poison cabinet: MMS, EMS, PMS, iPMS, MNNG, TEM, DMO, IMT and MC. The abbreviations suggest the connections and relations between the substances. Actually, most of them were alkylating agents, originally known for their use as chemical weapons (such as mustard gas) in World War I. In the 1970s the big family of alkylating agents became widely known as anti-cancer drugs. In 1979, when Bill Russell first tested the alkylating agent ENU in mice, he claimed sensationally: 'Specific locus test shows ENU to be the most potent mutagen in the mouse!'[52] Only a few months later Ehling reported on the induction of dominant mutations by ENU in own experiments.[53] Shortly thereafter, his group used the new supermutagen for the initiated comparative experiments.

ENU turned out to be so effective that Ehling's group used it in the design and refinement of mutagenicity tests throughout the 1980s. They also continued to test mutagens in the DLoT. In the course of these experiments, more than 500,000 mice were screened for cataract mutants. Of these, 170 were isolated and became the stock of the 'Neuherberg Cataract Mutant Collection'.[54]

When Ehling retired in 1993, the supervisory board of the GSF recommended that Ehling's unit be continued. It became an independent Institute for Mammalian Genetics in 1988, and work persisted on the quantification of genetic risks. However, Ehling's successor, Rudi Balling, was to turn the toxicogenetic experimental system upside down. Rather than apply ENU as the gold standard in the evaluation of mutagenicity tests, he used it as instrument to generate new mutants. As a developmental geneticist, Balling was interested in ENU-induced mutants as he understood their value for the investigation of the impact of genes on embryogenesis.[55] A prominent example was the successful genetic dissection of the segmentation process in *Drosophila melanogaster* by the embryologist Christiane Nüsslein-Volhard. The mutants critical to the success of these experiments originated from a systematic genome-wide screening for induced mutants with defined phenotypes. Notably, Nüsslein-Volhard had used ethyl methane sulphonate (EMS), a mutagen closely related to ENU, for the treatment of the fruit flies.[56] Of course, such mutant screens were time-consuming and expensive if one used subjects larger than flies.

The Neuherberg Cataract Mutant Collection proved that corresponding experiments with mammals were possible. In fact, the Biologikum of the GSF was probably the only place in Germany where a developmental geneticist could carry out mutagen-driven mutant screens with mice. First and foremost, the scale of the animal facility permitted the employment of large numbers of animals. Secondly, there existed the expertise to pursue such a project. Some of Ehling's former assistants experienced in managing ENU and mutation experiments, Jack Favor and Angelika Neuhäuser-Klaus, were still present. As Balling realized, what they had now been performing for many years was nothing less than one of 'the largest genome-wide screens'. Moreover, they had developed an improved protocol that allowed a 'very efficient mutagenesis rate in mice', more effective than the first protocol published by Russell in 1979.[57] The main methodological difference was that mice were no longer screened for well-defined standard mutants, but for completely new phenotypes.

At the end of 1996 Balling and his new co-worker, the embryologist Martin Hrabě de Angelis, launched a large-scale mutagenesis project. The goal of the Munich ENU Mouse Mutagenesis Screen was to systematically screen, analyse and maintain mutant mice for further research purposes. As the initiators explained, the goal was:

> the production of a large number of mouse mutants for genes which reflect models for inherited diseases in man. A better understanding of the molecular basis of inherited diseases requires suitable animal models ... The new mouse lines will be available to the scientific community for further analysis of gene function.[58]

Step by step, they brought together various clinical specialists and scientists skilled in subdivisions of murine zoology such as allergy, behaviour, immunology and steroid metabolism. By 2000 the project team had screened over 14,000 mice for clinically relevant parameters and discovered 182 new mutants.[59]

The GSF toxicogenetic programme had, finally, been transformed into a resource for genomics. Hence the Munich ENU Mutagenesis Screen Project was incorporated into the German Human Genome Project (DHGP). Since then the ENU Mouse Mutagenesis Screen serves as a 'platform' for systematic, genome-wide production and analysis of mouse mutants as model systems for hereditary human diseases. What Balling and Hrabě de Angelis offered was an approach that could compensate for the weak spot in the Human Genome Project: the focus on the mapping of the DNA code, they argued, had produced a 'phenotype gap', i.e. a lack of commensurate data representing the variability of clinical phenomena.[60] The ENU-driven transformation of the GSF programme turned the genotype-driven strategy of genomics upside down, into an approach oriented towards comparative phenotyping.

Conclusion: From Collections to Biobanks

The long-term history of human genetic animal modelling – what Nachtsheim had acclaimed to be comparative genetics – does not, of course, consist of *one* single research trajectory spanning from the 1920s to the present. There are many ruptures in this development. It shows continuity neither at the institutional level nor with respect to the research strategies and the experimental animals used. Protagonists changed, as did research interests, strategies and materials.

However, if one does not limit attention to one of these elements alone, one can see a chain of trajectories constituting a long-range story of comparative genetics. In the German context, discussed here, the transition from the first phase, with its focus on the genetics of human diseases, to the second phase, with its interest in mutation rates, was based on the commitment and work of one researcher. It was facilitated by the emergence of atomic energy, a powerful incentive for biological research. The journey from the Berlin comparative genetics project into the atomic energy programme proceeded from the use of radiation and radioisotopes for phenogenetic problems, to the genetics of radiation effects. The task of the mouse radiation project was to develop exact numbers for the comparative estimation of radiation threats. The transition from the second phase to the third phase of mass testing of chemical compounds was facilitated by knowledge of old-school comparative genetics and the provision of useful genetic strains for standard mutagenesis testing. The transition from the third phase to the fourth phase of genome phenotyping was possible only because the third phase had generated potent mutagens as instruments.

In this story, even the notion of 'comparison' in 'comparative genetics' comprised different meanings depending on its function within particular experimental rationales and political contexts. Comparative genetic pathology, as Nachtsheim conceived it in the 1930s, was different from the challenge facing geneticists in the late 1960s. The models for human diseases had been supplementary in character, i.e. they did not substitute research on human physiology, pathology and genetics, whereas the test models of the age of atomic and 'comparative toxicology' (Ehling) functioned as surrogates for research on humans.[61] The turn to comparative genomics retroactively realized Nachtsheim's older programmatic agenda, now with the mouse used as a model organism for ENU mutagenesis screens and phenotyping. But today's mouse models for inherited diseases in man do not fulfil the same experimental function as rabbits did seventy years before. First, mouse mutagenesis screens rely on chemical mutagens, and thereby on the scientific facilities created to support environmental politics. Second, from having been only a minor element in early medical genetics, developmental genetics has become dominant. Models are now designed to unravel the functional relation between DNA sequence and phenotype. Third, today's screens are not collections of natural phenomena, but systematically generated biobanks. Hence this story of comparative genetics describes a succession of different forms of comparative approaches.

The transformation of the GSF toxicogenetic programme into a resource within genomics emphasizes another aspect of scientific change. In 'boarding the mouse mutant express', the state-funded institutions turned out to be crucial.[62] Comparative genetics 'hibernated' in the structures generated by the concerns about atomic and chemical hazards. In the end, the former mutagenic tests facilities were converted into a post-genomic project intended to transcend the restrictions of mere genome sequencing in terms of function and development.[63] In 2001 the 'German Mouse Clinic' (GMC) at the GSF was founded as a core institution of a trans-European research consortium supported by the German National Genome Research Network (HGFN). This genealogy reflects a general pattern in the transformation of the life sciences in the last thirty years, as similar large-scale screening projects and mouse clinics have emerged in various countries. At almost the same time, the British Atomic Energy Research Establishment at Harwell launched a mouse mutagenesis screening project that was later turned into the Medical Research Council (MRC) Mouse Clinic.[64] Hence, in this long-term history of comparative genetics, state institutions such as the GSF and the AERE, usually regarded as inert and inflexible, appear as locations of scientific innovation.

Acknowledgements

Special thanks for numerous helpful comments and thorough editing go to Bernd Gausemeier and Ed Ramsden. The German Research Foundation (DFG) supported part of the research for this essay (project: 'Mutations and Mutagens. Biological and Risky Things in the Analytics of Biopolitics'). This essay is dedicated to Gerhard Baader.

9 CEREALS, CHROMOSOMES AND COLCHICINE: CROP VARIETIES AT THE ESTACIÓN EXPERIMENTAL AULA DEI AND HUMAN CYTOGENETICS, 1948–58

María Jesús Santesmases

In 1947 Enrique Sánchez-Monge, a young agronomic engineer from the Spanish city of Zaragoza, underwent a period of training at the Experimental Breeding Station of the Swedish Seed Association in Svalöf. In the laboratory, the bench next to his was occupied by the agronomist Joe Hin Tjio, a researcher from Java who had previously spent time in Denmark before meeting Sánchez-Monge at Svalöf (Figure 9.1). An invitation for Tjio to conduct research in Spain followed, initiating a decade of intersections between the two researchers, their research subjects and tools. Tjio continued his research at the Aula Dei Experimental Station in Zaragoza from 1948 until 1959, under contract as a cytologist and agronomist. The research agenda was to develop breeding and crop improvement in the middle of one of the poorest decades in twentieth-century Spain – wheat, rye and barley being basic food of both people and livestock in the first decade of the Franco dictatorship.[1]

At that time cytology was demonstrating great promise for agricultural research, and Svalöf was a renowned experimental station for agronomists to be trained in cytology techniques that could contribute to agricultural development. At Svalöf, both Sánchez-Monge and Tjio were working under the Swedish cytologist Albert Levan, and even after his appointment as head of the cytology unit at Aula Dei, Tjio would spend some months in Sweden each year in order to maintain his association with Levan. In 1956 Tjio and Levan would receive international fame for the exact determination of the normal number of human chromosomes.[2] Tjio's association with Sánchez-Monge and Aula Dei contributed to the spread of cytogenetic practices within the agronomic laboratories and clinics throughout Spain.[3] Sánchez-Monge, Tjio and Levan are representatives of an international network of researchers who, originating from agronomy and plant cytology, developed techniques that became diagnostic tools in the clinic, enabling medical genetics to emerge and expand from 1956 onwards.

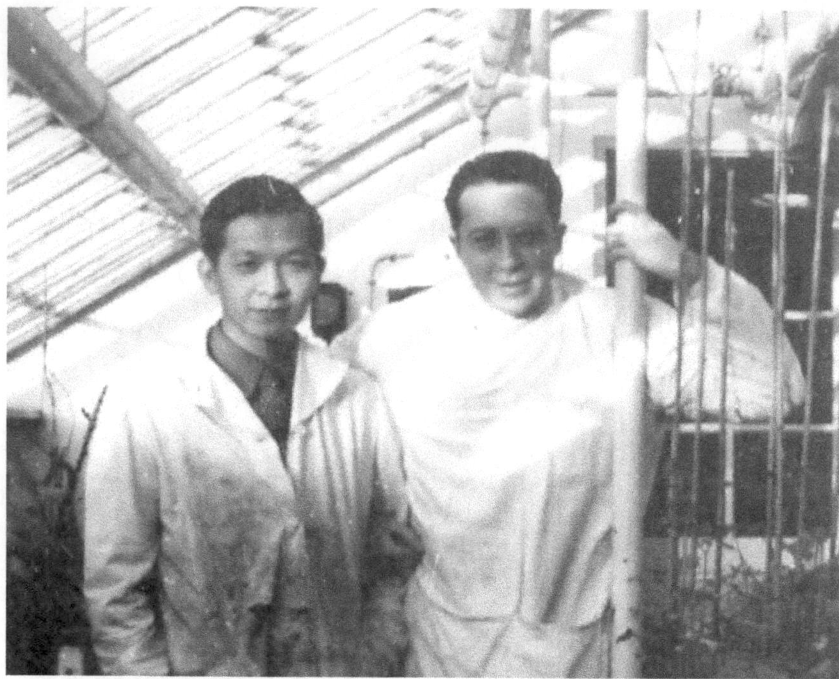

Figure 9.1: Joe Hin Tjio and Enrique Sánchez-Monge in Svalöf, 1947. Photograph reproduced courtesy of Rosa Sánchez-Monge.

At the conjunction of cereal and human research, a major role was played by the chemical substance colchicine, a product extracted from the meadow saffron (*Colchicum autumnale*) and a centuries-old therapy for gout. Colchicine has the ability to arrest mitotic cell division at metaphase. This made it useful for plant breeding, as arrested mitosis in plant tissues can lead to polyploidy, an increase in the normal number of chromosomes that is usually accompanied by an increase in the size and shape of plants as a whole, or of certain parts such as leaves, branches, flower parts, fruits or seeds.[4] 'While cell division is prevented', as one researcher explained in 1940, 'chromosomes continue to develop. They split into sister chromosomes but remain together and together go to the nuclear phase. In consequence chromosomes are doubled in number and the affected cells grow proportionately'.[5]

In contrast, polyploidy had not yet 'been observed in any appreciable extent in animals', and it was discovered a short time later to serve a rather different purpose in the cells of animals and humans.[6] Colchicine interferes with the formation of the mitotic spindle, which fails to form when a cell enters mitosis under the influence of the alkaloid. Adding colchicine to a culture of animal or human cells initiated a great deal of mitosis and 'a varying degree' of chromosome contraction, but it 'arrested' the affected cells in metaphase, hence increasing the number of cells in metaphase available for observation in a culture. With appropriate imaging techniques, such cultures could then be used for chromosome studies.[7]

As many authors suggested in the 1940s and 1950s, polyploidy and mitosis inhibition were part of the same phenomenon, in spite of their apparent differences. In both the breeding of new cereal strains and the visualization of human chromosomes, the use of colchicine introduced new production techniques for obtaining a new cereal variety that would from then on be included in agriculture statistics, and for obtaining high-quality slides for studying the chromosomes of human beings. The making of high-quality seed and human chromosomes thus affected the events of cell division very differently, while jointly contributing to the creation of a geography of cells and chromosomes that would become the locus of biological heredity.[8]

This explains why, in the early days of cytogenetics – the study of cell division by observing what happens to chromosomes during the process – plant cytogenetics and human cytogenetics developed in such close interaction, as demonstrated by the careers of Levan, Tjio and Sánchez-Monge. These fields, although pursuing very different aims, shared what can be called a manufacturing agent, colchicine, a substance that circulated from plants to human tissue cells and back to plants. The products of this interaction – high-quality slides of human somatic chromosomes, and a new variety of wheat and rye (*Triticale*) – may appear strikingly different, but the methods required to obtain them were stabilized in mutual interaction. In this essay I will investigate the relationship between Tjio and Sánchez-Monge as part of the early history of genetics, paying special attention to the exchange of laboratory practices and experimental materials between cereal and human cytogenetics. Human cytogenetics initially borrowed its practices from plant cytology, but by the late 1940s these areas of biological research were developing in parallel. Both research and knowledge spaces shared researchers as well as laboratory materials, experimental methods and styles of presenting evidence.

The Role of Agricultural Stations

Joe Hin Tjio was born in 1919 in Soemedang, Java. The island was then part of the Dutch East Indies, and he was educated in Dutch elementary and high schools. He went on to graduate from the School of Agronomy in Bogor, Indonesia in 1941, as an agronomic engineer. He then worked at the Botanical Institute in Bogor on the cytogenetics of tuber-bearing *Solanum* species, in a breeding programme searching for blight-resistant potato varieties. In 1942, following the Japanese invasion, Tjio was interned in a concentration camp in

Bandung, the capital of West Java. After his release, Tjio left the island in 1946 for Denmark, and with a fellowship from the Dutch government he continued his specialization in cytogenetics at the Royal Veterinary and Agricultural College of Copenhagen and, during the latter half of 1948, at the laboratory of the Swedish Seed Association in Svalöf, Sweden, and at the Institute for Genetics of the University of Lund. As previously stated, it was during this period that he met Enrique Sánchez-Monge.[9]

Also an agronomy engineer, Sánchez-Monge had been born in 1921 in Melilla, a Spanish region of North Africa, where his father had served in the army. He graduated with honours from the Madrid School of Agronomy in 1946. His family originated from Zaragoza, where he returned after graduation to work as a junior researcher at a new experimental station, the Estación de Biología Experimental de Cogullada, later renamed the Estación Experimental Aula Dei, created on the outskirts of the city in 1946. The research agenda of the station's director, Ramón Esteruelas, also an agronomist, led to Sánchez-Monge being trained abroad in cytology and cereal breeding.[10] Provided with a Portuguese grant, he spent a training period at the Elvas Plant Breeding Experimental Station. A later grant from the Spanish Junta de Relaciones Culturales (an agency that awarded grants for researchers, engineers and university professors to spend time abroad) led him to Svalöf for four months in 1947.[11]

At that time, Svalöf was internationally renowned among agronomy engineers as a reference point for productive seeds and successful plant breeders, and for a system of 'scientific' plant breeding that retained its connection with farmers' needs and expectations.[12] Created as an experimental breeding station in 1886 at the service of the Swedish Association for Seed Improvement, it was funded by farmers and entrepreneurs, with support from the state, to test imported seeds under Swedish climate conditions in order to improve cultivars. After the best plants and seeds had been selected, they were sown collectively for the next year's harvest, a method that had been used by farmers for many years.[13] The journal of the Swedish Seed Association (*Sveriges Utsädesförenings Tidskrift*) was created in 1891 for the publication of records and reports on the breeding experiments. Sowing and harvesting methods were as carefully repetitive and mechanical as harvesting had been for centuries: women and children, who soon gained experience, were employed to carry out these methods.

What would soon be known as the Svalöf Experimental Station received international recognition from both farmers and agronomists. Breeding programmes for the improvement of cereal crops were established for wheat, oat, barley and, towards the turn of the century, rye as well as for clover, potatoes, other vegetables and flowers. The station's 'agricultural programme', as a Spanish reporter called it in 1919, created a huge collection of seeds and a variety of systematic procedures for evaluating seeds and cultivars on the experimental land surrounding the station's building. An association with the Swedish firm that put the seeds on the market (Allmänna Svenska Utsädesaktiebolaget) provided the station with a highly practical and commercial character, the purpose of which, according to the Spanish report, was to provide Swedish farmers and agriculture with the best seeds.[14] An early adoption of pedigree-breeding for the production of 'pure lines' meant the station was receptive as well to the application of Mendelian genetics to breeding in the first decade of the twentieth century.[15]

A cytogenetic department began its activities at Svalöf in 1931, funded by the Knut and Alice Wallenberg Foundation. The first head of this department was Arne Müntzing, widely cited as a cereals cytologist who carried out research on maize, wheat, rye and hybrid cereals and was also editor of the Swedish journal *Hereditas*. The department was associated with the Institute of Genetics at the nearby University of Lund. Both Müntzing and Levan were faculty members of the university institute.[16] A cytologist himself, Levan developed methods for testing the effect of different chemicals on the number and shape of chromosomes. During their stay at the cytogenetic department in Svalöf, both Sánchez-Monge and Tjio developed an informal collaboration on chromosome fragmentation by the action of phenols and some other chemical substances.[17] At Svalöf, practices of experimental agronomy were systematically combined with chemistry and cell biology. Sánchez-Monge did cytological work on speltoid and compactoid forms of wheat, attempting to determine the chromosomal basis for their particular ear shapes. Chromosomes at meiosis were studied on pollen mother cells from anthers previously fixed in a solution of glacial acetic acid. The cells were stained with orcein, and the slide squashed with a thumb before the chromosome was viewed under a microscope (Figure 9.2). 'I lost the skin of my thumb fingertip after all this squashing', Sánchez-Monge later remembered.[18] This laboratory work was complemented by observations in the field. Sánchez-Monge went out to visit the experimental plots of the station with the agronomy engineer James MacKey, in order to learn about the cereal breeding sowing procedures employed at Svalöf: seeds were hand-sown in holes left by marked boards, made with the aid of large rakes.[19] The systematic way in which data about crop varieties were produced and collected at Svalöf strongly influenced Sánchez-Monge's approach to crop improvement, while his increasing skills in cytology led him to learn about cytology and genetics as the biological basis of crop heredity and breeding.

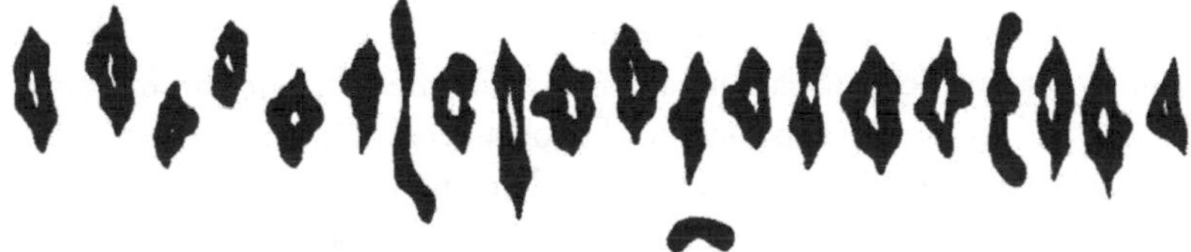

Figure 9.2: Metaphase chromosomes of speltoid wheat, from E. Sánchez-Monge and J. MacKey, 'On the Origin of Subcompactoids in Triticum Vulgare', *Anales de la Estación Experimental Aula Dei*, 1 (1949), pp. 33–64; plate 1. Image reproduced with kind permission by Estación Experimental de Aula Dei, Zaragoza.

Sánchez-Monge returned to Aula Dei from the Swedish station in 1948, after a short sojourn at the Estaçao Agronomica Nacional in Sacavem, Portugal. In the same year, Esteruelas suggested that Tjio be appointed as a cytologist for the cytological unit that would eventually be created at Aula Dei. Sánchez-Monge would become head of the cereal breeding unit. At that time the Estación Experimental Aula Dei was just five years old. It appears an agreement between three local authorities – the agronomist Ramón Esteruelas, the secretary general of the Consejo Superior de Investigaciones Científicas (CSIC) José M. Albareda, and the regional bank (Caja de Ahorros y Monte de Piedad de Aragón y Rioja) – enabled the creation of this experimental station. It was located in an agricultural region devoted to cereal crops, those grown on both irrigated and dry lands.[20] The main purpose of the station was to conduct research on biological problems that could affect agriculture, including those relevant to the Ebro valley region, cereal crops and blights, and also local fruits.[21]

In 1946 a new project was approved that led to the station's name, Estación Experimental Aula Dei, a name shared with the neighbouring monastery. A cytogenetics unit was among the first created in the Estación, with the plan for a new building including rooms in the ground floor for the cytogenetics of tree plants, of cereals and of fodder plants together with other botanical laboratories. The main working space for experimental cultivars was outdoors, but plans for indoor facilities supporting cytological work demonstrate that this area had been part of the research agenda of Aula Dei since its inception. By 1948 provisional facilities had been established at the School of Engineering in Zaragoza while the new building was constructed. Tjio's contract in Denmark finished that year, and thus he was free to accept the grant awarded by CSIC for the first year of his collaboration at Aula Dei.[22]

Colchicine as Agricultural Tool: The Triticale Project, 1949–58

During the decade that Tjio worked as a cytologist at Aula Dei, he spent three to six months each year as a visiting scientist in Lund; he also maintained his collaboration with Levan, sharing authorship of some publications until 1956. During the period of their collaboration, their research shifted from the chromosomes of barley to the chromosome cytology of healthy and malignant tissues in mice and rats, and of human tissues. Tjio's publications also referred to the effects on chromosomes of chemicals and drugs, such as penicillin, phenols and oxyquinoline, and of X-rays.[23]

Levan's work on plant genetics and colchicine began during the summer of 1937, when he visited genetics laboratories in the eastern United States and collaborated with B. R. Nebel at the New York State Agronomic Experimental Station. Their research was inspired by the early, striking results of Albert F. Blakeslee and Amos Avery regarding the action of colchicine on the chromosomes of Jimson weed (*Datura*).[24] Blakeslee's colchicine experiments resulted in varieties with double the number of chromosomes (tetraploids), producing bigger specimens. Unusually large plant size was thus causally correlated with an unusual multiplication of the normal number of chromosomes. Although polyploidy had long been detected in wild species, this was the first artificial method – that is, through the action of a chemical compound – to obtain polyploid species.[25] On his return to Sweden, Levan began experiments with colchicine and made basic contributions to the concept of polyploidy and colchicine mitosis from 1938 onwards (Figure 9.3).[26]

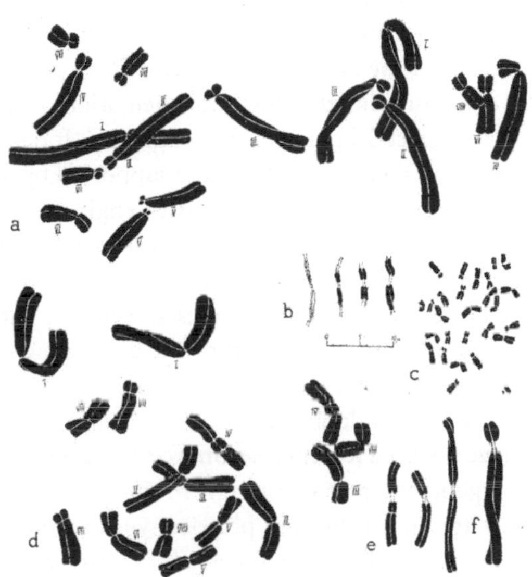

Figure 9.3: Polyploidy and colchicine mitosis, from J. H. Tjio and A. Levan, 'The Use of Oxyquinoline in Chromosome Analysis', ***Anales de la Estación Experimental Aula Dei*** **(1950), pp. 21–62, on p. 33. Image reproduced with kind permission by Estación Experimental de Aula Dei, Zaragoza.**

Apart from his continued collaboration with Levan, and closer to his duties at Aula Dei, Tjio performed research into the effects of pyrogallol in broad beans (*Vicia faba*); *Phleum echinatum*, a grass used for feeding horses; the cytology of a barley mutant; X-ray mutants of barley; and tetraploid rye.[27] Following a 1949 visit to Aula Dei by Danish plant biologist C. A. Jørgensen of the Royal Agricultural and Veterinary College in Copenhagen, Jørgensen suggested that Sánchez-Monge produce a forty-two-chromosome *Triticale* variety by crossing tetraploid wheat (*Triticum*) and rye (*Secale*) strains. *Triticale* varieties had long been regarded as useful for obtaining better cereal for milling and baking. It was believed the new variety would exhibit the drought resistance of rye, enabling it to grow on poor sandy soil, while at the same time retaining the grain qualities of wheat.[28]

In the 1940s, during the post-Spanish Civil War decade of hunger and poverty, resistance to drought was a much sought-after feature for cereals, intended to contribute to the autarchic policy of the Franco dictatorship.[29] Sánchez-Monge and Tjio's attempt to produce a forty-two-chromosome *Triticale* must be seen as part of this political culture, imposed by the Franco regime to promote the improvement of national production. This political rhetoric, however, was contradictory. In the case of the *Triticale* project, it initially included travel abroad to learn new techniques; and secondly, it involved the importation of a foreign researcher, Tjio, to develop what was then named a 'national' project of crop improvement, no matter how modest. Sánchez-Monge's role as a circulator of the practices of the agricultural development programme of Svalöf was instrumental, demonstrating that the implementation of any improvement was dependent on foreign collaboration. Although such foreign scientific relations often began on a personal basis, they were supported by Spanish research policy, which was granting a number of scientists, engineers and industrialists permission to travel abroad and learn about innovations produced during World War II. The case of the *Triticale* project also shows the transition taking place in Spain by the early 1950s, when relationships established by national firms and scientists with foreign projects contributed to the development of the Spanish economy, industry and research system, while at the same time leading to the end of the autarchic policy, undermining its rhetoric and forcing Franco's government to recognize the need for international connections.[30]

This political regime was part of the environment in which genetics as a term, and as a space for knowledge and practices with the meaning we give to it today, was then being established in a Spanish experimental agricultural station. Studies of heredity in plants, especially cereals, were mainly carried out by breeder-scientists like Sánchez-Monge, including the selection of seeds according to phenotypic features – the traditional duty of plant breeders and farmers. Following the discovery of polyploidy, and the artificial inducement of polyploidy in 1937, intervention in the production of seeds took a step forward. It was now possible to create varieties with more chromosomes than usual to obtain plants of larger size and weight. In the case of *Triticale* varieties, polyploidy had an additional, crucial advantage: an enhanced number of chromosomes appeared to increase successful cultivation. Cytogenetics thus appeared a promising domain to not only produce better or, at the very least, bigger cereal varieties, but also to stabilize, reproduce and multiply hybrids between distinct species.

By the late 1940s most of the *Triticale* varieties available possessed fifty-six chromosomes. From 1949 Sánchez-Monge tested the fifty-six-chromosome *Triticale* varieties, but they demonstrated the usual problems of low fertility and grain-shrivelling.[31] In his search for the forty-two-chromosome variety that Jørgensen had suggested, Sánchez-Monge collaborated with Tjio to obtain a strain that might substitute the rye-wheat hybrids already widely cultivated in some Spanish regions. The first step was to obtain hybrids by pollinating tetraploid wheat varieties, by hand, with diploid rye pollen. The result of this hybridization was a triploid *Triticale*, the hope being that the chromosome doubling of its hybrids by the action of colchicine would bring about hexaploid *Triticale*. From the 300 triploid hybrids tested, fifty-four produced seed.

To obtain specimens with double chromosome sets, tillers of the wheat and rye hybrids were treated with solutions of colchicine at different concentrations (0.1, 0.2 and 0.3 per cent during seventy-two hours). Treatment with colchicine included cutting back the tillers (*vástagos*) and capping each of them with an inverted vial filled with the colchicine solution in order to obtain fertile ears (*espigas*). These techniques, described in 1950 by British agricultural botanist George Bell, had produced the best results in wheat varieties.[32] For the colchicine treatment itself, Sánchez-Monge and Tjio carried out the majority of tiller and solution handling.[33] For sowing and harvesting there were many workers, many of them women, at the Estación.[34]

Out of 150 plants treated this way, sixty-nine produced fertile ears. Further testing by Sánchez-Monge resulted in three forty-two-chromosome *Triticale* varieties that demonstrated 'good vegetative vigour' when compared to their parent varieties. They exhibited neck hairiness and naked grains from the rye parent stock, and rachis fracture like wheat. In addition, the *Triticale* plants were higher than their parents and displayed increased grain weight.[35] The results were presented by Sánchez-Monge at the first International Wheat Genetics Symposium in 1958, held at the University of Manitoba, Winnipeg. Leonard H. Shebeski had recently initiated a research programme on *Triticale* at the university's Faculty of Agriculture.[36] This became the beginning of a long career in developing improved varieties by Sánchez-Monge, one of the best known being *Triticale cachirulo*.[37]

Colchicine and the Human Body: Tjio's Collaboration with Levan

Tjio's visits to Sweden were regarded by the director of Aula Dei as a convenient opportunity to receive more training, and therefore for the station to have a more highly skilled cytologist.[38] By the late 1940s Levan and Tjio had worked together on the fragmentation of plant chromosomes by the action of phenols and some other chemical substances.[39] They also attempted to use the staining product orcein in animal tissue, suggesting a shifting of their focus.[40] This move was developed further following a period that Levan had spent in the USA, at the Sloan-Kettering Institute in New York in the summer of 1955. As a guest at the laboratory of John J. Biesele, Levan's aim had been to obtain 'good' chromosomes in mammalian tissue cultures.[41]

When returning to Lund from New York in 1956, Levan co-authored a paper with Tjio presenting the results from their research on somatic chromosomes in human tissue. The publication included the reproduction of a slide showing a complete set of human chromosomes. In it, the chromosomes were not superimposed upon each other, but separated in a way that enabled their counting by a non-specialist reader.[42] Importantly, this image provided clear evidence that humans possessed forty-six chromosomes, unequivocally challenging the previously accepted number of forty-eight.

To produce this slide, Tjio and Levan had used primary explants taken from human embryonic fibroblasts. The tissue samples were provided by a laboratory at the Institute of Bacteriology in Lund, using tissues from embryos obtained from legal abortions. The method Tjio and Levan had used to obtain the slide included hypotonic pre-treatment. This pre-treatment consisted of washing the culture in a hypotonic salt solution less concentrated than was usual for rinsing cultures. It was this detail that helped reveal 'beautifully scattered chromosomes, pretty mitotic chromosomes', as the cytologist T. C. Hsu phrased it in the late 1970s.[43] After this pre-treatment, a colchicine dose was added to the culture medium. Manual 'mild squashing' was then done with the thumb so as to 'keep the chromosomes in metaphase groups', although for ideogram studies a more thorough squashing was preferable, according to the reconstruction of the experiments made by Hsu, the inventor of the hypotonic pre-treatment, in 1979. The slide produced by this method was to be observed through a microscope.

Tjio and Levan's slide created a new space for knowledge about the human body. It represented the body from which the sample had originally been extracted; but it also replaced this body. The slide had been manufactured through a technology that involved processes of extracting, rinsing, separating and differential staining. Most importantly, however, the technology involved arresting body cells in that stage of their normal development at which chromosomes could best be observed. The number, size and shape of a set of chromosomes became iconic of the whole body: chromosomes thus began to be seen as ontologically prior to the body and its anatomy. Human chromosomes began to carry specificity and scientific knowledge, and the 1956 slide was soon joined by a whole series of other slides of human chromosomes.[44] Tjio and Levan's method enabled the arrangement and rearrangement of human chromosomes, and the description of their shape, relative size and each one's place when arranged in a linear order according to size. This had been done before for plants in breeding research, to characterize new varieties, and also in *Drosophila*.[45]

The results were also communicated by Tjio to his fellow scientists at Aula Dei. He sent images of human chromosomes as postcards from Svalöf to the station director, and some of his original slides are still kept at the station's Cytology and Genetics Department. As evidence of the skills Tjio had developed at Svalöf, he and his wife carried some slides with them when returning to Zaragoza, and some of his research results were published in Aula Dei's journal. Through this circulation, the use of colchicines in human tissues became known and practised, even though, from the 1960s onwards, peripheral blood, rather than embryonic tissue, became the main source for human chromosome studies.

Early Human Genetics in Spain

Tjio left Aula Dei for two visits to the University of Colorado Medical Center in Denver to collaborate with Theodore T. Puck in 1958 and 1959, and, finally and definitively, for the National Institutes of Health campus in Bethesda, Maryland. Sánchez-Monge also left in 1958 for the University of Madrid; he was appointed at the School of Agronomy and the Faculty of Science, and in both academic settings he was the first full professor teaching genetics at the university. He continued to develop his skills with polyploids at an experimental station near the School of Agronomy and trained generations of agronomists.[46] There had been distinguished geneticists in Spain before the Civil War, among the most recognized being Antonio de Zulueta at the Museum of Natural Sciences in Madrid; Cruz Gallástegui at the Misión Biológica de Galicia, who was also very active after the war; and Jimena Fernández de la Vega at the University of Madrid Medical School.[47]

Throughout his career, Sánchez-Monge had been more interested in seed improvement than in genetics per se. For him cytogenetics was a tool, an easily handled one that contributed to his aim and expertise. However, initially in Svalöf and later with Tjio, Sánchez-Monge accumulated the skills to perform cytological explorations into chromosomes, whether stemming from cereals or from human tissues and blood. These skills and the associated knowledge enabled him to author many books and receive recognition from medical geneticists in Madrid. His academic trajectory shows his growing scholarship in genetics.

Sánchez-Monge was appointed professor of genetics, in the first university chair created in Spain with this name, in 1960.[48] The creation of this chair illustrates the origins of genetic practices in agronomy, selective breeding, and the improvement of seeds and livestock.[49] At that time genetics was a promising area of knowledge associated with agronomy, but it had begun to make a huge impact in clinical and medical practice. To give but one example of this, Tjio was awarded the first International Prize of the Joseph P. Kennedy, Jr Foundation in December 1962 'for his discovery of the exact number of chromosome in man'. Tjio shared the award with Murray L. Barr, whose discovery of the Barr body was used to determine the true sex where doubt existed, and Jerome Lejeune, for his discovery of the extra chromosome in Down syndrome. At the ceremony at the Stattler Hilton Hotel in Washington, DC on 6 December, according to the note released by the press office of the NIH, US president John F. Kennedy read the citation at 'a celebrity-studded banquet'.[50]

Sánchez-Monge's 1968 election to the Spanish Academy of Science (Real Academia de Ciencias Exactas, Físicas y Naturales) demonstrates the regard that both genetics and he himself were held in by scholars from other scientific disciplines. At a meeting on human genetics held in Madrid in 1975, Sánchez-Monge was invited to give the opening lecture, a general introduction to 'genetics and society', showing his symbolic authority in a field that had by then earned medical space in the clinic as a diagnostic tool.[51] 'They listened to me because I had worked beside Tjio', he remembered, suggesting that Tjio's fame both favoured and overshadowed his own.[52] 'The application of biological knowledge in the human clinic has been an achievement of the last two decades', he proclaimed at the 1975 meeting. Agriculture had been the first laboratory of genetics, but by that time medicine was reaping the benefits.[53] By emphasizing the practical value of genetics in both medicine and agronomy, Sánchez-Monge reinforced the image of agronomy as the origin of modern genetics, with himself participating in one of the earliest intersections of the fields.

His most well-known books on genetics were published during this early period of the 1950s and 1960s: *Genética General y Agrícola*, in collaboration with Ramón Esteruelas (Barcelona: Salvat, 1952); *Fitogenética, Mejora de Plantas* (Barcelona: Salvat, 1955, 2nd edn 1974); *Catálogo Genético de Trigos Españoles* (Madrid: Ministerio de Agricultura, 1955); the handbook *Genética* (Madrid: Dossat, 1966, 1972); *Diccionario de Genética* (Madrid: Instituto Nacional de Investigaciones Agronómicas, 1962, 1970); and *Razas de Maíz en España* (Madrid: Ministerio de Agricultura, 1962). The chronology of his published books displays both his early interest in plants and agriculture, and the transition that occurred as general genetics became an academic and scientific area, dominated by his own knowledge and expertise.

Sánchez-Monge's earliest publications on genetics came out during the 1950s, a period in which genetics was perceived as showing promise in both agriculture and medicine. His collaboration with Tjio demonstrates the exchange of cytogenetic practices between plant and human genetics. It was at the experimental station in Zaragoza where these two approaches and lines of research met, in the cytological laboratory in which cereal chromosomes and practices of polyploidy were the main research subjects. At that time, cereal cytology and human cytology developed in parallel. I would suggest that not only were the practices of human genetics at that time based on the earlier practices of plant genetics, but also that the techniques and tools, such as colchicine, were shared for different uses: to induce polyploidy in plants in order to invigorate them, and to arrest human chromosomes in metaphase in order to characterize them.

These practices developed in parallel to those of clinical cytogenetics. In Madrid a unit for cytogenetics was established at one of the general hospitals in 1962. Colchicine was still in use for arresting metaphase in chromosome division, following treatment of the sample with phytohemagglutinin, a mucoprotein from bean extract originally used to separate leucocytes within peripheral blood samples. Biopsy had been used for cytogenetic tests until 1960, and bone marrow was also a source of samples for a short while. Following the 1960 publication of Peter Nowell's findings at the Department of Pathology of the University of Pennsylvania, biopsy was replaced by peripheral blood extraction. In his studies on human leukaemia, Nowell had observed chromosomes in lymphocytes using phytohemagglutinin, and he began to utilize the substance to promote mitosis. Following the dissemination of his publications, blood samples became an easily accessible source for human cytological analysis.[54] This led to a widespread expansion of human cytology practices, venepuncture being far easier to perform, and less painful to experience, than biopsy and tissue extraction in general.

Conclusion

The material object at the crossroads between agricultural and medical applications that genetics was becoming in the late 1950s and early 1960s was colchicine, which remains to this day a fundamental tool in the search for polyploidy in cereals and for human chromosomes in the clinic. Researchers, materials and tools frequently crossed boundaries between the two fields. In the case studied in this essay, Tjio and Levan made the transition from plant cytology to human tissues, while Sánchez-Monge, even though remaining a plant breeding scientist, became a cytologist and mentor to a generation of geneticists and biotechnologists in Madrid.

The interventions made possible by drugs such as colchicine carried toxicity detectable in chromosomes in a wide variety of forms: polyploidy in plants (by colchicine), fragmentation (by phenols) and contraction at metaphase (by oxyquinoline).[55] The toxic effects of colchicine in human chromosomes led to clearer, separated images, making them visible and countable. In botanical applications, they led to larger plants and the promise of alleviating world hunger. Such toxicity was somehow hidden by the quality of the images of human chromosomes and the size of plants: the results were convenient, efficient and had no known side effects. This situation illustrates the contingent meaning of toxicity. Just as radiation became a source of mutations in *Drosophila*, so important in genetic studies of the fly, colchicine became an important tool in the study of cereal and human genetics in the 1950s.

Acknowledgements

I gratefully acknowledge the comments and suggestions from Staffan Müller-Wille in an earlier version of this essay, which was presented at the workshop Human Heredity in the Twentieth Century in Exeter in September 2010. For the location of archival resources, I would like to thank José M. Lasa and librarian José Carlos Martínez at the Estación Experimental Aula Dei (Zaragoza, Spain); David Cantor and the archivists at the Office for NIH History, NIH, Bethesda (Maryland, USA); and Steven Eidelman at the Joseph P. Kennedy, Jr Foundation. Enrique Sánchez-Monge's daughter, Rosa Sánchez-Monge, gave me access to the photograph collection preserved by her family. The late Enrique Sánchez-Monge granted me a long interview at his home in Madrid in 2007. The research for this essay was funded by the Spanish Ministry of Science and Innovation (FFI2009-07522).

10 PUTTING HUMAN GENETICS ON A SOLID BASIS: HUMAN CHROMOSOME RESEARCH, 1950s–1970s

Soraya de Chadarevian

In the post-World War II era one technique raised particularly high hopes to advance the study of human heredity. This was the technique of human karyotyping, which made it possible to visualize and analyse human chromosomes. Following this tool and the practices that accompanied it, we can gain insights into a broad range of developments and discussions around human heredity and the cultural concerns in which they were embedded. Chromosome research has been largely neglected in historical accounts of post-war genetics, in which molecular biology has taken much of the limelight.[1] This essay aims at redressing this situation arguing that human chromosome research was a high-profile subject that responded to urgent questions and attracted much funding and attention at the time. It suggests that the history of human cytogenetics provides a crucial chapter to understand how genetics has gained its dominant position in the late twentieth and early twenty-first century and points to important continuities to current genomic practices. The essay will review the political and scientific concerns that propelled the study of human cytogenetics after World War II and reconstruct the hopes and expectations that were put into the new techniques to visualize human chromosomes. It will then survey some of the fields – from radiobiology and cancer research to medical genetics, gender testing, criminology and worldwide population studies – in which karyotyping made an entry, providing new answers to existing questions and opening up new areas of investigation and debate.

Atomic Concerns and the Recount of Human Chromosomes

Chromosomes had long been an active area of genetic research. In the 1920s scientists agreed that humans had forty-eight chromosomes. However, human chromosomes were difficult to work with, as were chromosomes from animal cells more generally. The giant chromosomes in the salivary glands of the larvae of the fruit fly, first described in the 1930s, represented an exception. Thus most research on chromosomes was performed on plant cells, both because of the ease of working with that material and in view of its potential use for plant breeding.

After World War II, widespread efforts to establish the effects of radiation in humans as well as a continuing interest in the role of chromosomes in the aetiology of cancer provided new incentives to develop methods to study human chromosomes. The two strands of radiobiology and cancer research would become increasingly intertwined. Indeed, many researchers working in the cancer field came from radiation research, and many radiobiologists became engaged in cancer research. Similarly, much of the funding in cancer chromosome research came from sources funding radiation research at a time when the induction of cancer through the ever-expanding clinical use of radiation and through the effects of radioactive fallout became a growing concern of the nuclear age.[2]

We find this picture confirmed when we look at some of the key developments in human karyotyping in the middle decades of the twentieth century and follow the careers of some of the protagonists. Joe-Hin Tjio and Albert Levan from the University of Lund, who in 1956 first suggested that the number of human chromosomes was forty-six and not forty-eight, as had been believed for a long time, were trying to establish a standard against which to compare the bewildering changes in chromosome number and size observed in cancer cells and to establish if these were the cause or the effect of cancer. Levan, who headed the cancer chromosome laboratory at the Institute of Genetics in Lund, had worked on radiation-induced mutations in onion root tips, before moving to the study of cancer induction in humans. Tjio and Levan's conclusions regarding the new chromosome count were rather cautious, yet in the course of a few months the observation was confirmed by two researchers, Charles Ford and John Hamerton, at the Radiobiological Research Unit that was attached to the Atomic Energy Research Establishment at Harwell, one of the two key sites of the British atomic bomb project. The Swedish group had made their observation on cultured cells of the lung tissue of aborted foetuses, which were available to the Swedish researchers following the new abortion law in their country. Ford and Hamerton's use of fresh tissue of human testes, supplied to them by an Oxford surgeon, provided decisive evidence for the general applicability of the new chromosome count.[3]

Ford became a pivotal figure in the establishment of human cytogenetics in Britain, as other investigators turned to him for his expertise in cell preparation techniques. His career was in many ways emblematic of the new opportunities for research in human cytogenetics in the atomic age.[4] A trained botanist, he had spent a three-year stint at the Department of Atomic Energy at Chalk River in Canada to study the biological hazards of radiation using plant material, before he was called to head the cytogenetics section at the newly established Radiobiological Research Unit at Harwell, funded by the Medical Research Council. There his goal was to develop techniques to study radiation-damaged chromosomes in mammalian cells.

Advances in chromosome preparation at the time depended on a combination of new techniques. These included the development of tissue culture; the use of colchicine to arrest cell division in metaphase when chromosomes were condensed and organized on a central plate in the cell; the use of hypotonic medium to swell the cells; and squash techniques to spread the chromosomes on the microscopic slide. Ford's contribution consisted in further developing the squash technique and in adapting the whole set of techniques to work with the most difficult of tissues such as the testes and bone marrow that were crucial for genetic research. The bone marrow technique developed at Harwell, as well as the peripheral blood method developed by David A. Hungerford and his colleagues in the USA that eventually superseded it, were both originally devised to study the chromosomes of patients or experimental animals with radiation-induced leukaemia. By offering a less intrusive method to gain human tissue for karyotyping, the peripheral blood method opened the way for chromosome analysis to be performed on a much larger scale, both in the clinic and on the population level.

As indicated by these brief remarks, many of the human cytogeneticists in the 1950s worked on radiation-related problems or were funded by atomic energy funding agencies. In many of these studies, radiation was not just used as a tool for genetic research. Rather, the effects of radiation itself were the object of research. The chronology of events is significant here too: in 1954 the American test explosion of a hydrogen bomb on Bikini Island raised concerns over the biological effects of worldwide fallout from atomic testing; in 1956 the US and the UK governments issued reports that raised the alarm on rising cases of cancer through the clinical use of radiation;[5] in 1956 the number of human chromosomes was revised and improved protocols for human karyotyping became available. Thus karyotyping appeared as the right tool at the right moment to address a host of urgent political and scientific questions and debates surrounding the use of radiation in the post-war era.

Concerns surrounding radiation remained at the centre of much chromosome research throughout the 1950s and 1960s and provided new legitimization for human heredity research after the subject had been tarnished by eugenic and racial practices. Yet human cytogenetics also developed a life of its own and expanded into new territories.

Karyotyping and the Clinic

The confirmation of the new chromosome count was followed by a string of spectacular observations that linked unusual chromosome pictures with particular syndromes, including, most famously, the presence of an extra chromosome 21 in patients with Down syndrome, or 'mongolism' as it was still called at the time.[6] Other observations regarded sex chromosome-linked anomalies, like in the case of patients with Turner and Klinefelter syndromes that were identified as having an XO and XXY karyotype respectively. Excitement was also produced by the observation of an unusually small chromosome in the marrow cells of patients that suffered from a specific form of leukaemia known as chronic myeloid leukaemia, confirming the potential of chromosome research for the study of the aetiology of cancer. Participants described it as a 'wonderland of new discoveries'.[7]

The possibility of tracing complex clinical syndromes to a change in shape or number of chromosomes that was detectable under the microscope very much impressed clinicians at the time. However, it is important to note that this was not a one-way traffic from the laboratory to the clinic. Rather, clinicians who had become interested in genetics initiated many of the early chromosome studies of human diseases. There was especially a growing interest in hereditary diseases among paediatricians. Clinicians provided the samples and brought their clinical knowledge to the studies, while cytogeneticists performed the karyotype analyses. Thus, shortly after the recount of human chromosomes, Ford at Harwell was approached by Paul Polani, a physician at Guy's Hospital in London, who had for a while been studying women patients with Turner syndrome and had come to the conclusion that they might only have one X chromosome. Ford and his collaborators were able to confirm this prediction.[8] Polani as well as Lazlo G. Lajtha, a haematologist at Churchill Hospital in Oxford, later supplied Ford with tissue from Klinefelter patients.[9] Patricia Jacobs, based at the MRC Clinical Effects of Radiation Research Unit in Edinburgh, who beat Ford at establishing the Klinefelter case, collaborated with a local physician, John A. Strong.[10] The Edinburgh unit, headed by the radiologist and epidemiologist Michael Court Brown, was situated at the Western General Hospital. The collaboration with clinical staff became instrumental for much of the work developed at the unit that quickly established itself as one of the key centres for human cytogenetics. Following the results of the Klinefelter case, the medical geneticist and Galton Professor at University College London, Lionel Penrose, provided Ford with the bone marrow cells of a Klinefelter Down patient.

In Paris the initiative to study the karyotype of patients with Down syndrome came from Raymond Turpin, the senior clinician of the team at the Hôpital Trousseau credited with the discovery of the additional chromosome. In the 1930s Turpin had already pointed to the possibility that Down syndrome was a chromosome disease, brought about by environmental influences. Tjio's display of his chromosome images at the first International Congress of Human Genetics in Copenhagen in 1956 inspired Turpin to follow up on his intuition. The other two researchers on the team, Marthe Gautier and Jérôme Léjeune, also had a medical background.[11]

Penrose famously found 'the photograph of the cell from the man with two extra chromosomes from which the intelligence level, the behaviour and sexual character can be confidently predicted, just about as astonishing as a photograph of the back of the moon' (the reference is historic, as the first images of the 'far' side of the moon, taken by a Soviet satellite, had just appeared in the press).[12] Penrose also described the impression the chromosome images made on people who were never exposed to them before. He hoped it would raise interest in the field of human genetics and 'usher in a period of plenty' in respect to funding.[13] An important part of Penrose's excitement was that the new techniques at last 'put human genetics on a very solid basis'.[14] Concerning 'mongolism', that he described as 'one of the most baffling problems in paediatrics', he believed that it was now 'on the way to solution' – although the journey would still be long.[15] The following longer quote from his 1959 lecture powerfully summarizes the high expectations placed on the new technical approaches:

> It is evident from all this that there has been, during the last year, a major break through in the science of human genetics which will lead to a spate of new discoveries. We can now confidently look forward to the time when genes with known effects can be assigned to their correct locations on the chromosomes. We can also expect a great advance in our knowledge of how genes deliver their instructions to the cells both during development and in adult life. We may even expect to contribute to the problems relating chromosome anomalies to the problems of abnormal growth as in tumors. In fact it is a very encouraging period for those of us who have pursued the subject of human genetics for many years.[16]

Theodore Puck, one of the pioneers of cytogenetics in the USA, also highlighted the novelty of the findings, while at the same time making a strong link to the radiation context. He wrote:

> The current value of the maximum allowable dose was adopted in 1959. Since then we have become aware of a whole new group of human diseases which appear to be capable of being induced by radiation but whose importance and indeed very existence was unknown at the time the currently employed standards were adopted. These diseases constitute the genetic diseases due to chromosomal aberrations ... This set of diseases is so costly to man and to society that a re-examination of the permissible dose of radiation for large populations must be carried out as soon as possible.[17]

The initial euphoria of some of the early practitioners about the diagnostic power of the new tool was tempered by contradictory observations, as for instance a count of forty-six chromosomes in some cases of Down syndrome. The more precise characterization and standardization of the human karyotype achieved in the early 1960s helped to resolve some, but not all, disputes.[18] Nonetheless, with the establishment of amniocentesis and the passing of abortion laws, karyotyping became routine practice in prenatal screening. In the late 1960s new chromosome banding technologies significantly increased the resolving power of cytogenetics and with it the scope of the technique in clinical diagnosis and modern reproductive medicine.

Chromosomes and Sex

Many of the early observations on unusual chromosome pictures concerned the number of sex chromosomes. Next to the Turner and Klinefelter cases mentioned above, the case of a woman with a triple-X chromosome was reported. The case was described as a 'super female'.[19] The report was followed closely by the first description of an (asymptomatic) XYY man.[20]

A combination of technical, biomedical and cultural reasons were responsible for the first string of observations of sex chromosome anomalies and for the continuing focus of research on these cases. Trisonomies – or, as in the case of Turner syndrome, a monosomy – were easy to detect. A whole array of trisonomies could be expected, yet in fact only a handful of different cases were found. As became clear, only trisonomies of gene-poor chromosomes, namely chromosomes 13, 18, 21 and the sex chromosomes, were viable. Another factor driving research on sex chromosome anomalies was the broad application of the sex chromatin or Barr body test. This was an easy test introduced in the late 1940s that allowed researchers to test for the presence or absence of so-called Barr bodies, dark round structures in the cell nucleus that could be viewed under the microscope. The interpretation of the Barr bodies was uncertain, but as they were only found in cells of females, they were thought to form when two X chromosomes were present.[21] Originally performed on skin biopsies, it was later shown that the Barr body test could also be applied to buccal smears, prepared by scraping a few cells from the inner lining of the cheek. The Barr body test attracted much attention and stimulated much research, as recently shown by Fiona Miller, who has argued that the technique found its place in a burgeoning field of sex research.[22] Human cytogenetic research followed in its steps. Even once human karyotyping techniques became more widely established, the Barr body test continued to be applied in the clinical context and in population surveys. If an unusual number of Barr bodies was found, a full karyotype analysis that demanded much more time and skill could be performed.[23]

The application of the Barr body technique in the clinic had dramatic effects in the case of Turner and Klinefelter patients as it led to a reversal of their usual sex assignment. While a morphological description had assigned a female gender to Turner patients and a male gender to Klinefelter, the Barr body test indicated that Turner patients had to be regarded as males and Klinefelter – as they displayed a Barr body – as females. Because of the controversy surrounding these patients, clinicians were keen to provide cytogeneticists like Ford with samples to be tested with the new karyotyping techniques, only to see the gender assignment of Turner and Klinefelter patients turned on the head again.

The cytogenetic study of Turner and Klinefelter patients had another important effect on the understanding of the function of sex chromosomes. Until 1959 it was believed that – like in *Drosophila* – the Y chromosome was inert. Male sex was believed to be determined by autosomal genes that in females were checked by the two X chromosomes. According to this theory, XXY individuals should be females; the fact that they showed predominantly male characteristics – Barr body analysis notwithstanding – meant that the Y chromosome played a decisive role in the male sex determination.

Buccal smear tests followed by chromosome analysis were applied not only in the clinical context but also in the competitive sports context. Compulsory gender verification in female athletes was introduced by the International Association of Athletics Federation at the European Championships in Budapest in 1966, apparently because of increasing competition between East and West in the context of the Cold War and growing suspicions in the West that Eastern female athletes were outperforming their Western counterparts because they were, in fact, men.[24] The test introduced in 1966 required female athletes to parade naked in front of a panel of physicians. From this practice it seemed a step forward when buccal smear testing was introduced at the 1968 Olympic Games in Mexico City. Compulsory gender verification in the form of buccal smear testing, followed by a full chromosome analysis and measuring of blood hormone levels in negative or inconclusive cases, remained in place until 1991, when increasing pressure led to the discontinuation of the practice. It was re-introduced at the 1996 Olympics in Atlanta but again suspended shortly before the games in Sydney in 2000. The reasons for the elimination of the screening rested on changing sensibilities as well as on the increasing realization of the limitations of the genetic test in view of the descriptions of new syndromes like androgen insensitivity. Nevertheless, chromosome tests still play a role in the array of gender verification tests that is applied in specific cases.

Chromosomes and Crime

A high-profile case that gave karyotyping a lot of not necessarily welcome press concerned a survey of the population of the Scottish high-security hospital in Carstairs. The survey, performed by researchers from the Edinburgh unit, found an increased incidence of XYY cases in this institution. The results were published in the journal *Nature* under the title 'Aggressive Behaviour, Mental Sub-Normality and the XYY Male'.[25] As the title indicated, the paper suggested that the additional Y chromosome (whose function in male sex determination had only recently been clarified) predisposed its carrier to overly manly and therefore aggressive and criminal behaviour. In the words of its main author, the paper 'immediately caused a mayhem'.[26]

The postulated link between aggressive behaviour and the XYY chromosomes picture did not stand up to scrutiny. A follow-up study by the Edinburgh group that surveyed the cytogenetic status of about 2,500 males in a variety of penal institutions and approved schools in Scotland did not show an increased incidence of XYY males.[27] The higher incidence of XYY cases in high-security hospitals was confirmed, but the phenomenon was explained with the lower intelligence level in some individuals with XYY karyotypes. Further investigations revealed that men with an XYY karyotype that did not show any particular behavioural characteristics were also found in the general population. Nevertheless, the Edinburgh group suggested that only neonatal screening programmes, which did not suffer from the ascertainment biases of studies of institutionalized populations, and prospective studies of infants that were found to carry the XYY karyotype could determine the developmental and behavioural implications of the extra Y chromosome.[28] Such studies were started in Edinburgh as well as in a series of other cities. They continued into the 1990s amidst considerable controversy.

The XYY case is notorious in the history of human genetics. It can serve here as a window into the contemporary debates about human heredity and the cultural concerns to which the case responded. From the start, because of the association of aggression with crime and delinquency, the story attracted considerable media attention, catapulting chromosome research on the front pages of various media outlets.[29] In the midst of the civil rights and student protest movements, the association of chromosomes and aggression resonated with ongoing debates and anxieties over increasing aggression and violence in the public sphere. In addition, the prospective studies coincided with incipient debates about ethical guidelines for medical research and the rights of patients. Vocal critics, including the newly formed advocacy group Science for the People, exposed the neonatal screening and prospective studies as unethical, unreliable and politically wrong.[30] Together these aspects go some way to explain the length and vehemence of the debate around the XYY karyotype.

Despite widespread resistance to a genetic explanation of social behaviour – a question that was high on the agenda because of the raging IQ debate[31] – and the general tendency at the time to privilege the role of the social environment over hereditary dispositions, the question of reduced responsibility of XYY individuals was repeatedly raised. Already in 1962, Michael Court Brown, the director of the MRC unit in Edinburgh and an energetic promoter of the possibilities of karyotyping, suggested that legal authorities should give consideration to the findings of cytogenetics. He pointed to the question of the legal responsibility of people whose genotype might predispose them to delinquent behaviour as well as to possible consequences for the legal status of certain marriages, as for instance in the case of phenotypical women with a male karyotype.[32] In the wake of the XYY controversy, these considerations gained new valency. In at least a handful of widely publicized cases, the argument of diminished responsibility was used by defence teams in criminal courts to exonerate the accused. Although the courts were cautious in accepting the argument, the cases fuelled the popular imagination regarding the XYY man and his over-manly if not monstrous powers. They also provided the material for books and film adaptations, most notably the *XYY Man* series by English thriller writer Kenneth Royce, the first volume of which appeared in 1970. The fictional hero of the series, William 'Spider' Scott, although intelligent and non-violent, was unable to leave his criminal past fully behind him, presumably because of the extra Y chromosome that he carried.[33]

Human Population Studies

A review of the XYY controversy reveals the staggering amount of screening that was undertaken to investigate the questions relating to this specific karyotype. Many studies reported results from thousands or even ten thousands of individuals. These studies were part of an expanding series of population studies undertaken with the new cytogenetic tools in the wake of the first reports about chromosome anomalies. Neonatal studies were of special importance. At the MRC Unit in Edinburgh, which became one of the key centres for population cytogenetics, the first neonatal screening programme was set up in 1959. It was based on buccal smears, followed by full karyotype analysis in cases where an unusual picture was found. The aim of the neonatal studies was to establish the frequency of abnormalities in the general population and thus provide a point of reference for other population studies. The long-term aim was to correlate anomalies in the children with parental age, social class and ethnicity and thus to study the causes of the anomalies. In addition, the newborn screening programme was aimed at identifying the individuals that might need special attention and at providing data for genetic counselling.

The screening revealed an unexpectedly large number of chromosomal anomalies, or what was then more carefully described as genetic variation. Findings indicated that about 1 per cent of children showed a chromosome anomaly in their mitotic cells. One quarter of these regarded a sex chromosome anomaly; one quarter showed other kinds of trisonomies, with the majority being cases of trisonomy 21; the rest showed detectable structural rearrangements. This quite certainly represented an underestimation of the chromosomal variation present in the general population because of the various difficulties connected to visualizing chromosomal changes.[34]

In the wake of the XYY controversy, a new neonatal screening programme was set up based on full chromosome analyses. It was specifically designed to identify infants with XXX, XXY and XYY karyotypes for enrolment into the prospective studies. The screening programme soon comprised all children born in the two major Edinburgh maternity hospitals. Between 1967 and 1979, when screening stopped, 34,380 newborns were screened.

Other population subgroups studied at the Edinburgh unit included the inmates of institutions for the mentally retarded; mentally ill patients; long-stay prisoners; infertile or subfertile males and women; repeat aborters; and subjects exposed to ionizing radiation, such as cancer patients, industrial workers, people involved in the refuelling of depleted uranium or people exposed to radiation leaks at the Windscale accident of 1957, when a fire erupted at Britain's first plutonium factory. Subjects exposed to other toxic substances like aromatic hydrocarbons, herbicides and pesticides were also screened. As this list indicates, the use of karyotyping techniques to study the effects of radiation as well as the aetiology of cancer remained an important but far from the only concern.

At the Edinburgh unit two tools were set up to help the population studies: a registry of abnormal chromosomes and a computer-based effort to automate karyotyping. The registry was started parallel to the neonatal screening programme. It combined chromosome, medical, physiological and family data supplied or collected by collaborating physicians, social workers and pedigree researchers. By the mid-1960s it contained the data of more than 800 individuals and was perceived as a central tool for the unit's work on population cytogenetics, clinical cytogenetics, human reproduction and cancer.

The time needed to count and analyse chromosomes represented the most serious restriction for the clinical development of cytogenetics and for the development of population cytogenetics as Court Brown envisaged it. An ambitious and costly programme aimed at harnessing computers to do the job was put in place in the mid-1960s. Yet pattern recognition proved a difficult problem to solve with machines. The solution was found in an 'interactive system' that combined the scanning capacities of the computer with the pattern recognition capacity of the human operator, thus speeding up the work of karyotyping.

The Edinburgh unit was not the only institution involved in population karyotyping. From the late 1950s the World Health Organization (WHO) supported large-scale genetic surveys of newborn babies across various continents as well as genetic studies of 'primitive' or 'vanishing populations'. One such genetic survey of newborn babies involving twenty countries was for instance undertaken by the Population Genetics Research Unit in Oxford under the direction of Alan Stevenson. The aim of the survey, which involved about 400,000 babies, was to establish the rate at which hereditary defects were occurring in different parts of the world and, if possible, to relate the frequencies to such factors as ethnic affiliation, diet and geographical situation. These and other such studies at the time were based on the analysis of developmental malformations and on the study of variants and frequencies of haemoglobins or other serum proteins. They also included pedigree analyses and consanguinity studies. Yet from the 1960s karyotyping increasingly found its place among the tools deployed in these worldwide surveys that linked anthropological approaches with genetic and public health issues. It was for instance included in the guide to field methods issued as part of the human adaptability component of the International Biological Program launched in the early 1960s. The programme entailed provisions for 'genetic surveys on a world scale' that were also supported by the WHO.[35] The interest of the WHO in human genetics and in karyotyping stemmed from the same concerns about the mutational effects of radiation to which patients and the population at large were exposed in the atomic age, and it expanded from there. The WHO organized cytogenetic courses for researchers starting from the late 1950s.

Conclusion

The quick expansion of human karyotyping projects in the 1960s and 1970s shows that human cytogenetics, which developed in parallel to molecular genetics, was a very active area of research tightly bound to an intersecting set of scientific, clinical and political concerns, including especially the radiation context. Indeed, well into the 1970s, if not later, chromosome images were the most recognizable images of genetics. Only much more recently has the double helix taken the upper hand, but chromosome images still have a strong public appeal, as indicated for instance by Gina Glover's Chromosomal Stripy Socks artwork that received the 2008 Visions of Science DNA award.[36] This is only one of many art works using chromosome imagery. The human X and Y chromosomes in particular have acquired iconic status.

Following the karyotyping techniques from the laboratory to the clinic, the Olympic competition, the courtroom and the worldwide population studies provided insights into a broad range of arenas where human heredity came to matter and genetic knowledge was embraced, controversially debated or rejected. The XYY controversy in particular highlighted the scientific and ethical issues surrounding the production and use of genetic knowledge in respect to humans and the value various actors attached to it. Reviewing the cytogenetic studies of the 1960s and 1970s, it is surprising how much of it became controversial. Besides the multifaceted debate around the XYY karyotype, data archives such as the registry have also become controversial because of changes in medical consent and privacy rules. Today genomic research seems to follow many of the same trails as karyotyping, especially in respect to the focus on genetic medicine and population genomics, and in relation to data gathering and processing practices.

Lessons have certainly been learnt, especially in respect to ethical protocols. Yet to what extent the ethical problems of genetic screening and data gathering programmes have really been solved remains an open question. Resisting too narrow (molecular) genealogies and studying the whole spectrum of genetic practices in the preceding decades – including the broad range of projects and discussions around human cytogenetics in the 1950s to 1970s, before molecular approaches were slowly taking the upper hand – can help us gain a better understanding of current genomic practices and the changing cultural concerns in which they are embedded. It may also provide a cautionary tale about getting all too excited about new technological tools and their possibilities for solving questions surrounding human heredity, disease and identity, then and now.

Acknowledgements

I thank seminar participants in Edinburgh, Exeter, London, Paris and San Diego as well as Nathan Ha at UCLA and the editors and referees of this volume for many insightful comments.

11 THE DISAPPEARANCE OF THE CONCEPT OF ANTICIPATION IN THE POST-WAR WORLD

Judith E. Friedman

In the decade following World War II, a theory that some human hereditary illnesses appeared earlier and often more severely in succeeding generations went from being 'almost universally accepted' to being 'generally believed to be erroneous'.[1] This phenomenon, known as 'anticipation' from the early years of the twentieth century, had its origins in mid-nineteenth-century French degeneration theory and was noted in the works of such prominent scholars as Charles Darwin and Francis Galton.[2] Although theoretically controversial, physicians and psychiatrists routinely used anticipation to describe patterns of heredity that they clinically observed in families. One paper, published in 1948 by Lionel Penrose, the new Galton Chair of Eugenics at University College London (UCL), stands out as having firmly disproved earlier findings of anticipation.[3]

The arguments Penrose put forward against anticipation were so persuasive and influential that it took almost forty years until a Dutch neurologist began to question them.[4] Not until the discovery of a novel form of dynamic mutation in 1991 were most geneticists persuaded of the validity of earlier findings of anticipation.[5] But it was not merely Penrose's argument in 1948 that put findings of anticipation beyond the pale of accepted genetic practice for forty years. Instead, as I will argue, it was a combination of scientific, political and institutional factors that set the concept of anticipation outside the accepted bounds of human and medical genetics in the post-war period. In turn, the story of anticipation provides a lens through which to view developments in the field of human heredity that would be obscured if attention were paid only to mainstream scientific discourse.[6] In what follows, I will first present the main argument of Penrose's 1948 paper, and then sketch out the concurrent scientific, political and institutional developments that lent it so much weight.

Lionel Penrose and the Rejection of Anticipation

Before World War II clinically oriented researchers had observed anticipation in a variety of diseases, including Leber's hereditary optic neuropathy, cataract, familial jaundice, diabetes, mental illness, dementia praecox, Huntington's disease and, most notably, myotonic dystrophy (a disease characterized by muscle wasting and stiffness).[7] More theoretically oriented researchers, such as Karl Pearson, head of the Galton Laboratory for National Eugenics and the first Galton Chair of Eugenics at UCL, were sceptical and held that anticipation was a statistical artefact brought about by selection bias. Researchers had been examining families in which parents had been affected late enough in life that they were able to marry and have children, whereas there was no such restriction on age of onset in their children. Indeed, as others observed, early onset in children was even more likely to come to the attention of researchers.[8] Despite these theoretical objections, physicians continued to find anticipation in a variety of diseases.

In Britain, the Galton Laboratory of National Eugenics at UCL was a bastion of statistical research on human heredity. Julia Bell, a researcher at the Galton Laboratory, was well aware of the statistical arguments against anticipation. As part of her analytical work in the Galton Laboratory's monumental study *The Treasury of Human Inheritance*, she attempted to control for variables that might cause statistical errors, including findings of anticipation. Bell initially began to compare the differences in ages of onset between parents and offspring on the one hand, and aunts/uncles and nephews/nieces on the other, in order to test the hypothesis of generational selection bias. Despite the inclusion of individuals who were not directly related, Bell continued to note a tendency for decreased age of onset between generations in several diseases, particularly in the case of myotonic dystrophy. Sometimes, as in the case of peroneal atrophy (also known as Charcot-Marie-Tooth disease, which results in nerve damage and muscle wasting), this difference was relatively small (not quite five years) but in other cases, notably myotonic dystrophy, the difference was large (over twenty-three years).[9]

Lionel Penrose, a Quaker-raised conscientious objector with psychiatric and medical training, was among the fiercest opponents of the concept of anticipation. He had been refining his arguments against anticipation since the early 1930s, when he classed it with other non-Mendelian concepts of heredity like germ-plasm poisoning and the inheritance of acquired characteristics. He felt that such concepts should be discarded in favour of the mathematically based form of Mendelism being developed in England by Lancelot Hogben and J. B. S. Haldane.[10] I would suggest that Penrose's arguments against anticipation were a form of 'boundary-work', and that he wished to establish the notion of anticipation as 'non-science' in his endeavour to demarcate the boundaries of acceptable practice in human genetics.[11] However, he was not successful in achieving closure on the question until the publication of his pivotal essay in 1948.[12] Penrose tackled the issue of anticipation head-on, analysing the evidence in the case of myotonic dystrophy, the disease with the strongest evidence for anticipation. What was new in Penrose's study was a persuasive thought experiment that suggested that what appeared to be anticipation was merely an artefact caused by poor experimental design, selection bias and variable age of onset of disease.

To make this point, Penrose produced a table from Bell's data that visually juxtaposed the ages of onset of fifty-one pairs of parents and children who suffered from myotonic dystrophy (Figure 11.1). The table showed that the distribution of ages of onset in parent-child pairs was not symmetrical. In the majority of pairs, the child developed the disease twenty to forty years before their parent had. These were just the sorts of findings, Penrose noted, which were easily observed 'simultaneously' in parent and child, i.e. within the usual time frame in which studies like this were undertaken. The empty regions of the table, he felt, should have contained what he called 'complementary cases' in which the disease occurred at a later age in the child than in the parent – but these were cases that were likely to be missed in short-term family studies.[13]

Child

Parent

Years	0	10	20	30	40	50	Total
50		4	3	2	—	—	9
40	8	5	5	—	—	—	18
30	3	9	1	1	—	—	14
20	3	1	—	—	—	—	4
10	2	4	—	—	—	—	6
0	—	—	—	—	—	—	—
Total	16	23	9	3	—	—	51

Figure 11.1: Age of onset in dystrophia myotonica, from L. Penrose, 'The Problem of Anticipation in Pedigrees of Dystrophia Myotonica', *Annals of Eugenics*, 14 (1948), pp. 125–132, on p. 128. Image reproduced by permission of John Wiley and Sons.

Penrose's next table graphically portrayed the expected correlation of ages of onset between parents and children in cases where the child was affected earlier than the parent, where there was simultaneous onset in parents and children, and where the child was affected twenty, forty and sixty years after the parent

(Figure 11.2). It is notable how persuasively this table suggests the existence of individuals that had escaped the attention of clinical researchers. The vast majority of parent-child pairs in the observed data fall within the 'child earlier' and 'simultaneous onset' sections of the correlation table. By making the assumption that the correlation of ages of onset between parent and child should in fact be a symmetrical one, Penrose concluded that a significant amount of data was missing. It was, Penrose claimed, 'perhaps not an unreasonable assumption' that 'at least as many pedigrees had been missed as had been recorded'.[14]

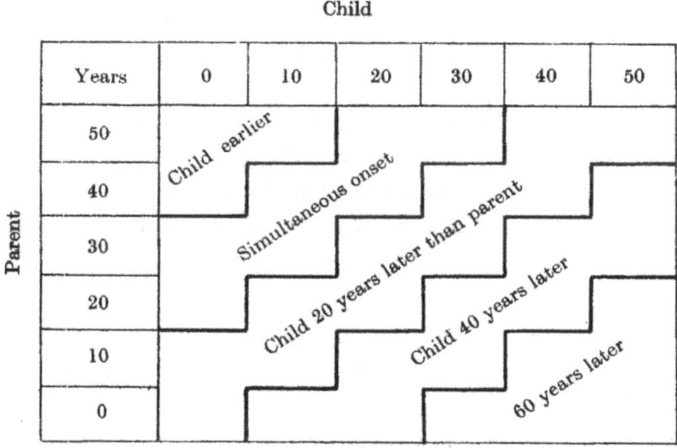

Figure 11.2: Age of onset correlation table showing relationship of dates of onset, from L. Penrose, 'The Problem of Anticipation in Pedigrees of Dystrophia Myotonica', *Annals of Eugenics*, 14 (1948), pp. 125–132, on p. 129. Image reproduced by permission of John Wiley and Sons.

Penrose made this assumption because of his genetic hypothesis of the cause of variation in age of onset. It had always been difficult to propose a genetic cause for anticipation. For one thing, there seemed to be no plant or animal model demonstrating this pattern of heredity.[15] Additionally, there was no real way to explain the phenomenon directly within the framework of Mendelian genetics, which left no room for a mutation that somehow increased in severity over succeeding generations. Allelic modification, according to which the onset of disease is determined by two genes, one modifying the effect of the other, was the only logical explanation for the variable manifestation of an autosomal dominant disease like myotonic dystrophy. This was also the explanation Penrose adopted, but it implied a symmetric distribution of onset of disease: an equal number of cases of early-onset disease in parents with late-onset disease in children, as cases of late-onset disease in parents with early-onset disease in children.[16]

Penrose therefore turned his attention to the researcher's ability to ascertain and count differences in the age of onset between parents and offspring to explain anticipation. He argued there would be complete ascertainment of cases if there were 'simultaneous' onset of the disease in parent and child, that is if the child developed the disease at an earlier age but in almost the same calendar year as their parent. If the disease appeared at the same age in parent and child, it would be separated by one generation or thirty calendar years. In these cases, Penrose argued, the likelihood of the researcher ascertaining the case would be reduced by 50 per cent. He felt that there would be almost no chance of ascertainment if the disease manifested late in the child (sixty years from the age of onset in the parent).[17] When one considers the relatively short work life of an individual researcher and the difficulties inherent in family studies, particularly of ascertaining the state of health of individuals long dead or who might not develop the disease for decades to come, Penrose's arguments appear quite reasonable.

With these assumptions in mind, Penrose assigned frequencies to his hypothetical alleles and, assuming the posited rates of incomplete ascertainment, calculated values that were very close to those observed by Bell in the case of myotonic dystrophy. The observed correlation coefficient of ages of onset between parent and child was 0.32 (as compared to Penrose's calculated 0.33), and the observed correlation coefficient of ages of onset between siblings was 0.67 (compared to Penrose's calculated 0.71).[18] This strongly suggested that his hypothesis was valid. Penrose added weight to these theoretical calculations by comparing the multi-allelic situation that he posited for myotonic dystrophy with similar multi-allelic loci in fruit flies and in humans, allowing him to conclude that 'the hypothesis that the peculiarities of inheritance of dystrophia myotonica are due to modification by one or more genes is not biologically improbable'.[19]

Consolidation of Human Genetics in the Post-War Period

There is a great deal of rhetorical strength to Penrose's 1948 paper. The scientific and medical community clearly found Penrose's assumption of missed 'complementary pairs' and his genetic hypothesis of allelic modification compelling. Most practitioners found it so compelling, in fact, that they just assumed Penrose's complementary pairs existed without ever seeing proof of their existence.[20] His argument thus stood unopposed for decades. The Dutch neurologist Chris Höweler, who challenged Penrose's hypothesis in 1986, later reflected that it took him 'four years of thinking and rereading Penrose's paper about fifteen times' before he identified the problems with the argument.[21] But the persuasiveness of Penrose's paper alone cannot explain the impact it had on the scientific and medical community. Arguments along similar lines had, after all, been developed in the decades before World War II, and yet findings of anticipation continued to be published. So the question remains how a thought experiment based on unproven assumptions, no matter how elegant and persuasive, could sway opinion on the question of anticipation after World War II. In order to answer this question, one has to look at the confluence of a variety of scientific, political and institutional factors that occurred at the time of Penrose's publication.

Some recent historical work has emphasized the continuity of medical genetics in the pre-war and post-war periods, particularly in the United States.[22] Others, including many human geneticists, have placed the critical period for the field in the decade between 1955 and 1965.[23] There is good evidence to support both claims. Nevertheless, I want to argue that the decade immediately following World War II was crucial in the history of human genetics. It was in this decade that membership in the field began to shift from enthusiasts with mixed backgrounds to those specifically trained in human genetics, thus leading to the consolidation and professionalization of the discipline. In the process, the boundaries of disciplinary research agendas were defined, canonical texts were written, and a new generation was trained that would dominate the field during the 1960s and 1970s. It was the adoption of Penrose's hypothesis about anticipation, among others, as part of the canon of human and medical genetics at this critical juncture that ensured its dominance for decades.

In North America these developments included the founding of a professional association, the American Society of Human Genetics, in 1948, and the creation of a professional journal, the *American Journal of Human Genetics*, the following year.[24] The difficulties facing this new field were clear to H. J. Muller, the first president of the American Society of Human Genetics. He argued that human genetics had to make its way between the errors of the past (the fascist eugenics of the Nazis) and the errors of the present (Soviet Lysenkoism).[25] He stressed the importance of the application of statistical analysis to the principles of Mendelian inheritance, and raised the hope that the mapping of the human genome through linkage analysis and chromosome mapping might one day be possible.[26]

At the same time, the science of genetics was experiencing its molecularization. Key developments included the discovery that DNA formed the genetic material in bacteria (1944) and viruses (1952), the elucidation of the molecular structure of DNA (1953), and the formulation of the central dogma of molecular biology (1957).[27] These discoveries, and the development and elaboration of the experimental systems in which they were made, fundamentally changed the field. The understanding of human heredity became increasingly mechanistic and quantitative. Post-war institutional expansion was aided by increased government funding and by direct funding from private organizations, such as the Rockefeller Foundation, which supported this new molecular and quantifiable approach to genetics.[28] Non-Mendelian forms of heredity, including cytoplasmic inheritance and neo-Lamarckian forms of heredity, were discredited because they did not fit into the dominant Mendelian paradigm.[29] Moreover, as the Cold War heated up, support for these controversial ideas became risky as they were linked to Communism, Soviet Lysenkoism and the destruction of the field of classical genetics in the USSR.[30] The association of Lamarckian notions of heredity with

Communist ideology could result in the possible loss of grants from funding agencies.[31] Those with unconventional views brought their scientific findings into line with standard thinking or found their work marginalized.[32]

When Penrose returned to England from Canada at the end of World War II, he stepped into perhaps the most prestigious position in the country for the study of human heredity. As the newly appointed Galton Chair of Eugenics at UCL, Penrose was also the head of the Galton Laboratory for National Eugenics and became chief editor of the Laboratory's journal *Annals of Eugenics* and its long-running monograph series *The Treasury of Human Inheritance*. An ardent anti-eugenicist, Penrose worked tirelessly to set the study of human heredity in Britain on more mathematically informed Mendelian principles. From the outset Penrose sought to separate the position that he occupied from its eugenic origins. As he informed one of his contacts at the Rockefeller Foundation in 1946, 'we are now mainly interested in specific problems of human heredity rather than in the general question of eugenics'.[33] He never liked the term 'eugenics' in his title, so he had 'The Galton Laboratory, University College' printed on his letterhead until 1963, when, after much effort, Penrose finally succeeded in having the name of the Galton Chair itself changed from the Chair of Eugenics to the Chair of Human Genetics. Changing the name of the journal published by the Galton Laboratory proved to be an easier task. Under his editorship the subtitle of the *Annals of Eugenics* changed to 'A Journal of Human Genetics', and the title of the journal itself became the *Annals of Human Genetics* in 1954.[34]

Penrose thus occupied a prominent role in the post-war Anglo-American community of human geneticists. Muller singled out the material published in the *Annals of Eugenics* under R. A. Fisher and Penrose as 'having set a very high standard' for statistically based genetic analysis.[35] And J. B. S. Haldane – one of Britain's most important geneticists and the individual who had recommended him for the post – called Penrose 'the greatest living authority on human genetics'.[36] Research at the Galton Laboratory under Penrose's leadership was supported by repeated operating grants from the Rockefeller Foundation from 1945 until his retirement in 1965.[37] The Galton Laboratory thus became one of the most prominent sites for training and research in human genetics after World War II. Penrose's students were not just from Britain but also from Canada, the United States, New Zealand and Australia. Many important figures in the field of human genetics during the second half of the twentieth century either trained or worked at the Galton. The list reads like a *Who's Who* of the field, including, among others, Barton Childs, Harry Harris, David Hsia, Ursula Mittwoch, Jan Mohr, Arno Motulsky, James Renwick, Edith Rüdin and Curt Stern.[38]

In his landmark book *The Structure of Scientific Revolutions*, Thomas Kuhn discussed the importance of textbooks in establishing and defining 'the legitimate problems and methods of a research field for succeeding generations of practitioners'.[39] It is in textbooks, also, that one can see most readily how quickly anticipation was rejected. Between 1930 and 1948 many textbooks dealing with human hereditary disease dealt with anticipation, whether or not the author(s) agreed with the concept.[40] After 1948 the situation changed dramatically, even as the number of textbooks on human and medical genetics published rapidly increased. Of the thirty textbooks surveyed in Table 11.1 that were published between 1949 and 1970, fully 50 per cent do not mention anticipation at all. The remaining 50 per cent discuss it in a negative fashion, explaining away findings of anticipation using some or all of the arguments made by Penrose in his 1948 paper. Penrose's explanation for anticipation was thus adopted into early human genetics textbooks as a paradigmatic achievement, which helps to account for the rejection or disappearance of anticipation in the writings of those trained in human and medical genetics.

Table 11.1: Human or medical genetics textbooks, 1949–70

Date	Author(s)	Title	Discussion of Anticipation		
			Negative	Unlikely	No Mention
1949	C. Stern	*Principles of Human Genetics*	✓		
1951	T. Kemp	*Genetics and Disease*		✓	
1953	A. Sorsby	*Clinical Genetics*		✓	
1954	J. Neel and W. Schull	*Human Heredity*			✓
1955	S. Reed	*Counseling in Medical Genetics*			✓
1956	E. Colin	*Elements of Genetics*			✓
1959	A. Montagu	*Human Heredity*			✓
	L. Penrose	*Outline of Human Genetics*	✓		
	J. A. F. Roberts	*An Introduction to Medical Genetics*			✓
1960	C. Stern	*Principles of Human Genetics*			✓
1961	L. Penrose	*Recent Advances in Human Genetics*			✓
1962	C. Clarke	*Genetics for the Clinician*			✓
1963	W. Lenz	*Medical Genetics*	✓		
	L. Penrose	*Outline of Human Genetics*	✓		
	J. A. F. Roberts	*An Introduction to Medical Genetics*			✓
1964	C. Clarke	*Genetics for the Clinician*	✓		
	V. McKusick	*Human Genetics*			✓
1965	M. Whittinghill	*Human Genetics and its Foundations*	✓		
1966	D. Y.-Y. Hsia	*Lectures in Medical Genetics*			✓
	J. and M. Thompson	*Genetics in Medicine*		✓	
1967	R. Pratt	*The Genetics of Neurological Disorders*	✓		
	J. A. F. Roberts	*An Introduction to Medical Genetics*			✓
1968	A. Emery	*Heredity, Disease, and Man*	✓		
1969	C. Carter	*An ABC of Medical Genetics*			✓
	C. Clarke	*Selected Topics in Medical Genetics*	✓		
	H. Lynch	*Dynamic Genetic Counseling*			✓
	V. McKusick	*Human Genetics*	✓		
1970	A. Emery	*Modern Trends in Human Genetics*			✓
	R. Goodman	*Genetic Disorders of Man*	✓		
	J. A. F. Roberts	*An Introduction to Medical Genetics*			✓

A brief examination of the first of these textbooks, Curt Stern's *Principles of Human Genetics*, illustrates both the small size of the human genetics community, Penrose's influence within it during this early period, and the importance of these textbooks in setting the foundation for the education and training of human geneticists in the 1950s and beyond. Stern was a German-born geneticist who had first trained with Richard Goldschmidt at the Kaiser Wilhelm Institute for Biology in Berlin, before receiving additional training in genetics in the Morgan group's 'fly room' at Columbia under the auspices of a Rockefeller Foundation fellowship. Unable to return to Germany with the rise to power of the Nazi Party in 1933, Stern was fortunate to obtain a position at the University of Rochester, where he taught courses in general and human genetics.[41] Stern wrote his textbook 'in an attempt to fill the need for an introduction to the study of human genetics'.[42]

Stern and Penrose appear to have met and formed a collegial relationship during the latter's sojourn in North America during World War II. By January 1941 the two had begun a correspondence and arranged for an ongoing exchange of reprints of their articles.[43] Their correspondence would continue until Penrose's death in 1972.[44] As a geneticist with statistical training, Stern already had cause to be cautious of anticipation, noting that 'the concept of anticipation does not readily fit in with the system of genetic facts and interpretations'.[45] He agreed that ascertainment bias likely lay behind findings of anticipation and felt that Penrose's theory of allelic modification offered an explanation for the observed differences of ages of onset from one generation to the next.[46]

The German human geneticist Eberhard Passarge called Stern's *Principles of Human Genetics* 'the first textbook of human genetics'.[47] James Neel, one of Stern's most famous and influential students, called it 'the most successful textbook on human genetics ever written'; large numbers of the three English-language editions were sold, and it was translated into seven foreign languages.[48] Victor McKusick, another pioneer in the field of human and medical genetics, called Stern's work 'the most influential textbook' of those that he read during his own education in human genetics during the early 1950s.[49] The impact of this text was pervasive in the field, and many of the papers published between 1948 and 1970 that discussed anticipation cited Penrose's influential paper, Stern's textbook or both in their criticisms of anticipation.

The influence of Penrose's explanation of anticipation went beyond the confines of human genetics proper. Before World War II, most advocates of anticipation had been clinically oriented researchers. They reported findings of decreasing age of onset of disease over successive generations within the families that they studied, even if they could not explain the cause of their observations. After Penrose's influential paper, however, discussion of anticipation in the clinical literature became increasingly uncommon. Where anticipation was discussed, it was generally only to dismiss findings of decreasing age of onset in succeeding generations as statistical artefacts.[50] Only in the case of myotonic dystrophy did two researchers, both trained during the 1930s, continue to put forward the argument that anticipation was indeed taking place. Their findings were essentially ignored.[51]

This shift in clinically oriented literature was due in part to the development and expansion of the field of human and medical genetics. The descriptive clinical papers of the pre-war period were giving way to more analytical papers that relied increasingly on statistical and genetic analysis. Clinical specialists did not often receive much statistical or genetic training as part of their medical education. Those specifically trained in genetic and statistical analysis became the acknowledged experts, and physicians tended to defer to their opinions. The experience of the British neurologist Dr John Walton, now Baron Walton of Detchant, provides an illuminating example of the changes taking place in the study of human heredity in the 1950s and how these developments helped in the disappearance of the concept of anticipation.

Walton finished his medical training at Newcastle Medical School in 1945. He served in the British Army from 1947 to 1949, and he began his neurological research as an assistant to Professor F. J. Nattras at Durham University.[52] During his medical training Walton had received only 'rudimentary' training in human genetics.[53] When it came to analysing the results of his neurological studies, Walton sought the advice of experts. He consulted with the animal geneticist Dr Ursula Philip (King's College, Newcastle upon Tyne) and Dr Cedric Smith, a statistician and geneticist at the Galton Laboratory.[54] One of Walton's papers dealt with various forms of muscular dystrophies and sought to determine their genetic mode of inheritance. Walton also, rather unsuccessfully, attempted a linkage analysis between the muscular dystrophy genes and other genetic markers.[55] He submitted his paper to the *Annals of Human Genetics*, and Penrose, as editor, invited him to the Galton Laboratory to discuss it. In his submission, Walton had included a brief discussion of reported findings of anticipation. Penrose disagreed with this 'and argued that this was an artefact of identification' and that 'the offspring of affected individuals were identified earlier as suffering from the disease'.[56] As a result, there was no discussion of myotonic dystrophy or findings of anticipation in the published version of this paper, or in a follow-up paper published the following year.[57] In this way Penrose was able to directly police the boundary he sought to mark between acceptable and unacceptable practice in human genetics.

Walton's research and his experience in publishing his results illustrates several of the changes outlined above, including the decline of descriptive clinical observation in favour of genetic and statistical analysis, and the rising authority of geneticists and statisticians who were specifically trained to undertake such analyses. The example also graphically reveals Penrose's role as a scientific gatekeeper. As a young neurologist, Walton sought to publish the results of his research in an important scientific journal. As the editor of the journal, Penrose sought to ensure that the papers published in the *Annals of Human Genetics* met his standards of scientific excellence. Penrose believed that anticipation was an artefact, Walton readily removed its discussion from his paper, and anticipation vanished from the scientific literature.

Conclusion

In the years following World War II, the concept of anticipation in hereditary disease, once used to describe findings of decreasing age of onset of illness in succeeding generations, all but vanished from the scientific and medical literature. Where anticipation was discussed, it was now almost universally dismissed as having been caused by statistical error and ascertainment bias. The key turning point in the reception of anticipation was the publication in 1948 of a paper on the subject by Lionel Penrose. A number of factors, scientific, political and institutional, facilitated the spread and acceptance of Penrose's theories. This period saw the rise to dominance of a Mendelian and increasingly mechanistic framework for understanding heredity. Unconventional interpretations of genetic phenomena, both eugenic and Lamarckian, were suppressed by political and social pressures. Penrose's prestige, social capital and connections, as well as the scientific value of his arguments, all helped to ensure the rapid spread of his ideas and their inclusion in a significant proportion of the textbooks used to train the rapidly increasing ranks of human and medical geneticists. These developments helped Penrose achieve a long-sought goal of placing anticipation beyond the bounds of accepted scientific discourse. Anticipation had become a textbook case of a notion of human heredity that became outmoded and was discarded because it did not fit within the boundaries of contemporary developments in human genetics. Such observations remained beyond the pale until the early 1990s, when the discovery of a new form of dynamic mutation allowed researchers to relate the development of earlier-onset forms of disease directly to genetic changes that occurred from one generation to the next.

Acknowledgements

I am grateful for the suggestions and comments to this essay made by the editors of this volume, Bernd Gausemeier, Ed Ramsden and, in particular, Staffan Müller-Wille. Research on this subject would not have been possible without the help of the archivists at the Rockefeller Archive Center, the University College London Library Special Collections and the American Philosophical Society Library. I cannot thank Chris Höweler and Lord Walton of Detchant enough for being willing to share their recollections with me; their contributions were invaluable. Earlier versions of this essay were presented at the Human Heredity in the Twentieth Century (A Cultural History of Heredity V) Workshop and the NIH Office of History Works in Progress Seminar. I am grateful for the feedback given at these meetings and from the Fellows of the NIH Office of History, Director Robert Martensen and Deputy Director David Cantor. Special thanks go to Hank Grasso of the NIH Office of History for his help in preparing the images used. My work has been supported by funding from the Social Sciences and Humanities Research Council of Canada, the Rockefeller Archive Center, the Max Planck Institute for the History of Science and the National Institute of Neurological Disorders and Stroke.

12 'THE MOST HEREDITARY OF ALL DISEASES': HAEMOPHILIA AND THE UTILITY OF GENETICS FOR HAEMATOLOGY, 1930–70

Stephen Pemberton

What dimensions of twentieth-century experience made medicine 'genetic' and genetics 'medical'? This question, deftly addressed in Nathaniel Comfort's *The Science of Human Perfection: How Genes Became the Heart of American Medicine* (2012), is a multifaceted problem. In consolidating his book's broader argument, Comfort explains how cytogenetics gave medical geneticists their 'organ' in the 1960s. The 'gene' then became to medical genetics what the heart already was to cardiology – a way of marking and legitimating professional identity. Yet, as Comfort also makes clear, medical geneticists' 'getting their organ' only meant at this stage that physicians could deliver greater diagnostic accuracy and more refined preventive measures.[1] Not until the 1980s and 1990s, with the rise of molecular medicine and gene transfer experimentation, did gene-based therapies emerge as a viable and sustained preoccupation for experimental physicians. Comfort's historical treatment of medical genetics confronts such conundrums by localizing medical interest in genetics in a much longer time frame – the long twentieth century (1890s to the present). Most contentiously, Comfort also challenges the 'disingenuous' idea among most practitioners of genetic medicine as well as a few of its historians that the eras of DNA (1950s–1960s), genomics (1970s–2000s) and post-genomics (2000s–present) have little in common with the expressly eugenic eras that preceded them.[2] Comfort's interpretive framing of the problem makes clear why the histories of physicians' long-standing interest in hereditary disorders should matter to scholars interested in the histories of human genetics and medicine. The histories of human genetics and medical progress have long been interwoven, and to a degree that our historical narratives have still not adequately articulated.

A localized focus on the histories of well-recognized 'hereditary' diseases can aid historians in clarifying what is 'genetic' in medicine and 'medical' in genetics. As Peter Harper highlights in his *Short History of Medical Genetics* (2008), even though medical genetics is usually situated as a development of the late

1950s onwards, any account of this 'specific field of research and practice' will be misleading if it ignores the substantial attention that physicians devoted to hereditary diseases and their transmission in preceding decades and even centuries.[3] Harper suggests it is somewhat arbitrary to treat the heyday of classical genetics as the definitive period of gestation for medical genetics, because 'writings on the medical aspects of inheritance, chiefly in the form of information on hereditary disorders, stretch back not only to the beginning of modern genetics in 1900 but a century earlier, thanks to the interest and careful reports of physicians'.[4] Harper and Comfort each explain in their own fashion that our histories of human and medical genetics must undoubtedly account for the considerable attention that inquisitive physicians devoted to knowledge of hereditary maladies before the mid-twentieth century. A good starting point is haemophilia, a disease that physicians regularly characterized as 'the most hereditary of all diseases' between 1855 and 1965.[5]

This essay utilizes haemophilia – the archetypal hereditary bleeding disorder – as a reference point for interpreting the rise of genetic medicine; it does so by localizing how genetics mattered to experimental haematologists from the 1930s through the 1960s in their primary mission to manage haemophilia and other bleeding disorders among patients and their families.[6] Experimental physicians who made haemophilia and other hereditary bleeding disorders a focus in the mid-twentieth century were among the first doctors in the United States to feel the pull of both classical and molecular genetics and try to integrate these 'allied' sciences into their ongoing efforts to advance medical research and education as well as manage disease in the clinic. The story I tell here is based on the standard narrative of development that experimental haematologists working on hereditary bleeding disorders themselves tell about the evolution of their field. My point here is not to get to the essential truth of that story – either to validate its perspective or to problematize its assumptions – but to emphasize that the geneticization of haemophilia in the mid-twentieth century was advanced not by geneticists or researchers *tout court* but specifically by experimental physicians who were primarily focused on the haematological dimensions of the disease. These physicians were working in the tradition of experimental pathophysiology, and they came to embrace genetics in the mid-twentieth century for its perceived relevance to the clinic – well before it was fashionable to do so.

Such integration of genetics into experimental haematology came naturally to many of its practitioners because, in their way of thinking, medical knowledge of haemophilia was *always already* 'genetic' in the sense that some concept of heredity had long been perceived as a critical aspect of this disease. Medicine was effectively transforming haemophilia into a manageable disease in the decades immediately following World War II. This therapeutic revolution was largely haematological in its orientation, meaning that advances in genetics were at best secondary to the principal aim of identifying and controlling the mechanisms that were most immediately responsible for prolonged bleeding in patients. Yet even as leading experimental physicians privileged haematological over genetic understandings of hereditary bleeding in the post-war decades, advances in genetics were usually interpreted as complementing the medical community's preferred, haematological strategies of control. In this particular context, that is, the importation of genetics into clinical settings was possible because it did not represent a radical challenge to traditional concepts, methods or institutional arrangements.

Hereditary Bleeding in the Longue Durée

Haemophilia has been the subject of continuous medical and scientific concern since the beginning of the nineteenth century, and heredity has been integral to the concept of haemophilia from its inception.[7] The concept of haemophilia was effectively born in 1803, the year that Philadelphia physician John Conrad Otto (1774–1844) published 'An Account of an Hemorrhagic Disposition Existing in Certain Families' in New York's *Medical Repository*. The 'Account' related the plight of the descendants of a woman named Smith, who settled in Plymouth, New Hampshire, in the late 1720s. Many of Mrs Smith's descendants exhibited what Otto called a 'hemorrhagic idiosyncrasy' or 'disposition'; yet the condition did not afflict Smith herself or any of her female kin. This 'surprising circumstance' indicated to Otto that females were capable of 'transmitting' the disease to their sons, although they were themselves not affected by it.[8]

Following a relatively short period between 1803 and 1817, when American physicians played a critical role in shaping medical conceptions of the disease, English, French and German physicians proved to be far more interested in advancing the science of hereditary bleeding.[9] The medical literature on haemophilia was already considerable by the 1860s, and much of it highlighted the overwhelming evidence of familial inheritance and the preponderance of cases among males, which some estimated to be as much as fourteen male cases for every reported case in a female.[10]

German physicians were especially effective in advancing knowledge of the disease beginning in the 1820s; collectively, their approach to the problem of hereditary bleeding helped establish standards for clinical thinking about haemophilia.[11] Christian Friedrich Nasse (1778–1851), a medical professor at the University of Bonn, published the first comprehensive clinical investigation of the 'hereditary disposition to fatal bleeding' in 1820. His clinical studies confirmed that this hereditary disposition only occurred in males, that these males showed no signs of transmitting the disease themselves, and that it was their unaffected female relations – mothers and sisters – who transmitted the condition through marriages with men who exhibited neither symptoms nor a familial history of bleeding. Nasse elevated this finding into a principle of clinical practice when he maintained that observance of this inheritance pattern was a necessary condition for any diagnosis of this hereditary disease. The principle was known in medical circles as 'Nasse's law' well into the twentieth century.[12] Yet Nasse's law was not universally observed among doctors treating bleeder patients. There were many physicians who believed that haemophilia could occur in females, or that the condition was transmissible directly through the male as well as female line. There was also considerable debate about how to explain *de novo* cases of haemophilia – i.e. the appearance of classic haemophilia symptoms among males who had no family history of the disorder.

Although it may be hard to imagine that physicians ever doubted that haemophilia was a blood disease, not until the 1890s did clear evidence emerge from experimental laboratories showing that patients with haemophilia suffered from impaired blood coagulation. If haemophilia's relevance for nineteenth-century medicine centred on its conceptualization as a constitutional and hereditary malady, its medical profile changed considerably once haematological enthusiasts cast haemophilia as a veritable blood disease in the opening decades of the twentieth century.[13]

Haemophilia's reputation as a hereditary disorder of the first order continued to matter among American physicians even as its status as a blood disease grew between 1900 and World War I. Nowhere was this reputation more apparent than in the ubiquity with which Progressive-era medical literature recommended that sisters of haemophilic boys and men refrain from having children or even marry. Such females were identified by a variety of names – most commonly, in English, as 'carriers', 'transmitters' or 'conductors'.[14] Eugenicists and geneticists spurred physicians as well as the public to emphasize haemophilia's hereditary dimensions even as the disease's haematological dimensions became the practical as well as experimental focus by the late 1910s. A critical year was 1911, the year that British physicians William Bulloch and Paul Fildes published an unprecedented study of the hereditary features of haemophilia as part of the *Treasury of Human Inheritance*, edited by Karl Pearson and authorized by the Francis Galton National Laboratory for Eugenics.

Bulloch and Fildes gave precedence to the hereditary dimensions of haemophilia by defining the malady quite simply as 'an *inherited* tendency in *males* to *bleed*'. This definition emphasized what they described as the disease's three cardinal characteristics, and reinforced their self-described 'opinion' that haemophilia should be known as a 'chronic liability to immoderate haemorrhage' that was essentially 'hereditary' and 'confined to the male sex'.[15] Accepting that medical experts had always disagreed about whether a haemophilia diagnosis should be reserved only for male patients, Bulloch and Fildes reviewed and annotated the 949 known cases of haemophilia that had been identified since 1519, and effectively mapped out 607 family pedigrees of hereditary bleeding on this basis. They found only forty-four families that exhibited indisputable histories of haemophilia. Ten of these forty-four families reported female bleeders among them (nineteen individual cases in all). But Bulloch and Fildes determined that the available evidence in each case was too limited, too circumstantial or too easily explained by other, more prevalent disorders to be true haemophilia in a female.[16] They therefore concluded that transmission of haemophilia followed the pattern predicted by Nasse – namely, that it passed exclusively through the unaffected mothers and sisters of haemophilic males, whom they called 'conductors'. Importantly, Bulloch and Fildes also sought clarification in the literature as to whether affected males could pass on the disorder to their offspring after 'skipping' a generation. They concluded that the literature did not support this notion.[17]

The idea that only males got haemophilia rose to the level of orthodoxy following the rise of Mendelian thinking in the 1910s. While Pearson's emphasis on descriptive science prohibited Bulloch and Fildes from employing a Mendelian perspective in their haemophilia study, many of their readers found confirmation of Mendel's relevance there.[18] The publication of Bulloch and Fildes's research followed on the heels of Thomas Hunt Morgan's 1911 discovery (using fruit flies) that certain heritable traits are linked to sex characteristics and transmitted in accordance with Mendelian principles. Geneticists soon deduced that the well-documented hereditary defect for haemophilia was located on the X chromosome and conformed perfectly to a Mendelian understanding of sex-linked recessive inheritance, and the interwar years witnessed haemophilia's rise as an exemplary X-linked recessive disorder.[19] By the 1930s haemophilia was widely cited as a sex-linked recessive genetic defect by experts seeking to educate the public about the relevance of heredity to their lives.[20]

While physicians invested in haemophilia research remained generally supportive of the new genetic understandings of haemophilia, these dimensions of the disease eventually became secondary in the 1910s, particularly after the rise of transfusion medicine in World War I. William Henry Howell, the influential physiologist at Johns Hopkins Medical School, went so far in 1914 as to declare Bulloch and Fildes's hereditarian definition of haemophilia 'unsatisfactory'. 'All recent works agree ... that this delayed or deficient coagulability ... is the characteristic feature of hemophilia', he stressed, and that 'attempts to explain the proximate or ultimate cause of the condition [should] start from this point'.[21] As anyone paying attention understood, the science of heredity provided a principle for preventing haemophilia's transmission, while the haematological perspective yielded the possibility of its clinical control. Physicians who encountered haemophilia in the era almost always did so in a clinical setting, where transmission was a far less pressing problem than stopping a bleed, ameliorating pain, or preventing a death. The practical benefits of framing haemophilia as a blood disorder were far more evident to physicians by the 1920s than the eugenicist's emphasis on its hereditary dimensions; and yet there remained plenty of occasions – e.g. confirming a diagnosis or curtailing familial transmission – where physicians happily embraced the hereditarian orthodoxy.

Haematology and the Hereditarian Orthodoxy in the 1930s

While haemophilia was widely described as a sex-linked hereditary disease during the 1930s, physicians invested in experimental medicine remained primarily interested in clarifying the defect responsible for delayed clotting. Haemophilia's status as a haematological disorder was no longer in question, although there was little agreement among investigators regarding what pathophysiological mechanism was the culprit. The dominant theory in the early 1930s held that a platelet defect was responsible. Another theory held that an inhibitory substance in the blood prevented prompt clotting. A third proposed that haemophilic bleeding was due to a missing clotting factor (a globulin) in the blood plasma. Not until the late 1930s did growing evidence from the hematologic laboratory point to the general correctness of the third theory. Thus, between 1939 and 1947, classical haemophilia was collectively redefined as a plasma clotting factor deficiency (a deficiency of antihaemophilic factor, today known as clotting factor VIII). What I would like to stress in this section, before moving on to the 1950s, is how the science of heredity factored into this ongoing discussion among leading haemophilia researchers.

The physicians who were at the leading edge of haemophilia research in the 1930s were not trained in the science of heredity; indeed, very few practitioners knew enough about genetics before the late 1940s to qualify as experts. In 1930, for instance, the *Journal of the American Medical Association* reported indirect transmission of haemophilia through the male as a novel find, suggesting that Mendelism took a while to penetrate into the medical field (in the USA at least).[22] The 1920s were a transitional decade in which inquisitive haemophilia doctors were aware of the hereditarian study of Bulloch and Fildes as well as Mendelism, but not yet prepared to deploy their understanding of haemophilia's genetic features in ways that substantially advanced their experimental or therapeutic practice.

As was true in the 1920s, the 1930s witnessed haematologists largely observing the hereditarian orthodoxy that Bulloch and Fildes had laid out in 1911, i.e. they were fairly uniform in reserving the haemophilia diagnosis for male patients with congenital bleeding.[23] But even if haematologists increasingly relied on Mendelian concepts in their thinking about haemophilia, they appear to have done so rather superficially. In fact, haematologists had ample justification to downplay the importance of these concepts vis-à-vis the emerging potential of medicine to utilize blood and plasma transfusions to manage the severest of bleeds.

Mendelism did not tell clinicians much more about hereditary haemophilia than was already evident in the extant medical literature. In a sense it told them even less, since there was confounding variability of symptoms, severity and health histories to be found among patients exhibiting hereditary bleeding. Experienced clinicians were experts in such diversity, and the clinical usefulness of genetics was minimal when it came to improving the diagnosis, treatment and prognosis of individual bleeder patients. As far as the cardinal clinical criteria for haemophilia went, knowledgeable clinicians of this era only entertained questions of heredity once they had established that the patient had a prolonged clotting time and symptoms consistent with a congenital bleeding disorder.[24] The hereditary profile was less critical, particularly since a large minority of haemophilia cases lacked a family history to confirm a pattern of inheritance. In fact, geneticist J. B. S. Haldane reported in 1935 that a full third of haemophilia cases were the result of mutation.[25]

The only area where genetics had practical import was in preventing familial transmission of the bleeding disorder. Thus as more clinicians gained fluency with Mendelism, they learned that they could tell patients and their families the actual probability that female carriers of the malady would have a haemophilic son (25 per cent) or a carrier daughter (25 per cent). Even here, however, the gain in knowledge did not substantially alter the clinician's approach. What experimental haematologists knew about classical genetics in this decade mostly just confirmed the correctness of the preventive approach that medical doctors had endorsed since the early nineteenth century: namely, that sexually mature members of haemophilia families should be discouraged from procreating (especially the females).

Even though physicians working on haemophilia in the 1930s did not substantially alter their views on the basis of work in genetics, some of the more inquisitive investigators among them did endorse the possibility that the sciences of heredity might one day be critical to the clinical management of haemophilia. In the USA this debate centred around the work of one haemophilia specialist in particular – a young haematologist at the University of Illinois named Carroll LaFleur Birch (1895–1969) who was unique for being the first female physician in the United States to gain an international reputation as a haemophilia researcher. In the 1930s she agreed with the new hereditarian-genetic orthodoxy that characterized haemophilia as 'recessive, sex-linked character'. Interestingly, however, Birch would soon become a leading advocate for saying that haemophilia might best be characterized as a 'sex-limited disease' (i.e. as occurring only in males on the basis of non-genetic factors) on the grounds that this characterization better served the purposes of clinical management. Biological sex, she theorized in 1931, potentially held the key to controlling haemophilic bleeding, but not through the mechanisms of sex-linked heredity; she posited a relationship between sex hormones and the control of blood clotting. Her theory built upon the idea that female transmitters of haemophilia were somehow immune to the disease.[26] Oxford University's Robert Gwyn Macfarlane later described her intriguing thesis thus: 'Women don't get hemophilia; therefore, if you feminize a male by means of a sex hormone, he will stop having hemophilia'.[27]

Birch's work first garnered significant professional and media attention in the spring of 1931, when she reported some initial success in alleviating bleeding in two 'high-grade hemophiliacs' following treatments by ovarian extract.[28] Journalists were quick to report the idea that sex hormones might hold the key to controlling haemophilia. Even before Birch's first paper appeared, the Associated Press identified her patients as brothers from a 'family of hemophiliacs in Southern Illinois'. Birch told the AP reporter that an 'injection of the extract on one of them resulted in no symptoms of the disease for eleven months'.[29] The older brother, whose haemophilia was more severe, reportedly had no bleeding for five and half months following a transplant of the ovarian extract to his abdominal wall.[30] The full results of her experimental hormone treatments appeared in the *Journal of the American Medical Association* in late 1932. Nineteen of the haemophilia patients she had treated with ovarian extract had a 'good response', while nine others had shown 'definite but less marked improvement'. She was nevertheless cautious and did not recommend ovarian extract as a substitute for blood transfusion.[31]

Although there was a good deal of enthusiasm for Birch's findings in 1931 and 1932, subsequent study of her sex hormone thesis failed to confirm her claims that ovarian extract reduced the frequency or severity of bleeding episodes in haemophilia patients.[32] Birch's work on sex hormones did not end as she hoped, but it did generate medical interest in the possibility that haemophilia might not be an exclusively genetic disorder.[33] Birch continued to maintain throughout the 1930s that haemophilia was possibly a 'sex-limited disorder' (i.e. the result of epigenetic factors) as well as being a 'sex-linked disorder' (i.e. a genetic phenomenon).[34] By the late 1930s physicians treating haemophilia patients were thus still seeing very little knowledge coming directly from genetic studies that contributed substantially to the pressing need to improve clinical management of the condition. Yet Birch's work had also given haemophilia investigators an opportunity to consider the relevance of genetics to their haematological strategies of control.

Genetics among Post-War Haemophilia Researchers, 1947–65

The years between 1947 and 1965 were a particularly important era in the medical effort to understand and manage haemophilia and other hereditary bleeding disorders. The principal focus of haemophilia research in the era was overwhelmingly upon improving clinical management of interminable bleeding. When physicians treating patients with hereditary bleeding spoke of 'prophylaxis', they were more often referencing transfusion practices or behavioural techniques for preventing or alleviating bleeds rather than dwelling on how to curb the transmission of the disorder. Advances in transfusion medicine and the wartime innovation of plasma fractionation convinced many physicians that experimental haematology was capable of bringing haemophilic bleeding under increasing degrees of control. In the United States, print, radio and television discussions of haemophilia often conveyed that promise to the public beginning in the early 1950s. More importantly, advances in transfusion medicine spurred patients and families to join physicians in rendering haemophilia management. The rise of haemophilia advocacy after 1947 embodied this movement.[35]

Among the post-war experimental haematologists studying haemophilia and other bleeding disorders were a handful of enterprising investigators who saw a need to integrate state-of-the-art haematology with the advancing science of human genetics. A striking and early example was the era's debate about the possibility of 'true' haemophilia in female patients. The question of whether or not 'true' sex-linked haemophilia could occur in a female was still unresolved in the late 1940s. The 1930s and 1940s witnessed the occasional report in the medical literature of females experiencing moderate to severe hereditary bleeding. Cases of female bleeders so far were all questionable haemophilia because none met the Mendelian requirement of being homozygous – a female offspring of a male haemophiliac (X^HY) and a female carrier (X^HX). A few scientists theorized that the X^HX^H combination was lethal.[36] Others, like Birch, suggested the X^HX^H genotype might exist, but not manifest as a bleeding tendency because of non-hereditary factors.

This debate about the X^HX^H genotype was not settled until two key discoveries in the early 1950s. In the first, pathologists Kenneth Brinkhous (1908–2000) and John Graham (1918–2004) bred haemophilic dogs at the University of North Carolina (UNC) to determine what were the practical consequences of mating a male haemophiliac with a female carrier. The beauty of the laboratory had always been its capacity for creating conditions that were improbable in the everyday world, and the new availability of haemophilic dogs allowed Graham and Brinkhous to breed female dogs that were homozygous for haemophilia in 1949 and thereby demonstrate the viability of this 'theoretical genotype'.[37] British investigators resolved the debate for good in 1951 when they confirmed the 'nigh impossible' X^HX^H genotype in a clinical setting by discovering two female patients with classical haemophilia (factor VIII deficiency).[38]

The haemophilia dog studies engineered by Brinkhous and Graham at UNC in the late 1940s and early 1950s were an initial effort by experimental haematologists focused on haemophilia to make genetics a formal part of their laboratory-based approach to hereditary bleeding disorders. As I have detailed elsewhere, Brinkhous acquired a pair of female Irish setters with a hereditary bleeding disorder to study haemophilia in the human.[39] Brinkhous saw the existence of these bleeder dogs as an unparalleled opportunity to advance haemophilia research if he could only render them into a sustainable animal model of human haemophilia. Ironically, the bleeding episodes in the dogs needed to be managed if they were to become a viable colony of experimental animals. Not only did these bleeder dogs require regular transfusions from normal, healthy dogs so that they could grow into sexual maturity, but these potential 'canine hemophiliacs' also had to feel well enough to engage in sex when researchers sought to breed them. Keeping the dogs healthy and happy enough to reproduce involved advanced medical as well as animal care, but it also entailed a thorough understanding of the genetics involved if the animals were to be experimentally useful. At the end of the day, Brinkhous and Graham embraced human genetics as an allied science of haematology because their earliest experiences trying to create and sustain of colony of bleeder dogs had shown them that genetic knowledge was a practical necessity for advancing haematological control of haemophilia and other bleeding disorders.

As early as 1953 this canine haemophilia research helped Brinkhous's research team develop an important new assay for measuring clotting defects in patients with hereditary bleeding (the partial thromboplastin time). And in the 1960s the dogs were the initial test subjects for what was to become the first antihaemophilic clotting factor (VIII) concentrate to be approved by the FDA and marketed to the public. By the mid-1970s the productivity of this medical animal model was widely known in medical circles (especially among haematologists). In fact the National Institutes of Health funded this dog colony continuously between 1947 and 1998, making Kenneth Brinkhous the first medical researcher to receive fifty years of extra-mural funding from the NIH.[40]

As previously suggested, Brinkhous's colony of dogs with hereditary bleeding gave researchers affiliated with UNC diverse incentives to make genetics central to their understanding of haemophilia and its management. In fact dog research depended on it, initially because it was necessary for Brinkhous, Graham and their colleagues to demonstrate that the hereditary bleeding in these dogs was not only a canine form of haemophilia, but also one that was largely indistinguishable from that found in human patients with classical haemophilia (factor VIII deficiency). The genetic studies on the dogs thus had at least three purposes. First, they helped Brinkhous and Graham create a sustainable colony of bleeder dogs for research. Second, they helped reify these bleeder dogs as true canine haemophiliacs wherever the dog's condition was confirmed to be an X-linked recessive disorder. And third, the UNC dog studies ultimately helped haemophilia researchers to understand that the clinical variability seen in the blood of haemophilia patients and carriers had its roots in genetic mechanisms. Later, when haemophilia research went molecular in the 1980s and 1990s, these dogs became ready-made tools for testing the viability of genetic therapies as well as recombinant DNA therapies for clotting factor replacement.[41]

The career of John Graham is also telling of how Brinkhous and the UNC blood researchers embraced genetics in the 1950s. Graham had been a young pathologist in the late 1940s, and Brinkhous (who was the pathology department chair) insisted that Graham get some formal training in genetics for the betterment of both research and teaching at the medical school. Brinkhous sent Graham to Michigan's Heredity Clinic (at Lee Dice's Institute of Human Variation) to learn some formal genetics for three months in 1954 from James Neel and others. Then when Graham returned to North Carolina, Brinkhous directed him to teach human genetics to the medical students regularly. For the next fifteen years Graham was given full autonomy to teach human genetics to the medical students, and he always stressed the importance of obtaining genetic information from their patients, and how to go about collecting and analysing it. Graham also initiated and ran the Medical School's genetics graduate research programme from 1961 to 1985. Later, he liked to brag that the distinguished paediatrician Dr Neil Kirkman had told him that 'he had never encountered clinical clerks as adept at taking pedigrees as those he had found on his arrival at Chapel Hill in 1965. Not at the [Johns] Hopkins, not at Emory, not at Oklahoma'.[42]

But it is Graham's growing reputation as an expert in the genetics of hereditary bleeding and the work that he did in conjunction with Brinkhous's research group that best illustrates how genetics mattered for post-war physicians engaged in experimental haematology. Graham was the lead investigator in all of the department's work involving the biochemical genetics of blood coagulation, and his contributions helped usher in an age where physicians were increasingly familiar with the science of genetics and geneticists became increasingly educated by physicians about practical as well as experimental medicine.[43]

Finally, while the haemophilia research programme at UNC was unusual in its relatively early embrace of genetics, it is pretty clear that the high productivity and reputation of this programme was directly related to the fact that Brinkhous embraced genetics and made it integral to the core project of finding ways to understand and control the blood coagulation defects in haemophilia and other hereditary bleeding disorders. It was the novel opportunity to do canine studies of hereditary bleeding that gave Brinkhous, Graham and other haematological researchers considerable incentives to care about genetics and make it central to their concept of haemophilia and other hereditary bleeding disorders.

Beyond UNC, experimental haematologists in the 1950s and 1960s were also trying in a more concerted way to integrate genetic understanding into their pathophysiological investigations of hereditary bleeding disorders. In *The Bleeding Disease* (2011), I detailed how vibrant the field of blood coagulation research was in the 1950s. Various changes and innovations in how experimental haematologists identified human patients with bleeding disorders and analysed their blood brought about a serious reconsideration in how haematologists and other physicians should classify haemophilia and other forms of hereditary bleeding. There was a growing awareness in the 1950s of the diverse mechanisms underlying hereditary bleeding after three research groups independently reported what is today called factor IX deficiency in 1952.[44] Haemophilia C (factor XI deficiency) and other autosomal forms of hereditary bleeding were also coming to light. By 1954 experimental haematologists had discovered so many real and imagined variations on hereditary bleeding that William Dameshek, the editor of the journal *Blood*, issued a special issue devoted to debating the question, 'What is Hemophilia?' The 'hematologic rialto', Dameshek complained in 1954, now included 'not only haemophilia, but pseudo-haemophilia, haemophilia-like disease, para-haemophilia, deuteron-haemophilia, haemophilia A, B, C, haemophiliod disease A, B, C, Christmas disease, and the "literature" knows what else!'[45] Such clarification seemed necessary to haematologists because the clinicians among them were being overwhelmed by the growing experimental literature on blood coagulation.[46]

The hereditarian principle of linking haemophilia to the sex characteristics was brought into play by influential haematologists at this critical moment. Some experimental haematologists advocated a more liberal interpretation of the haemophilia concept (a few going so far as to say that haemophilia was not a disease but a syndrome), but they did not prevail.[47] Haemophilia researchers from Oxford (like Robert Gywn MacFarlane) as well as UNC (John Graham) were among those experts who insisted that haematologists and physicians pay attention to inheritance patterns. In particular, they appealed to the principles of Mendelian genetics as a key to differentiating classical haemophilia and haemophilia B (then called PTC deficiency or Christmas disease) from the other forms of hereditary bleeding whose inheritance patterns indicated autosomal forms of transmission (factor XI deficiency, sometimes called haemophilia C, being among the most controversial). In effect, these leading haemophilia researchers were arguing that the principles of Mendelian genetics provided the critical rationale for linking observations about the relative incidence of hereditary bleeding among males and females to a truly causal explanation for the pathologies. From the late 1950s forward, if one wanted to speak of haemophilia truthfully – to be within the bounds of truthful scientific discourse regarding this pathology – one had to acknowledge that sex-linked inheritance was an essential aspect of haemophilia's identity.[48]

Conclusion: Haemophilia Management and the Rise of Medical Genetics

As far as medical concepts go, haemophilia's long-standing reputation as a hereditary disease provides historians with an opportunity to gauge what was old and new in medicine's embrace of genetics across the long twentieth century. I have tried in my overview of the history of haemophilia research to suggest how a few post-war physicians sought to integrate genetics into the broader haematological programme that medical practitioners as well as medical historians usually credit with bringing haemophilic bleeding under control. Again, the broader relevance of this history is to frame haemophilia among other widely acknowledged hereditary diseases as a lens onto the local conditions under which medicine became genetic and genetics medical, and to emphasize that clinical concerns infused the experimental haematologist's interest in and early embrace of medical genetics in the post-World War II decades.

What, then, did these high-profile medical advances in post-World War II haematology and haemophilia management have to do with genetics? As detailed here, there was a long and storied tradition that conceptualized haemophilia as a hereditary disease. That medical tradition began in the early nineteenth century, and it preceded haemophilia's widespread characterization as a potentially tractable blood disease by no less than nine decades. While there were modest attempts among physicians in the first half of the twentieth century to relate the clinical and genetic aspects of haemophilia to one another, serious talk of genetics in its relation to the medical management of haemophilic bleeding largely entered clinical settings at the same time that blood coagulation research was enjoying its so-called 'golden age' (between 1947 and 1964).[49] Thus even as post-war haematologists constituted haemophilia management primarily in terms of clotting science and transfusion medicine, leading investigators were also increasingly keen to embrace what genetics and geneticists offered to the mix.

If advances in genetics from the 1950s forward complemented the medical community's preferred, haematological strategies for controlling haemophilic bleeding, that was also because the importation of genetics into clinical settings did not represent a radical challenge to the traditional concepts, methods or institutional arrangements of organized medicine. When genetic counselling as a formal aspect of haemophilia management in the United States appeared in the mid- to late 1960s, it was immediately integrated by leading haematologists with other specialty approaches in what became known as the comprehensive care model for treating bleeding disorders.[50] Thus genetics was formally integrated into haemophilia care at the same time that concentrated blood products brought the promises of post-war haematology to fruition and helped solidify the concept that the best approach to treating haemophilia was a comprehensive approach – i.e. one that involved a multidisciplinary team of medical experts and health workers.

The relevance of haemophilia's history to the broader story of how genetics became medical and medicine genetic runs against the grain of the standard narrative among practitioners of genetic medicine that stresses that medical genetics had very limited clinical relevance in therapeutic terms before the molecular turn of the 1980s and 1990s made gene-based interventions a promising and occasionally effective tool in the clinicians' therapeutic armamentarium. Among haemophilia specialists, specifically, the late 1980s and 1990s witnessed the first truly promising therapeutic applications of molecular biology in the form of recombinant DNA clotting factor concentrates. Yet as I have suggested in this essay, leading experimental haematologists had long regarded haemophilia as both a haematological and a genetic disease, and they had not only imagined these dimensions of the disease as complementary, but long viewed effective clinical management of the disease in terms of both heredity and blood. On the basis of what other historians of science and medicine are now uncovering, I suspect that haemophilia was not unique in this regard. In any case, it seems dubious today to call haemophilia 'the most hereditary of all diseases'; it is merely one among many prominent hereditary diseases in medical history that illustrates the actual as well as potential clinical rewards of explicitly framing medicine as genetic and genetics as medical.

Acknowledgements

The author thanks Staffan Müller-Wille and Ed Ramsden; the essay benefited greatly from their comments and editorial acumen.

13 HOW PKU BECAME A GENETIC DISEASE

Diane B. Paul

The problematic of this essay may strike some readers as odd. After all, phenylketonuria, or PKU as it is more commonly known, was understood to be inherited nearly from the time it was first identified as a disease entity by Norwegian physician and biochemist Asbjørn Følling in 1934. Indeed, by the mid-1940s its autosomal recessive pattern of inheritance had been well confirmed. But the genetic aetiology of PKU was not always a defining characteristic of the disease. Whether an inherited condition is characterized as 'genetic', and, if so, the meaning and importance attached to that designation, is context dependent, varying with place, time, the specific features of the disease that are of greatest salience to patients, researchers and clinicians, and the general visibility of genetics in the culture. Thus Jean-Paul Gaudillière has shown that for Lionel Penrose and his British peers, the characterization of Down syndrome as a genetic (chromosomal) abnormality had very different implications than it did for Jérôme Lejeune and many of his compatriots in France.[1] And writing of cystic fibrosis, Keith Wailoo and Stephen Pemberton explain that in the 1960s and 1970s, 'neither families nor experts emphasized the "genetic" features of the disease. To be sure, they understood it to be a "hereditary" disorder, but this way of thinking did not capture what they saw as its fundamental biological underpinnings'.[2] This essay asks: when and why did the inherited nature of PKU come to seem a crucial feature of the disease, and with what consequences? Before tackling this cluster of questions, it might be useful to take note of a few essential facts about the nature of the metabolic error in PKU and how it is diagnosed and treated.

The Nature, Diagnosis and Control of PKU

PKU is a rare autosomal disorder of phenylalanine metabolism. Phenylalanine, an essential amino acid that is found in all dietary proteins, is necessary for protein synthesis and other biological functions. Because humans do not synthesize it endogenously, they must obtain it from the foods they eat. However, only some of the ingested phenylalanine is necessary for normal growth and development, with the rest ordinarily converted to another amino acid, tyrosine. In PKU, a deficiency of the hepatic enzyme phenylalanine hydroxylase (PAH) results in an insufficiency of tyrosine and, more importantly, an excess of phenylalanine. In some way that is still not well understood, the accumulation of phenylalanine and its metabolites damages the developing brain. Before newborns were routinely screened for the disease, affected children typically experienced profound cognitive impairment and often other abnormalities, including small head size, hyperactivity, seizures and behavioural disruptions. In severe cases, children might lose interest in their surroundings and never learn to talk, walk, sit up by themselves, or control their bowels or bladder. Most such children were eventually institutionalized.

As early as the 1930s it was hypothesized that since humans only obtain phenylalanine from the foods they ingest, the effects of the disease might be ameliorated if affected infants were placed on a diet from which most of the phenylalanine was eliminated. This goal could not be achieved simply by avoiding dietary protein, since the result would be severe malnutrition. (Lionel Penrose had tried this approach in the 1930s with disastrous results.[3]) However, in the 1950s researchers succeeded in developing amino acid mixtures from which the phenylalanine had been removed through a charcoal filtering process, and experiments seemed to indicate that nutritional therapy could at least ameliorate some symptoms of the disease. Those experiments converged with the development of a urine test that could be used to detect the disease in infants, and some physicians, hospitals and public health programmes in the USA, UK and elsewhere began to screen asymptomatic newborns. But screening really took off in the 1960s with the invention by Robert Guthrie and his assistant Ada Susi of a bacterial inhibition assay for PKU that was simpler, cheaper and far more sensitive than the urine test, and that could administered just a few days after birth, before brain damage had occurred. At least equally important was the choice of blood – obtained by sticking the heel of the newborn – as the analyte. Unlike urine, blood is highly stable, making it possible for results to be sent to central laboratories where they could be processed in batches. By 1965 thirty-two American states had enacted screening laws, and by the end of the decade, blood spot screening for PKU had become routine in most US states and Canadian provinces, the UK, Australia, New Zealand, Israel, France and Germany. By the mid-1970s the practice was near universal in Central and Northern Europe.

As a result thousands of children and their families have been spared the devastating effects of this disease. Today many individuals who once would have been institutionalized can attend school, hold jobs, and marry and raise families. But the dietary regimen is arduous. A typical adult ingests about 3,500–5,100 mg of dietary phenylalanine each day. Adults with PKU are ordinarily advised to ingest no more than about 350–500 mg, and those with the most severe forms of the disease even less. To achieve a reduction on the scale suggested even in moderate cases requires not only the exclusion of obvious high-protein foods like meat, fish, nuts and dairy products, but also severe restrictions on such staples as wheat flour, rice (one-half cup cooked: 59 mg), pasta (one-quarter cup cooked spaghetti: 103 mg), potatoes and beans. Even many fruits and particularly vegetables contain substantial amounts of phenylalanine. For example, a medium banana contains 58 mg, a single medium Portobello mushroom 64, a quarter cup of raw peas 73, and a quarter cup of cooked spinach 164.[4] One plain bagel or a single slice of cheese pizza would exceed the total daily phenylalanine allowance for most people with PKU. Although there are low-protein substitutes for wheat flour, rice, pasta, bread and other food items, high manufacturing costs and small markets combine to make these products expensive, the costs are often not covered by insurance, and these artificial foods do not have either the consistency or taste of their natural counterparts.

Moreover, to ensure sufficient protein intake as well as calories, therapy for PKU must include substantial amounts of a special 'medical food' or 'formula' that contains all the necessary amino acids except phenylalanine, plus extra tyrosine, calories and often vitamins and minerals. The formula consists of free amino acids, which in contrast to intact proteins have an unpleasant taste and smell. To avoid large fluctuations in blood phenylalanine, the formula should be consumed in at least three servings spaced roughly evenly throughout the day.

In the 1960s, when blood screening for PKU began, it was generally assumed that the diet could be discontinued around the age of five, when gross brain development was complete. In reality, the need for treatment turned out to be perpetual. Controlling the phenylalanine intake of infants and small children, whose diets are largely determined by others, is a very different matter than it is for older children, and especially adolescents and adults, who make their own choices and who need to cope with the challenges of managing diet in the context of school, work and social activities. Food is central to the way we develop and maintain social relationships, but the extraordinarily restrictive PKU diet creates profound barriers to sharing meals with others. The diet is onerous for other reasons as well. People with PKU must calculate the phenylalanine content of everything they eat and factor it into their daily allowance. They can never be spontaneous about going to restaurants or to a friend's house for dinner. The medical food and low-protein substitutes are costly; the costs may not be covered by insurance, or if so only for children, up to a certain amount or with other limitations. For these and other reasons, few adolescents and adults rigorously adhere to the diet.[5] The multiple obstacles to adherence to the diet help explain why people with PKU often experience neuropsychological deficits, such as difficulties concentrating and generalized anxiety, and why they are twice as likely as their peers to experience problems in school.[6]

PKU as Paradigm

Nevertheless, dietary treatment for PKU has indisputably been a success, even if, as with many medical accomplishments, it is incomplete. That success has come to serve as the premier illustration of the point that 'genetic' should not be equated with 'fixed'. A typical example: 'There is a tendency among the lay public to believe that genetic means unchangeable. This belief is false. For example, the invariably serious neurological effects of phenylketonuria ... can be largely prevented by providing the affected newborn with a phenylalanine-restricted diet'.[7] In particular, the case of PKU has come to serve as a model of successful intervention in the course of a genetic disease. Indeed, it is often referred to as a paradigm for thinking about such diseases. Thus the Canadian biochemical geneticist Charles Scriver writes that '*PKU is now celebrated as one of the first human genetic diseases to have an effective rational therapy*. Such recognition constituted a "paradigm shift" in medical thinking about genetic disease in general'.[8] Today, in the discourse of biomedicine, the successful alteration of the course of PKU is used to illustrate the unique contribution of genetic research to the improvement of clinical outcomes and also to legitimate the expansion of newborn screening to other conditions and of other kinds of genetic testing. As British geneticist Angus Clarke notes, the PKU case has 'accumulated a large store of goodwill and of ethical credit in favour of genetic screening programmes' in general.[9]

However, before PKU could serve these purposes, the fact that it was *inherited* had to be emphasized to a much greater degree than had been the case in the 1960s, when most state screening programmes were established. To those politicians, parent advocates and others involved in the campaign to legislate screening for the disease, its hereditary character was of little importance. Similarly, while popular articles almost always noted that the disease was hereditary and occasionally described its recessive mode of transmission, the focus was elsewhere: on the ability to prevent mental retardation, thus sparing parents suffering and saving taxpayers money, and the possibility that a similar approach would prove effective against other retarding disorders. That the devastating effects of the disease had far more salience than its aetiology is reflected in the US state legislative hearings on mandated testing, where the fact that PKU was inherited received virtually no attention. None of the US statutes establishing newborn screening programmes even mentioned genetics. A committee that analysed the passage of those laws concluded that at the time, 'There was little recognition of the implications for public policy, or for the impact on individuals who were screened, of the fact that PKU is a *genetic* disease'.[10]

However, in the period when most US newborn screening programmes were established, the implications of that fact would anyway not have been obvious. A majority of US states had launched programmes by 1965, before prenatal diagnosis for the disease existed.[11] The PAH gene was only cloned in 1983, and in any case, access to abortion was highly restricted in the 1960s. PKU testing did incidentally provide information on carrier status since the parents of affected infants would be obligate heterozygotes. But in the 1960s the question of what difference it might make, if any, that a disease was genetic – and associated issues of genetic discrimination, confidentiality and privacy – did not yet appear on the policy agenda. (That is one reason for the lack of informed consent requirements in most newborn screening programmes.) These issues would only emerge in 1970s as the result of developments in both molecular and medical genetics.

Genetics in the Wider Culture: The 1970s

The mid-1970s witnessed an explosion of controversy over the use and regulation of genetic technology. One catalyst was the advance in molecular biology, which, even before the development of recombinant DNA (rDNA) techniques, prompted predictions of the 'genetic engineering' of new genes and human qualities. Already in 1969, California Institute of Technology molecular biologist Robert Sinsheimer eagerly anticipated the emergence of a 'new eugenics' that would overcome the limitations of the old variety. In his view, attempts to manipulate human breeding, a slow and clumsy process, would soon be replaced by direct genetic interventions – a prospect applauded by some commentators and deplored by others.

Then in 1973 Herbert Boyer and Stanley Cohen created the first transgenic organism by splicing frog DNA into a plasmid for an *E. coli* bacterium, an achievement followed a year later by Rudolf Jaenisch's creation of the first transgenic animals with the introduction of a foreign DNA tumour virus into the genomes of mice. The rapidly increasing ability to join molecules from diverse sources generated concern as well as excitement among elite molecular biologists, several of whom warned of the possibility that recombinant organisms of an unpredictable nature could be created and prove harmful to laboratory workers or, should they escape from laboratory containment, the general public. Their calls for strict procedures to prevent escape from containment and a moratorium on very risky experiments culminated in the Asilomar Conference of February 1975, which produced a temporary consensus that there should be extreme caution in rDNA experiments. Concern soon expanded beyond the boundaries of the molecular biology community. The US Congress held hearings on rDNA research, and some localities implemented their own regulations. Whether the new technology presented a threat to health or the environment or would serve to revive eugenics became matters of intense public concern. With the rapid commercialization of the field, debates also swirled around the morality of 'patenting life'.[12]

Contemporaneous developments in medical genetics aroused a similar mix of enthusiasm and concern. Amniocentesis, the first practical method for detecting genetic disorders in pregnancy, was developed in the 1960s but was of little practical utility before abortion was decriminalized. Following passage of the 1967 Abortion Act in the UK and the 1973 US Supreme Court decision in *Roe v. Wade*, amniocentesis for the purpose of detecting Down syndrome increasingly became a routine aspect of clinical practice. But the use of prenatal diagnosis also provoked controversy, especially around the issue of whether policies designed to forestall the birth of affected children signified a new eugenics.

In the 1970s as well, national and state legislation was first enacted to support research on genetic diseases, as well as promote and regulate genetic screening programmes. Responding to pressure from black professionals, celebrities and community activists who argued that the incidence of sickle cell anaemia was much higher than that of diseases that received far more attention, and that the neglect was explained by the race of the sufferers, in 1972 the US Congress passed the National Sickle Cell Anemia Control Act, which provided funding for sickle cell research, educational activities, and screening and counselling programmes. In his signing statement, President Richard Nixon declared sickle cell anaemia to be an 'especially pernicious disease because it strikes only blacks and no one else'.[13] Four years later Congress enacted the National Sickle Cell Anemia, Cooley's Anemia, Tay-Sachs, and Genetic Diseases Act, which permitted public funds to be used for voluntary genetic screening and counselling programmes.

By the mid-1970s many screening programmes (under a variety of public and non-governmental auspices) had been established for sickle cell disease and carrier status and also, at the community level, for Tay-Sachs disease. As there was no effective treatment for either disease, the primary aim of such screening was necessarily to provide reproductive information. But sickle cell testing was soon engulfed in controversy when widespread confusion between the sickle cell trait and the disease sickle cell anaemia resulted in the stigmatization of carriers and sometimes discriminatory treatment in jobs and education.

PKU Screening as a Cautionary Tale

In this context of heightened awareness of potential pitfalls in screening for genetic conditions, the question arose of what could be learned for the development of other screening programmes from the relatively extensive experience of screening for PKU. The Committee on Inborn Errors of Metabolism of the National Academy of Sciences (NAS), chaired by distinguished paediatrician and geneticist Barton Childs, was charged with investigating the history, current standing and effectiveness of screening for PKU, and also with reviewing screening programmes for other genetic conditions such as the haemoglobinopathies (sickle cell disease and trait and Thalassemia) and Tay-Sachs disease.

In its 1975 report the committee concluded that PKU screening was justified, but it criticized the haste with which screening statutes were enacted in the mid-1960s when there existed unanswered questions regarding which infants needed to be treated and for how long and the efficacy of the low-phenylalanine diet. According to the report, 'mass screening and treatment were implemented on a broad scale before adequate data were available on the indications and necessity for such treatment', and the decision to mandate the test was characterized as 'ethically questionable because of failure to consider enough facts'.[14] Legislators, hoping to save money and responsive to intense pressure from local parent organizations, enacted statutes whose implications they did not fully understand. To avoid a repetition of this experience, there should be greater oversight of genetic screening programmes, and the committee proposed a set of ethical, legal and economic principles to govern their operation.

The history of newborn screening for PKU thus served as a cautionary tale for genetic testing in general.[15] The lesson drawn by the committee and other commentators was that genetic tests should be assessed by more stringent criteria than was applied in the case of PKU, where screening was mandated prematurely, with 'thousands of infants ... subjected to an incompletely validated and potentially hazardous intervention'. The point was that although we were lucky and narrowly dodged the bullet, we cannot count on being so fortunate and should not make that mistake again.[16] But history could only serve as a warning if the Guthrie-Susi bacterial assay was defined as a genetic test and the uncertainties, complexities and unintended consequences of screening and treatment for the disease emphasized.

However, in other contexts of genetic research and medicine, the PKU story was already taking a different and ultimately more consequential turn, one that would reinforce the geneticization of the disease but also result in a radical simplification of the account of life with the disease. That trend began in the 1970s with the controversy over the genetics of intelligence and intensified in the 1980s with the debates about whether to map and ultimately sequence all human genes.

PKU and the Critique of Genetic Determinism

In 1969 Berkeley psychologist Arthur Jensen famously asked: 'How much can we boost IQ and scholastic achievement?' His answer, in effect, was 'not much'. According to Jensen, genetic differences accounted for at least half of the black-white gap in IQ test scores, which explained why compensatory education schemes had failed.[17] His essay produced a storm of controversy, with Jensen criticized both for exaggerating the significance of heritability estimates and for inappropriately generalizing from statistics on the heritability of IQ differences within races to conclusions about differences between them. Two years later Harvard psychologist Richard Herrnstein published an analogous argument in respect to social class, which he soon expanded to a book, *I.Q. in the Meritocracy*.[18]

The IQ debate had initially focused on the validity of genetic explanations for group differences in intellectual performance. The heritability of *individual* differences was taken for granted. Studies published by British psychologist Cyril Burt had seemingly established a heritability of about 80 per cent for IQ. But in 1972 Princeton psychologist Leon Kamin charged that Burt's results were, statistically speaking, too good to be true. After reviewing Burt's and the four other classic studies of the heritability of IQ, Kamin concluded that, 'there exist no data which should lead a prudent man to accept the hypothesis that I.Q. test scores are in any degree heritable'.[19] A heated debate followed on both the standards required to demonstrate the heritability of intelligence and the scientific and social value of heritability estimates.

Proponents of such research argued that it was both possible and desirable to design experiments on the heritability of human cognitive and personality traits, including intellectual performance, that met 'reasonable' methodological criteria; that newer and better-designed studies had confirmed the existence of a substantial heritability of IQ, even if the new estimates were lower than Burt's; and that these results mattered for social policy. The message was typically that compensatory education and other policies designed to overcome the effects of poverty and racism have rested on a naive belief in the power of the environment; to succeed, interventionist strategies needed to take genetic differences (as reflected in heritability estimates) into account. Critics, on the other hand, generally argued that heritability estimates of human mental and behavioural traits were scientifically and socially meaningless. They stressed the methodological difficulties involved in designing experiments that would break the association of genotype and phenotype (a problem resulting from the fact that relatives generally share similar environments), and they insisted that the enormous efforts required to overcome this problem could not be justified by either the potential scientific or social interest of the results. Heritability estimates, they argued, lack any policy relevance since they are not a measure of the importance of genes in determining an individual's phenotype; they are not generalizable (since heritability estimates vary with the mix of populations and environments); and above all, they are not an index of plasticity.

In the context of this emotionally charged debate, the efficacy of treatment for PKU provided a dramatic, decisive and easily understood rejoinder to the argument that a high heritability of IQ would defeat efforts to boost scholastic performance. Critics stressed that PKU was a trait with a heritability of 1.0; that is, all the phenotypic variation among newborns is due to genetic variation. Yet an environmental intervention prevents otherwise severe neurological damage. The ability to intervene in PKU thus demonstrates that a trait may have a high heritability and still be extremely sensitive to environmental change. Because the PKU case provided such a clear illustration of the fact that biology is not destiny, it came to serve as the standard illustration of the flaws of genetic determinism. In the early 1970s critiques of Jensen and Herrnstein almost invariably invoked the ability to intervene in PKU in arguing that research on the heritability of IQ was misguided. Indeed, the editors of a 1976 compendium of critical readings on the IQ debate wrote, 'To use the standard example, consider phenylketonuria', in explaining how novel manipulations of the environment can not only improve the performance of a given population (in the PKU case, the IQ scores of treated children) but reduce individual differences as well (since the diet would raise the mean IQ of children with the disease but not of others).[20]

A few years later, when the sociobiology debate erupted, the case of PKU was again deployed to argue against genetic determinism. The following passage from a contemporaneous critique is typical:

> There is an allele that, on a common genetic background, makes a critical difference to the development of the infant in the normal environments encountered by our species. Fortunately, we can modify the environments ... and infants can grow to full health and physical vigor if they are kept on a diet that does not contain this amino acid. So it is true that there is a 'gene for PKU'. Happily, it is false that the developmental pattern associated with this gene in typical environments is unalterable by changing the environment.[21]

The same example was again invoked for the same purpose when the IQ debate re-emerged with the 1994 publication of Richard Herrnstein and Charles Murray's *The Bell Curve*, which argued that intelligence is highly heritable and that differences in intelligence largely explained individual and group differences in social and economic status in the USA. Like Arthur Jensen, the authors also maintained that environmental interventions to raise IQ scores had proved largely futile, and that to be successful, social policy needed to take facts about the genetics of intelligence into account. The debate resurrected all the arguments and counter-arguments of the 1970s, including the same use of PKU. For example, one trenchant review of *The Bell Curve* argued that its authors were wrong to conclude that 'equalizing environments will have no effect' on intellectual performance, for 'it turns out that if you put all infants on a diet low in the amino acid phenylalanine, the disease disappears'.[22]

PKU and the Human Genome Project

While critics in the sociobiology and IQ debates cited PKU to argue that the social order is 'not in our genes', others deployed PKU for a quite different and in some ways contradictory purpose: the defence of a genetic approach to medicine, and particularly the international effort to map and sequence the complete human genome. When the Human Genome Project was first proposed in the mid-1980s, many biologists expressed concern that it would siphon funds from other, more scientifically interesting efforts. Potential funders were also wary. Aiming to convince their peers, members of Congress and the general public that this expensive project represented a worthwhile expenditure of public money, proponents mounted an intense public relations campaign that involved expansive claims for the scientific, technological, economic, social and medical value of the project. The information gained would secure US leadership in biotechnology and promote economic competitiveness, produce technologies that would revolutionize many domains of biology, and generate 'deep insights into the nature of humanity and our relationships to the world of which we are a part'.[23] Above all, it would alleviate suffering. Thus, according to its supporters, the project would revolutionize medicine, resulting in cures for dread diseases – an aim with deep appeal to Congress. According to Harvard molecular biologist Walter Gilbert, a 1980 Nobelist in chemistry, co-inventor of a major technique for DNA sequencing, and co-founder of the biotech companies Biogen and Myriad Genetics: 'The possession of a genetic map and the DNA sequence of a human being will transform medicine'.[24] Biologist Leroy Hood, inventor of an instrument to automate DNA sequencing and co-founder of several biotech companies, agreed that 'access to the genetic and sequence maps will fundamentally change the practice of clinical medicine'.[25]

But *why* should it revolutionize medicine? The assumption was that locating disease-causing genes on chromosomes and determining their nucleotide sequence was requisite to a deep understanding of the causes of disease and hence to the development of truly effective interventions. As James D. Watson, first director of the project, explained in summarizing a conversation with a congressman, in the struggle against disease it is an enormous advantage to find that genetics is a contributing cause. 'Ignoring genes is like trying to solve a murder without finding the murderer', he claimed. 'All we have are victims'. According to Watson, 'if we find the genes for Alzheimer's disease and for manic depression, then less money will be wasted on research that goes nowhere'. We thus need to convince members of Congress 'that the best use for their money is DNA research'.[26]

Critics were unimpressed by such claims for the importance of genomic information for human health.[27] They maintained that the project advocates were overpromising, and typically cited the 'therapeutic gap' – the fact that genetic research had produced many more tests to diagnose or predict disease than means to effectively treat or prevent it, except by preventing births of affected individuals. They noted that 'causal stories are lacking and therapies do not yet exist; nor is it clear, when actual cases are considered, how therapies will flow from a knowledge of DNA sequences'.[28] They tended to be especially sceptical of promises that gene therapy aimed at curing rather than mitigating the symptoms of disease would follow from possession of mapping and sequencing data.

In the context of controversy over the genome project, the PKU story acquired immense appeal to geneticists. With few effective interventions to point to other than abortion, the success in treating PKU came to function as a standard rejoinder to critics of the project, and more generally as a way to legitimate both genetic research and the expansion of genetic testing. Already in the early 1980s a metabolic clinician-researcher had remarked that neonatal screening programmes for PKU 'have been widely cited in textbooks of biology and genetics and in lectures to the general public', since they represent 'one victory in the struggle against genetic factors, which are seen as being unalterable'. And he noted that 'PKU programs have become a showcase of the benefits to be derived from large-scale screening for genetic disorders'.[29] With the controversy over the genome project, the case of PKU acquired even greater value to advocates of a genetic approach to medicine in general, and the expansion of genetic testing in particular.

The legitimating role of PKU is nicely illustrated by a pair of National Public Radio (NPR) interviews conducted in the 1990s. In the first, a caller to a show on the Human Genome Project asked about the relevance of genomics to breast cancer. He noted that the popular press was full of stories 'about the magic of science and how genes are going to solve all of our problems', suggested that we should focus more on social context, and asked, 'Has anything ever been solved by genetic research?' His question was tackled by Robert Waterston, director of the Genome Sequencing Center at the Washington University School of Medicine, who replied: 'In terms of has it solved anything, there's a genetic disease called phenylketonuria – PKU – and just simply by testing infants at birth – and for those infants who test positive, if you give them a different kind of milk, you prevent brain damage. So this is clearly an instance'.[30] Three years later, Francis Collins, then director of the US Human Genome Project, was also interviewed on NPR. That interview was bookended by comments on PKU. At the beginning, after acknowledging that 'the clinical consequences of genetics have been largely in the diagnostic arena up until now', Collins stressed that there are also genetic diseases for which treatments have been developed, 'including the one that all newborns are screened for, the thing called PKU, where simply getting on the right diet prevents mental retardation'. At the close, responding to a question about BRCA testing, he replied: 'I would say lives have been saved from this sort of genetic effort, actually, extending back some 20 or 30 years. And again, PKU is the example where the paradigm was proven'.[31]

A Triumph for Genetic Research?

For PKU to legitimate the Human Genome Project, the success of screening had to be attributed to a 'genetic effort'. But screening and treatment for the disease had been routinized in North America and much of Europe two decades before the PAH gene was cloned. The ability to treat PKU rested on the biochemical insight that an excess of dietary phenylalanine was somehow connected to the mental retardation associated with the disease, and that the symptoms might thus be mitigated if exposure to phenylalanine were reduced – an insight dating back to the 1930s. The attribution of the ability to prevent mental retardation to *genetic* research is a product of the 1980s and the controversy over the genome project. But it has now become standard, repeated even by those with no stake in promoting a genetic approach to medicine. For example, under the heading 'Most Traits are Affected by Environmental Factors as well as by Genes', the authors of a well-respected genetics textbook write that as a result of dietary treatment, the capacities of children with PKU 'can be brought into the normal range', and that 'PKU serves as an example of what motivates geneticists to try to discover the molecular basis of inherited disease. The hope is that knowing the molecular basis of the disease will eventually make it possible to develop methods for clinical intervention through diet, medication, or other treatments that will ameliorate the severity of the disease'.[32]

Improved molecular understanding may well enable more effective or less burdensome clinical interventions in PKU. But to date genetics has contributed remarkably little to either diagnosis or therapy for the disease. Both carrier testing for at-risk relatives and prenatal diagnosis for pregnancies at increased risk are possible if the specific disease-causing mutations in the family have already been identified, but the required analysis is complex and expensive, and neither procedure is widely used.[33] The cloning of the PAH gene generated enormous excitement about the prospect of gene therapy – but as with gene therapy more generally, those hopes were eventually disappointed.

Mutation analysis is sometimes helpful in predicting the severity of disease and in tailoring individual treatments. There is great allelic variation in PKU, however, with over 500 mutations identified in the PAH gene, and most individuals with the disease are compound heterozygotes.[34] This complexity has hampered efforts to develop diagnostic procedures based on genotype-phenotype correlation.[35] In treating patients, it may be useful to know whether a particular mutation is mild, moderate or severe. In particular, genotyping may help predict which individuals will respond to a new therapy involving supplementation with sapropterin (otherwise known as BH4 or by its trade name, Kuvan), an enzymatic cofactor for phenylalanine hydroxylase. But these are recent developments. To claim that the prevention of brain damage in PKU is a clear instance of 'genetic research' mocks the historical record.

As PKU acquired symbolic meaning, the story of its diagnosis and treatment became progressively simpler. Its cultural transformation began with the IQ and sociobiology controversies, where it served to illustrate what was wrong with genetic determinism, and it intensified with the controversy over the Human

Genome Project, where it served to demonstrate the value of a genetic approach to medicine in general and to the expansion of genetic testing in particular. Of course it functioned most effectively for these symbolic purposes when shorn of complications. In the 1960s and 1970s uncertainties, mistakes and unintended consequences were widely acknowledged, at least among medical geneticists and professionals in public health. But as PKU acquired paradigmatic status, all nuances were lost. 'One can, in fact, have the gene, yet with proper dietary changes never show the manifestations', writes one author.[36] According to another, by limiting dietary phenylalanine, 'individuals with the two mutant alleles for processing phenylalanine can avoid the toxic buildup of the amino acid in their brain. In essence, they modify their environment so that it contains little or no phenylalanine. And in that environment, the PKU mutant alleles are harmless'.[37] In the now ubiquitous narrative, treatment appears effortless and the cure complete. Individuals with PKU and their families and clinicians could only wish that were so.

Acknowledgements

This essay was adapted from chapter six of D. B. Paul and J. P. Brosco, *The PKU Paradox: A Short History of a Genetic Disease* (Baltimore, MD: Johns Hopkins University Press, 2013).

14 THE EMERGENCE OF GENETIC COUNSELLING IN THE FEDERAL REPUBLIC OF GERMANY: CONTINUITY AND CHANGE IN THE NARRATIVES OF HUMAN GENETICISTS, *c.* 1968–80

Anne Cottebrune

Whereas modern genetic counselling was already established in the UK and the USA by the 1940s, it was not until the beginning of the 1970s that it became institutionalized in the Federal Republic of Germany (FRG). During the first decades after World War II, it was provided sporadically to single persons, families, couples and parents of unborn children, who asked for advice from human geneticists established at the universities. In the 1970s regular genetic counselling services were introduced, driven, in part, by the increased interest of public health authorities. By then genetic counselling had become an acknowledged medical service, receiving government support and public acceptance. This essay traces the emergence of a climate favourable to genetic counselling. In particular, it analyses how eugenic motives shaped the discourse of human geneticists involved in the institutionalization of genetic counselling.

Over the past decades, an increasing amount of historical research has identified the longevity of eugenic discourses and practices – from the turn of the last century, when eugenics emerged as a biopolitical concept defined by the aim of improving the 'hereditary health' of the 'national body' (*Volkskörper*), to well beyond 1945.[1] Although eugenicists propagated voluntary 'genetic marriage counselling' long before the political upheaval of 1933, eugenics is usually regarded as a political programme demanding authoritarian implementation, a nexus epitomized by Nazi racial hygiene. As various historians have emphasized, however, the development of reproductive medicine and genetic diagnostics in the course of the second half of the twentieth century produced a new kind of eugenics, usually labelled as 'new eugenics' or 'liberal eugenics', which was no longer aimed at improving the genotype of a whole population, but instead at ensuring the genetic health of individuals and their descendants.[2] According to this view, new methods of genetic profiling and karyotyping transformed reproduction into a matter of individual decision-making and planning. For historians and sociologists, genetic counselling seemed a paradigmatic case for this shift towards a new biopolitical constellation.[3] They saw the field developing after 1945, in opposition to earlier authoritarian practices of eugenic 'education', as a non-authoritarian way of providing genetic information to protect families from genetic disease. Practitioners similarly depicted genetic counselling in terms of helping individuals make responsible decisions.[4] However, historians and sociologists have also pointed out that the field embodies the emergence of a new eugenic practice that helped to disseminate a normative model of genetic health in the target group.[5] As I would like to highlight in this essay, counselling practices also entailed a notion of individual responsibility for the genetic health of society.

The investigation of the motivations of experts who promoted genetic counselling services in the FRG invites us to take a closer look at the fundamental ambiguity of the neo-eugenic discourse that combined the motive of individualized prevention with the aim of population betterment. The project of genetic counselling can certainly be regarded as a response to individual worries about genetic risks, but it is also associated with a health policy aiming to reduce both risks in the population and public expenses. This ambivalent purpose of genetic counselling is reflected in the statements of many of its proponents. Until the beginning of the 1980s, the discourse of West German human geneticists regarding 'individualized' human genetics was still permeated with concerns about the biological future of humankind. From this perspective, this essay will question the assumption that eugenic motives were completely discredited after 1945. First I describe the key features characterizing the institutionalization of genetic counselling in the FRG that was, in accordance with international developments, connected with its integration into preventive medicine. Then I discuss the complex and multilayered discourse of the human geneticists who played a key role in the emergence of genetic counselling in West Germany, identifying the intermingling of individual-oriented and population-oriented motives in genetic counselling.

Institutionalizing Genetic Counselling in West Germany

The term 'genetic counselling' was introduced by the American human geneticist Sheldon C. Reed (1910–2003), who had been giving genetic advice to families at the Dight Institute for Human Genetics at the University of Minnesota from 1947. As he described it in 1974, he chose the notion to distance himself from a concept introduced by the Danish human geneticist Tage Kemp (1896–1964):

> There was no generally accepted name for what I was doing, although the terms 'genetic consultation' and 'genetic advice' had been used in the Dight Institute Bulletin ... I did not like Kemp's term 'genetic hygiene', because the popular concept of

> the world 'hygiene' in the United States had to do with the use of toothpastes, deodorants, and other relevant items. The term 'genetic counselling' occurred to me as an appropriate description of the process which I thought of as a kind of genetic social work without eugenic connotations.[6]

Reed is today considered a pioneer of the new approach to the provision of genetic advice. In the United States there was rapid growth in the numbers of centres of genetic counselling or 'heredity clinics' in the 1950s and 1960s.[7] Between 1968 and 1980 the number of private heredity clinics increased from 115 to 500.[8] In 1974 there were 387 centres in the USA (with the worldwide number at 890).[9] In the United Kingdom the first genetic clinic was established in 1946 at the Hospital for Sick Children in London.[10] Similar to the USA, the UK witnessed a rapid expansion of genetic counselling services in the 1950s and 1960s.[11] Due to these developments, the organization of genetic counselling services became a matter of international debate by the end of the 1960s. The World Health Organization's (WHO) expert committee on human genetics discussed these issues during a meeting in Geneva in September 1968. As a result the WHO published recommendations on genetic counselling in its technical report series; therein, genetic counselling was defined as a medical service that 'should be devoted to the welfare of the individual or family seeking advice'.[12] The counsellor, the paper stipulated, 'should not pursue any genetic programme designed to benefit future generations if this programme conflicts with the immediate interests of his patients'.[13] The WHO's resolution on the topic became a central reference for the West German human geneticists involved in the creation of the first genetic counselling centres in their country. They adopted the definition of genetic counselling as a form of preventive medicine, with emphasis on public education and the need for better training in human genetics for physicians. The 'preventive' understanding of genetic counselling was leaning on a new generation of epidemiological studies that helped to establish the modern concept of risk in the 1950s. A well-known prototype of this kind of research was the so-called Framingham prospective study on chronic heart diseases that was aimed at identifying risk factors and their impact over a long period of time.[14] Epidemiological research soon extended to the field of human genetics, and both geographic areas and birth cohorts were examined in order to detect genetic disorders and to define risk factors. During the 1970s, however, it became increasingly clear that 'risk populations' were not easy to access by means of genetic counselling. Acceptance for counselling services remained limited to the upper social strata. In consequence, human geneticists tended to propagate the ideal of the responsible patient taking care of his or her own health, and they promoted relevant educational measures. Beyond this, they supported pilot experiments with health centres conceived to gain access to populations that were under-represented in genetic counselling services.

The first German handbook on genetic counselling, written by the human geneticists Walter Fuhrmann (1924–95) and Friedrich Vogel (1925–2006), appeared in 1968. The turning point at which genetic counselling emerged as a topic of public concern was a conference entitled *Genetik und Gesellschaft* (Genetics and Society) held at the University of Marburg in 1969. The event brought together a new generation of human geneticists who had been trained after World War II, and it offered the opportunity for a long-overdue reflection on the discipline's past. The main organizer of the conference, the Marburg human geneticist Gerhard Wendt (1921–87), took pains to dissociate post-war human genetics from Nazi racial hygiene. He stressed the possible benefits to be expected from the recent methodological advances of human genetics. He used the publicity to demand the setting up of genetic counselling centres, an appeal he would repeat the following year in another high-profile conference.[15] For three days, around 100 experts, politicians and journalists attended fourteen presentations and discussed the implications of progress in biomedicine and human genetics.[16] Talks and debates were covered extensively in the press.

Wendt's call for the institutionalization of genetic counselling was readily taken up by public health authorities. From 1970 the German Ministry of Health had been considering the possibility of sponsoring a pilot programme, and between 1972 and 1975 it sponsored the establishment of two model institutes for genetic counselling in Marburg and Frankfurt to spur the creation of other centres throughout Germany.[17] The Frankfurt project was focused on urban populations with the aid of chromosome analysis, whereas the Marburg centre attended to a rural population and concentrated on spreading information about genetic counselling through leaflets, newspaper articles and radio programmes.[18] In this campaign, basic principles of human genetics and its implications for genetic counselling were depicted in order to promote the understanding of genetic risk. Publications in the mass media emphasized the prevention of children born with genetic disorders, highlighting how counselling services could spare families of suffering caused by genetic defects.[19] Counselling interviews would advise couples with regards to their family planning and reproductive choices. However, it was underlined that any final decisions should be left to those counselled.[20]

For each project, the Ministry provided funds of 210,000 DM over three years. From 1972 the costs of genetic counselling were covered by health and social insurance schemes and expanded rapidly. In 1979 a survey conducted by two human geneticists, Eberhard Passarge (b. 1935) and Friedrich Vogel, revealed the existence of around twenty genetic counselling centres in the FRG.[21] The efforts of West German human geneticists in creating a dense network of counselling services were successful. Most of the centres were created through private funds, especially from foundations created to help disabled persons and their families. Their financial support can be explained partly by the participation of human geneticists in their managing committees, but also by the growing acceptance of prevention concepts in the aftermath of the Contergan scandal that had so shaken the West German public in the early 1960s.[22] It was not until the end of the 1970s that governmental support was more widely provided, thus enabling genetic counselling to become an integral part of standard medical services. In Heidelberg, for example, genetic counselling services were first institutionalized in 1977 through the financial support of the Stiftung Rehabilitation, a foundation devoted to the integration of disabled people. When the Stiftung withdrew from sponsorship in 1981, the state of Baden-Württemberg took its place. At a national level, the Aktion Sorgenkind (Problem Child Campaign), another foundation devoted to the support of disabled persons and especially handicapped children, was very active in sponsoring genetic counselling until the early 1990s. The board of the Aktion Sorgenkind started discussing activities in the field in 1979, after Gerhard Wendt had suggested funding the Stiftung für das behinderte Kind (Foundation for the Handicapped Child), over which he presided. A specific foundation was created in early 1980 to distribute funds from the Aktion Sorgenkind for the promotion of genetic counselling, providing grants for the advanced training of physicians. Yet the Aktion Sorgenkind never saw its role as funding regular posts; from the beginning its support was conceived as temporary, intended to help overcome initial difficulties. In the end, all private sponsors retreated from sponsorship and genetic counselling became a state-run affair. The implementation of genetic counselling in the FRG was, therefore, the result of a conjunction of foundation-based and political sponsorship.

Post-War Narratives of Human Geneticists

After 1945 the promotion of the science of human heredity in the FRG was extremely difficult. Renamed *Humangenetik*, the field received very little funding during the 1950s. It developed with an emerging generation of human geneticists who were trained in the field in the 1950s and 1960s. Most of them were trained either at the Max Planck Institute for Comparative Genetics and Pathological Genetics (Max-Planck-Institut für vergleichende Erbbiologie und Erbpathologie), directed by Hans Nachtsheim,[23] or at the Institute for Human Genetics and Anthropology in Münster, led by Otmar Freiherr von Verschuer from 1951.[24] Both men were part of the old establishment of German racial hygiene. Yet from the late 1960s, human genetics experienced an accelerated process of medicalization. In this context, the new generation of human geneticists advocated a form of counselling for the benefit of the individual – i.e. the parents of unborn children – rather than for the benefit of society. Most of them stressed that while the counsellor had to provide patients and clients with the most accurate estimation of genetic risks, the final decision had to be left to the concerned persons alone. Owing to the advances of aetiological research, the development of biochemical tests, especially in connection with metabolic diseases, the extended application of chromosome diagnostics, and the operationalization of prenatal diagnostics from the 1970s onwards, counsellors were no longer dependent on statistical estimations based on phenotypical observations of the client's family. Counsellors were also increasingly able to provide clients with laboratory-based test results.

At the same time, German human geneticists struggled to convince the public that modern human genetics had nothing to do with eugenics and National Socialist racial hygiene. This became especially obvious on the occasion of the aforementioned symposium, *Genetik und Gesellschaft*. The main organizer of the Marburg symposium, Gerhard Wendt, who had been trained at Nachtsheim's Max Planck Institute in the mid-1950s, hoped that the conference could contribute to the emergence of a new image for human genetics as a socially relevant discipline, freeing it from the burden of its past in Germany. Wendt called for an objective discussion of the new possibilities of human genetics, arguing that while the public was aware of the impact of technological improvements, it did not yet appreciate the importance of recent advances in biology. Furthermore, he underlined the contrast between National Socialist eugenic politics and post-war human genetics. The latter, he wrote in the conference volume, had nothing to do with the

> wishful thinking of the Nazis that forced sterilization could be used to eliminate hereditary diseases ... The presentations will also show that modern human genetics does not see its task for society in developing questionable plans to improve the human race or utopian ideas of manipulating human genes.[25]

Wendt was not the only geneticist at the Marburg symposium who dismissed National Socialist racial hygiene. Reflecting on the National Socialist experience, many scientists focused on assessing the effects of old eugenics on the genetic make-up of the population. They argued that eugenic measures were unnecessary because they were ineffective. Thus, remarkably, eugenics was rejected not on ethical grounds, but rather due to its unrealistic objectives. In an article published in 1956 entitled 'On the Limits of Practical Eugenics', the veteran eugenicist Fritz Lenz had already come to the conclusion that the frequency of hereditary diseases had most probably not been reduced during the National Socialist era. Pointing to the effects of increasing mutation rates and medical care, he admitted that the prospects of classical eugenics were limited. This kind of rationale shaped the background in which institutionalized genetic counselling emerged during the 1970s. The public image of genetic counselling as a medical service for the benefit of the individual was closely connected to the experts' discourse on the impractical nature of the old eugenics.

During the Marburg conference, human geneticists developed two arguments against eugenics, which were put forward in the first talk by the British human geneticist Lionel S. Penrose. On the one hand, they drew attention to the impossibility of classifying genes as good or bad and pointed to the changing perceptions of various diseases in both past and present times.[26] On the other, they underlined the fact that hereditary diseases could never be eliminated due to mutations and the increasing number of heterozygotes. According to the human geneticists Helmut Baitsch and Horst Ritter, each individual was, on average, the carrier of five harmful genes.[27] Therefore, they concluded, it was obviously impossible to eliminate all harmful genes. This did not imply that human geneticists completely renounced the objective to influence the gene pool. Even if the majority of them were convinced that progress in medicine would cause an increase of harmful genes because it facilitated the reproduction of their carriers, they reasoned that the dysgenic effects could be limited to an innocuous level. This limitation could be realized through genetic counselling and the systematic implementation of protective measures against mutations. The alleged unfavourable effects of medical care and therapeutic improvements served, therefore, as an argument to stress that genetic counselling was necessary in the modern world.

While West German human geneticists presented systematic counselling and protection against radiation and other mutagens as the only realistic means to safeguard the gene pool of humankind, they depicted genetic engineering as neither practicable nor desirable.[28] It was also regarded as incompatible with the self-image of modern human genetics as a medical discipline.[29] West German human geneticists usually distanced themselves from utopian ideas about the breeding and modelling of human stock. In this context, heterologous insemination was also criticized for ethical reasons.[30] Speculations on a possible manipulation of the genome were dismissed as an option with little direct relevance that should not be overstated. They were also considered to be potentially harmful to the mission that human genetics had yet to fulfil. As Friedrich Vogel emphasized, the sensation caused by debates surrounding the selective engineering of the genome was hardly helpful to the establishment of human genetics as a discipline that was primarily concerned with disease prevention.[31] In this regard, West German human geneticists clearly distanced themselves from the debates within the North American human genetics community, epitomized by the CIBA symposium 'Man and His Future' in 1962. Instead of supporting positive eugenic measures aimed at altering the gene pool, preferably within a short period of time, West German human geneticists adopted a pragmatic approach to the genetic problems supposedly caused by civilization and medical progress. Based on his conclusions regarding the limited impact of 'old' eugenics, Lenz presented himself as an advocate of *Erbhygiene*, or gene hygiene, as defined by the Danish human geneticist Tage Kemp.[32] In his talk at the Marburg conference, Baitsch pleaded that they confine themselves to the practical task of human genetics in the service of preventative medicine:

> What is left for us to do is not to wait for a utopian era but rather bring about a number of small realistic steps, an important one of which is mutation prophylaxis ... and reducing the pathological significance of affliction due to hereditary disease through early diagnosis and treatment. We will be able to improve and strengthen genetic counselling and the awareness of society.[33]

Creating a demand for genetic counselling was an issue that was largely discussed among scientists involved in the institutionalization of human genetics. A precondition was the improved education of the medical profession and the wider public, especially groups considered as 'risk populations'. In 1972 Fuhrmann pointed out the important role of general practitioners as mediators:

> A comprehensive and timely genetic consultation often fails due to the insufficient knowledge of the concerned patients. Here, the practitioner is in a key position. It depends on his attentiveness and information if a patient comes to know about the possibility of genetic counselling and if he recognizes its value for his family.[34]

In the ideal case envisioned by human geneticists, the practice of counselling would incite people to make rational decisions, avoid risky reproductive behaviour and, ultimately, internalize their 'responsibility' for the coming generation. A restrained optimism prevailed. Yet it was usually combined with the notion of pervasive threats to the gene pool, as, for example, in the contribution of Horst Ritter:

> In reviewing the entire complex, we can see that on the one hand, the number of hereditarily ill people will increase over the next few centuries due to our medical achievements and changes in living conditions. On the other hand, however, one can predict positive developments in therapy, preventive medicine, and through the extension of eugenic counselling, though certainly with less success in the latter field. Therefore it seems quite possible that the potential positive effects may actually even out the negative ones.[35]

Interestingly, Ritter's argument rested on the assumption that human genetic diseases were increasing in the modern world – an old eugenic argument. It is also noteworthy that he judged the present eugenic effect of genetic counselling as poor; but, like many of his colleagues, he held that once widely established, counselling would bear fruit in the long term. The fact that human geneticists constantly reflected on the possible long-term eugenic effects of genetic counselling is striking, as it clearly contradicted with their assertion that counselling was purely a medical service for the benefit of the individual families seeking advice. A closer look at the justifications for the need of genetic counselling reveals an inherent ambiguity in the experts' discourse. The statements of human geneticists reveal that while genetic counselling was depicted as a non-invasive form of medical advice for individuals, the objective of a eugenic improvement of the population continued to inform their arguments. On the one hand, they declared that the poor state of genetic counselling in Germany ruled out any significant effects on the spread of pathogenic genes in the population. As Vogel, a pioneer of genetic counselling in West Germany, stated in his contribution to the Marburg conference:

> If we look at the relatively low number of people that come to us for help, we must conclude: the effect of our family counselling, relative to the entire population, is relatively small. That demonstrates that we cannot follow a eugenic goal. Our focus is on helping individuals and individual families.[36]

This self-restraint, however, was followed by a reflection on the future viability of 'eugenic goals':

> Genetic counselling is a part of prophylactic medicine for the individual. However, I do believe that genetic counselling, when viewed across the entire population, will in the long term have some effect. As doctors gain more and more human genetic knowledge, more and more patients will be better counselled either by them or by referral to the counselling centres. The possibility of counselling will also become better known in the general population and as more people become aware of basic biological facts, more and more of them will decide to abstain from producing at-risk children.[37]

Although human geneticists were presumably serious about their publicly proclaimed opposition to the eugenic practices of the past, they were still arguing on the basis of older eugenic ideas. In the epilogue of the proceedings of the Marburg conference, Gerhard Wendt implicitly addressed the issue of the eugenic responsibility of the medical community:

> The increase in the rate of mutation and the reduction of natural selection most likely imply a risk to the genetic health and the ability of future generations. If we take this risk seriously, then doctors today, when treating and counselling patients with hereditary diseases, must take into account the impact on the health and ability of future generations. The self-image of the doctor, who also feels responsible to society in this spirit, must be reconsidered.[38]

In claiming for genetic counselling a central place in medicine, Wendt directly invoked the classical eugenic image of natural selection disturbed by modern medicine. A similar rationale can be found in a more cautious statement by Fuhrmann:

> Even if the deterioration of the genetic material, caused by the increase of certain pathological genes against which treatment is available, will advance but extremely slowly, we should not forget that practically any acceptable eugenic measure will only take effect in the same slow way. Hence, such efforts must run parallel to the development of therapies against hereditary ills, if they are not to arrive hopelessly late.[39]

Even though Fuhrmann, in contrast to other geneticists, did not point out the possible catastrophic consequences caused by the supposed reduction of natural selection, he nevertheless took it for granted that any progress in therapy for hereditary diseases had to be complemented by measures against the propagation of the respective genetic traits.

The Intertwining of Individual and Society-Oriented Genetic Counselling, 1968–80

Human geneticists did not react to a real demand for genetic counselling in the population, but rather sought to stimulate a need for it. As the enforced implementation of genetic counselling was out of the question, they concentrated on efforts to educate the population and to train the medical community. Institutes of human genetics offered numerous courses to train interested physicians in the basic principles of human genetics and to enable them to identify genetic defects. Funds from Aktion Sorgenkind were not only used for grants to medical researchers, but were also devoted to spreading advanced training in medical genetics in the medical community. In addition, we can identify a trend in the provision of genetic counselling through the formation of a seamless network of counselling centres, again meeting the postulated need of society. This goal was vindicated through a cost-benefit analysis that was openly discussed by human geneticists and adopted by public health authorities. In their proposals for genetic counselling services, human geneticists justified the costs of these services by comparing them with the costs of caring for a disabled person – always underlining the large financial benefit of genetic counselling services. This mode of argumentation proved to be very successful for obtaining state sponsorship and thus advancing the institutionalization of the field.

As noted before, the narratives of West German advocates of genetic counselling were characterized by a concurrence of 'new' and 'old' eugenic ideas. Interestingly, Vogel used the expressions 'eugenic counselling' or 'eugenic family counselling' until the end of the 1960s.[40] In his first text on the matter, jointly published with the paediatrician Walter Fuhrmann in 1968, Vogel began to develop an individual-centred approach to genetic counselling, in which psychological aspects were taken into consideration. Many human geneticists became more willing to attend to the individual problems of their patients, adapting their consultation by taking into account the patient's sociocultural background and mindset. Fuhrmann stressed the psychological constitution of the patient as an important factor in assisting them in their reproductive choices.[41] However, doctors retained a dominant role in the doctor-patient relationship. Vogel and Fuhrmann held that while the parents made the final decision on whether or not to have children, doctors should not evade their responsibility to give their own advice. This attitude was still expressed in the latest version of the guidebook published in 1982.[42] Even though Vogel and Fuhrmann described the application of human genetics as a form of prognostic assessment that helped maintain individual health, they still argued that genetic counselling was also an instrument to avoid the birth of children with genetic problems. In their understanding, individual-oriented and population-oriented aspects were closely intertwined: helping the individual or the family to identify and deal with genetic problems was connected with the hope to influence, in the long run, the genetic composition of the population.

A similar ambivalence can be found in the views of Nachtsheim's student Karl-Heinz Degenhardt, who became professor for human genetics and comparative genetic pathology at the University of Frankfurt am Main in 1961. According to Degenhardt, the main goal of genetic counselling was to prevent the transmission of pathological genes through targeted client counselling, but he maintained that the ultimate aim of genetic prevention went beyond the care for individual cases. Degenhardt explicitly pointed to the financial burden to the state caused by the costs of rehabilitating disabled persons. These growing expenses, he stated, could be reduced if each citizen took more personal responsibility for his or her own health.[43] While Degenhardt did not openly demand the systematic identification of genetic defects and state-run interventions in reproduction, the recourse to the well-known argument of costs caused by genetic defects gave the matter of counselling political urgency. The possibility of cost saving became a central motif when it came to the establishment of genetic counselling services. In the Scandinavian countries in particular, these arguments were used to boost state funding for prenatal diagnostics, but also for implementing more extensive sterilization policies.[44]

Besides Degenhardt, Wendt was one of the most prominent advocates of this type of preventative, state-supported counselling. In his writings, he compared the costs of creating counselling centres to the costs of caring for handicapped individuals, pointing to the massive savings that could be achieved by creating these centres. In a paper entitled 'Is the Number of Handicapped People Increasing?', for which he received an award from the Cornelius Helferich Foundation in 1978,[45] he wrote:

> We must be clear in finally recognizing that the solution to this problem is not to invest ever more money in caring for the ever increasing number of people with disabilities who are getting older and older. The current status of care for the handicapped can be compared to a person who is furiously pumping water out of his basement but who is completely ignoring the fact that he should also be stopping up the hole in the water pipe. This defective pipe is the daily stream of children with disabilities that are born.[46]

Both Wendt and Degenhardt based their arguments on a crude cost-benefit rationale that differed little from those that had characterized classical racial hygiene or eugenics.[47] By presenting disabilities as an unacceptable burden for family members and society in general, they implicitly supported an understanding of genetic counselling as a service not only for the health of the individual, but also for the good of the community.

Conclusion

The institutionalization of genetic counselling in the FRG began slowly following World War II. It was not until the 1970s that regular genetic counselling services were introduced, following a long-overdue reflection on the crimes committed in the name of eugenics after decades of a tacit continuity of eugenic ideals. However, the narratives of the West German human geneticists who promoted the institutionalization of genetic counselling demonstrate that many aspects of pre-1945 eugenic thinking were not completely discredited. In spite of their proclaimed opposition to 'old eugenics' – understood as a policy aiming to improve the genetic make-up of a population – they did not clearly distance themselves from eugenic objectives and rationales. The long-term eugenic effects of genetic counselling on the gene pool were a central argument in their efforts to win public acceptance for genetic counselling. Moreover, some of them openly used cost-benefit rationales in their campaign for a network of counselling centres in the FRG, thus falling back on a set of arguments already used by eugenicists in the first half of the twentieth century. It is true that they clearly distanced themselves from the principles of compulsory eugenics as practiced during the National Socialist era. Nevertheless, their emphasis on the need to prevent the birth of disabled children, by way of counselling and the systematic education of the public, raises doubts as to their claims that genetic counselling would preserve the individual's freedom of choice with respect to reproduction. Arguing along these lines, West German human geneticists were quite successful in promoting their discipline and popularizing their ideas of prevention. From the 1980s onwards, however, they met more and more resistance: genetic counselling and the increased application of prenatal diagnosis in form of amniocentesis came to be criticized by politically active disabled persons and by self-help groups as practices that violated the human rights of individuals.

15 PERFORMING ANGER: H. J. MULLER, JAMES V. NEEL AND RADIATION RISK

Susan Lindee

How did expert engagement with the security state shape quotidian professional scientific practice? In this essay, I explore a dispute in 1956 between two prominent geneticists in the United States about the proper way to apply results with *Drosophila* to human radiation risk. The disagreement ended with a hastily called summit meeting at Oak Ridge National Laboratory, but the views of the two key geneticists involved did not change much. Human geneticist James V. Neel (1915–2000) continued to believe that radiation risk could only be assessed through studies of human populations, and Drosophilist Herman J. Muller (1890–1967) continued to argue that results with *Drosophila* suggested alarming risks to people all over the world. The dispute itself is only one of many about radiation risk and certainly not even the most important one – though I do think that historians have been insufficiently interested in general in the logic of extrapolation across species. But I suggest here that this single argument provides a way to begin to explore the roles of anger as *professional practice* in mid-century genetics, and by implication in technical networks in general. The evolutionary biologist Ernst Mayr, observing a different dispute between H. J. Muller and Theodosius Dobzhansky, once asked 'what makes the geneticists such a bunch of emotional prima donnas?'[1] Indeed, what?

Drawing on well-established literatures in sociology and anthropology on the performance of emotion, I suggest that genetics was an emotional science, characterized by deep tensions that were about much more than genes or chromosomes or evolution. In the 1950s and 1960s it was a science implicated in the general militarization of natural knowledge, the legacies of eugenics and racial hygiene, the race science debate, the rise of a feminist critique of science, and public fears of the risks posed by atomic weapons. Its practitioners were engaged in a profound, almost existential, debate about the future, and about 'what it means to be human'.

Scientists' engagement with the state's monopoly on socially sanctioned violence – in Max Weber's terms – may have produced forms of anger that reflected new experiences of professional dissonance. Scientists trained in the 1930s and 1940s learned in the course of their training that science was open, universalistic and internationalist, an endeavour conducive to the welfare of mankind. These ideas about internationalism and openness were much repeated in textbooks, in writings by scientists, and even in the work of philosophers, historians and sociologists of science in the 1950s and 1960s, whose celebration of these scientific values at times reached an almost shrill tone. Yet in practice, in the heart of the Cold War, science was often not open but secret, not internationalist but nationalistic, and not conducive to the 'welfare of mankind' but focused on the sophisticated technical production of injury to human beings – on new weapons, new surveillance methods, new information systems, even new ways of bringing down economies or dictatorships. Experts from physics to sociology found their research calibrated to enhance the power of the security state, and scientists trained to see themselves as creating knowledge for the good of mankind often found themselves engaged in something that felt very different to them as the Cold War intensified.[2] Whether they spoke of this dissonance (some did) or not, it had consequences for the organization and culture of science. One of those consequences was anger.

At the height of the Cold War in the United States, scientists were angry at other scientists who did defence work, or who did not, who identified possible security risks, or who did not, who favoured the production of new weapons, or who did not. Many of the more unpleasant name-calling episodes are well known and well documented, though historians writing about them do not generally foreground anger or emotion as social performance. J. Robert Oppenheimer, Edward Teller, E. U. Condon, Linus Pauling and many other prominent scientists took sides in public debates about bombs and risks, and they faced censure from their colleagues on all sides of all issues.[3] There were also disputes in the social sciences, and of course in genetics and biology.[4] In many cases, technical details were part of the fight. Could the H-bomb work, and who said it could not?[5] Was there a linear response curve for radiation, and which scientists claimed that there was not?[6] Was democracy scientifically preferable, and who dared to say otherwise?[7] Anger and calibrated emotional display are a part of the history of science in the Cold War.

As the sociologist Arlie Hochschild taught us thirty years ago, emotions involve social performance: there are the feelings, whatever that might mean, and then there are the particular, often baroque, rules about how they can be expressed. These need not match – indeed, they often do not. Hochschild's path-breaking 1983 study of emotional labour in the workplace called attention particularly to inauthenticity in the performance of emotions in professional settings, for example in flight attendants, who must be cheerful no matter how they feel, and in bill collectors, who must be angry whether they are angry or not.

She later coined the term emotional dissonance to describe the experience of performing one feeling while experiencing another.[8] The rules shaping the performance of emotion reflect social consensus, and noticing these rules is part of understanding any social network, whether in Jane Austen's fictional but vivid estate at *Mansfield Park*, or in the meetings of the Atomic Energy Commission's Advisory Committee on Biology and Medicine.

Newer research grounded in Hochschild's work has focused less on inauthenticity and more on emotion as a feature of everyday life that reflects a cultural repertoire which people deploy to advance their situational agenda. Emotional expression, these scholars suggest, can be purposive and strategic, intended to produce a certain outcome. It can be 'analyzed as a domain in which culturally specific narratives and rhetorics are used to advance the situational agenda of actors'.[9] In addition, an increasingly sophisticated literature on social performance and gender has called our attention to the ways that professional life is a heavily coded and deeply gendered domain. University of Pennsylvania PhD student Whitney Laemmli has been exploring some of the ways that prominent male scientists in the 1960s, including James Watson, promoted a hyper-masculine image of science at a historical moment when science was under siege – from feminist critics, anti-war movement leaders, political observers and activist scientists who constituted a sort of fifth column within the community. Watson was not the only scientific figure who served as a lightning rod in the controversies of the 1960s and 1970s. E. O. Wilson, Arthur Jensen, Luca Cavalli-Sforza and of course Neel and Muller, as well as, in slightly different ways, Robin Fox, Lionel Tiger and Desmond Morris, all took part on some level in public controversies that involved negotiations of scientific identity, authority and legitimacy.[10]

In this context, the debate over the genetic effects of radiation evolved in a context of a 'New World' of nuclear risk.[11] Geneticists found that they had expertise crucial to the nuclear state. At the same time, the increasing importance of genetic knowledge, particularly genetic knowledge of human risk, posed problems for them. Geneticists on one side or the other of key questions about the threshold dose, appropriate risk, dosimetry at Hiroshima and Nagasaki, and genetic effects (if there were any) were often angry, emotional, frustrated and annoyed. Historians who work on this period know how angry experts became around these issues, but they commonly do not foreground the anger or necessarily even mention it. The anger is, so to speak, naturalized, understood as a normal part of scientific debate. It might be normal in some sense, but normality can nonetheless be historically informative and revealing. At least, this is what I propose here.

In this essay I am interested in one particularly emotional interaction, between the Nobel prize-winning fly geneticist H. J. Muller and the University of Michigan medical geneticist James V. Neel. We might call this essay a study of social performance in the micro-politics of the Cold War. Both Neel and Muller were major figures in the community in the post-war period, and they knew each other well. They do not seem to have been close or particularly friendly, and this could be because they disagreed about many questions raised by the genetic effects of radiation; but it could also be because both men were in one way or another independent thinkers, and both had a tendency to engage in the masculine performance of public anger, not just with each other.

Muller was a fly geneticist who was the first president of the American Society for Human Genetics, a eugenicist to the end, and Nobel Prize winner at Indiana University.[12] In the 1930s Muller's leftist politics made him a focus of FBI suspicion in the United States, and in 1934 he accepted an invitation to move to a genetics research institute in the USSR, where he stayed three years. He returned to the United States to hold positions at Amherst and finally at Indiana University in Bloomington. His general tendency to defend his ideas with considerable energy led to a series of public and scientific disputes, with T. H. Morgan, Theodosius Dobzhansky and many others. Neel was trained in both medicine and science, holding an MD and a PhD, and he ran an important programme in medical genetics at the University of Michigan. He was generously supported by the Atomic Energy Commission throughout his career and was more or less inside the fold of the AEC.[13] His work on the genetic effects of radiation with William J. Schull was commonly understood as 'reassuring'. Neel, however, carefully defended his distance from AEC oversight, sometimes seeming to see the issue in terms of institutional legitimacy and administrative firewalls.[14] Muller, conversely, published alarming reports for public consumption that called into question AEC standards for exposure and predicted a disturbing biological future. His ideas about a 'load of mutations' that would eventually cripple the species attracted journalistic interest, and he was at one point proclaimed to be 'the world's greatest scientist' in a magazine profile about radiation risk.[15] Muller had that kind of visibility and public edge. He was generally seen as a thorny adversary of the AEC, though he also received significant AEC support (like almost every prominent geneticist in this period), having been awarded $279,312 by the AEC from 1951 to 1962 – about $31,000 per year, at a time when the US average annual salary was less than $3,000.[16] This funding seemed to be uninflected by his sometimes florid public pronouncements about irresponsible medical uses of radiation or about the high risks of fallout and the disastrous future they were producing.

In this context, taking AEC money was aggravating and possibly contaminating, but everyone was getting AEC money (geneticists but also botanists, ecologists, biomedical researchers of all kinds) through a peer review system not unlike those of other federal funding agencies like the NIH. Some of the biggest critics of AEC standards and policies and practices either worked there (Knapp) or received significant, ongoing AEC support (Gofman).[17] Nonetheless, 'AEC' could be used as an accusation, in a sentence about bias – Muller identified some positions as 'AEC promoted', while Gofman said all the NAS reports on the genetic effects of radiation were biased in favour of AEC goals and perspectives and tainted by AEC interests. Much later, in 2000, when Neel was falsely accused by journalist Patrick Tierney of starting an epidemic in a Yanomami population to test a theory about fitness, Tierney invoked Neel's AEC support for the project to suggest its illegitimacy.[18] AEC support, in this narrative, provided evidence of contamination. The contrast between the institutional realities of the positive role of the AEC in modern biology and the emotional meanings of the 'AEC' as contamination, both then and now, do matter to this story. It provides part of the context for understanding the disagreement between Muller and Neel.

Neel and Muller participated together at virtually every important meeting focused on the genetic effects of radiation from about 1947 until Muller's death in 1967. They knew each other well, though they were not of equivalent age or status and they do not seem to have been particularly close. Muller was twenty-five years older and a Nobelist, in his mid-fifties when they began to interact, and Neel was thirty or so and a newly minted MD/PhD. Muller was a major figure in radiation genetics, with significant scientific capital. All the advantage should have been on his side in any debate about the genetic effects of radiation. Yet Neel had some advantages in terms of assessing the genetic risk to human populations from fallout, which is more or less what they were fighting about: he was a trained physician, and he knew the circumstances of data collection in Japan, where most of the data on human populations exposed to radiation was being collected as these debates unfolded. Neel ran the genetics programme of the Atomic Bomb Casualty Commission in Hiroshima in the 1940s and 1950s, and he wrestled for his entire professional life, until his death in 2000, with many of the complex problems that the genetics project in Hiroshima and Nagasaki posed. Muller visited the laboratory on Hijiyama Hill in Hiroshima once for two days, in 1951, and focused his work on flies. But he ran a remarkable programme of fly research at Indiana, and he had strong empirical data to back up every claim he made about genes and radiation – something Neel lacked despite decades of trying to pin it down in human populations.

What were Muller and Neel fighting about in the fall of 1956? They disagreed about what results with flies meant for human risk. Neel took the position that results with flies meant very little or even *nothing* and that more research with humans was crucial; Muller felt that the fly results meant a great deal for human exposure and more research with flies was crucial. The problem was not simply that flies might be inappropriate surrogates for calculating human risk. It was also that any conclusions reached were relevant to the institutional and policy constraints that could be placed on the development of atomic energy.

The dispute began at a consensus meeting, this one organized by the World Health Organization (WHO). The effects of radiation had been the subject of two earlier consensus meetings in a single twelve-month span, when three different (though sometimes overlapping) groups of scientists made an effort to weigh in on the genetic effects of radiation with high-profile reports for public consumption. (Still to come in 1958: the United Nations Scientific Committee on the Effects of Atomic Radiation report.[19]) The WHO Study Group on the Effect of Radiation on Human Heredity met on 7–11 August 1956 at the University of Copenhagen. Proposing that 'man's most precious trust is his genetic heritage', the WHO committee report was also an effort to map future directions for research that could 'increase our understanding of the genetic effects of ionizing radiations on man'.[20]

In general, the meeting was recalled as highly contentious.[21] Certainly both Neel and Muller were in fine form, and they left the meeting with an unresolved issue on the table. The issue was Neel's paper, which was a fully fledged attack on the idea that results with flies or mice could be applied to human problems. The paper that Muller found so disturbing opened by saying that extrapolation from experimental organisms (which is what Muller did) should not be attempted: 'We should prefer not to attempt to extrapolate from other species to man, but rather to base our thinking entirely on human data'.[22] One might ask, what human data? Neel by 1957 did have some human data, collected at Hiroshima and Nagasaki, though by his own calculus of the 'five factors' necessary to assess radiation effects, he did not have what he needed. Assessing radiation, he said, required a knowledge of the spontaneous mutation rate (in human populations, unknown); the induced mutation rate (in human populations, unknown); the total gene number (in human populations, unknown); the 'accumulation factor', which was the ratio of already present recessive genes to those arising spontaneously in each generation through mutation (in humans, unknown); and the 'manner in which selection operates on the total gene complex' (in all species, unknown).[23] Muller characterized the paper as taking 'my methods for granted [meaning not explaining them] and ... raising objections to them'.[24] He told Neel as their debate began, 'you criticized my data and conclusions without being familiar with the evidence that I had presented'.[25]

The confusion between them circled around the specific locus test that Muller used in his fly work – the strategy of crossing stock flies known to be homozygous for some known recessive allele or alleles, with irradiated 'wild type' flies. Any mutations induced by irradiations in the wild type flies in the known alleles would be presumed to be recognizable in the first generation.[26] Neel believed that the specific locus test would miss some mutations (but this was assumed in Muller's model), and that the rates at the known loci might be different from the 'general' rates of mutation; Muller was baffled by Neel's objections on this point:

> We must be thinking at cross-purposes for I do not see the relevancy of the points mentioned in your letter of October 30. I was not trying to find out the total number of mutations occurring at any particular locus, however that may be defined, in a Drosophila chromosome, but only the number that gave visible effects[27]

Perhaps a bit disingenuously, in discussing a paper that said in its opening salvo that extrapolation was unwise, Neel claimed to Muller that he 'did not feel myself so much attempting to undermine the principle of extrapolation from Drosophila and the mouse to man, as to point out the permissible limit of opinion as to where this extrapolation leads us. In this respect, I still find room for honest differences of viewpoint'.[28]

Their back and forth on the question meandered with reasonable collegiality through October and November, until Muller's four-page 7 December 1956 letter to Neel, which was a kind of Pearl Harbor (fifteen years to the day after the other Pearl Harbor) of their relationship. Neel did not respond to it. The 'Jim' of October had become Dr Neel, and Muller proposed that Neel's handling of the extrapolation problem would damage *Neel*: 'Although you yourself would in the end be the one most injured by publishing so demonstrably erroneous a set of points'. There were also serious public risks, because in the WHO publication, Muller said, there would be no opportunity for critique by other scientists.[29] Muller predicted a rapid, and devastating, downfall for Neel if the paper were published; it would soon be found to be incorrect, and this would embarrass the WHO. Even worse, Neel's claims about flies would:

> cast unjustified doubt in the minds of an enormous and influential audience on the value of the contribution which studies on the genetics of other organisms than man have made and can make, when taken in connection with the evidence from man, to the specific problems of spontaneous and radiation-induced mutation rate and mutational load in man.

Muller thus made explicit, in an intriguing way, how disagreement could cost the geneticists AEC support, including funding and public support from Congress. It would be better, Muller said, to argue the questions out in private.[30]

Muller even proposed a meeting. He would be willing to go to Ann Arbor to meet with Neel to 'lay these things before you'. Neel misunderstood the science, Muller said, and Neel's emphasis on variations in rates of mutation in different populations of *Drosophila* was a red herring, because while the rates did vary (something Muller's own work had explored in detail in the 1920s), the ratio between visible mutations and lethals tended to consistency. The absolute numbers were not relevant: 'The great variation in spontaneous mutation rate, on which you lay so much emphasis, and the resultant discrepancies between the absolute frequencies obtained by different Drosophila workers are beside the point, i.e. quite irrelevant to the extrapolation problem'.[31]

Presumably just after receiving this letter, on 11 December, Neel wrote a weary letter to Alexander Hollaender, director of the Division of Biology at Oak Ridge National Laboratory: 'I do not feel that the paper raises the public polemic which Dr. Muller insists it will, unless not to agree completely with all that Dr. Muller has written constitutes such a polemic'.[32] And to his mentor and friend Curt Stern, then in the Department of Zoology at the University of California, Berkeley, the same day: 'This paper of mine, which raised a number of questions concerning the mutation rate figures commonly quoted for a variety of species, upset Dr. Muller quite considerably'.[33]

Two weeks later, Muller told I. S. Eve, Medical Officer in Charge of Questions Dealing with the Atomic Energy and Health at WHO, that Neel had 'not answered my letter of December 7'. By this time the whole controversy was being shared – all the correspondence, the drafts of the papers, the draft discussion document – in Alexander Hollaender's lab at Oak Ridge. Hollaender had administrative and diplomatic skills and could navigate the tensions related to AEC expectations of the genetics community.[34] He also enrolled the head of the *Drosophila* genetics group, Ed Novitski, who had worked with both Alfred Sturtevant (first) and then Theodosius Dobzhansky.[35] Novitski – a skilled Drosophilist – wrote to Neel to say that he had been given everything and gone through it all carefully, and while he agreed with Neel's insistence that the final evaluation of radiation effects in man will depend on studies of human materials, 'I am inclined to agree with Muller in principle on several points', including Muller's concern that Neel's paper could be 'misconstrued by influential non-geneticists' and lead to a *reduction in support for work with experimental organisms.*[36]

Through Hollaender's Christmas intervention, on Sunday, 6 January 1957, Neel and Muller met in person at Oak Ridge, with Hollaender as the referee, and Novitski and perhaps one other Oak Ridge geneticist in on the discussion.[37] I have not found a direct account of these discussions, but they apparently ended well enough. Both Neel and Muller revised their papers, and in the published volume the papers seemed to be operating at two different domains, at cross-purposes, not in dialogue with each other. Muller explained why point mutations were a good way to track radiation effects, and included a short discussion of why any statements about specific loci in any publications in the past 'for the present writer' were 'only a short-cut mode of expression'.[38] Neel's published paper was a much more direct assault on extrapolation, pronouncing it a very bad idea, and explaining that mutation rates varied from fly to fly and from locus to locus.[39]

Neel's conclusion after his summit meeting with Muller at Oak Ridge was that Muller was threatened by human genetics:

> I think I appreciated for the first time some of the facets that I had not previously understood as to why Muller was so upset. For years some zoologists have made critical remarks on man as an object of genetic study; this despite the fact that in my

> opinion many of them really did not have a feeling for human material or appreciate its possibilities. Now a human geneticist has turned around and pointed out some of the difficulties in working with Drosophila. This almost comes under the category of 'man bites dog'.[40]

Later in January he sent Muller his revised paper with a conciliatory note, expressing respect and also doubts about all the numbers floating around relating to radiation risk.[41] Neel said he was expecting 'to devote much of my remaining scientific life to providing data relevant to reaching a decision on this matter', and he believed that 'we are on the threshold of a new era in the study of human genetics, with every prospect of advancing our knowledge of man as rapidly in the next 30 years as we have of Drosophila in the past 30'.[42] Muller, for his part, complained about Neel in various letters that spring, telling correspondents that Neel's paper for the WHO volume had been both erroneous and invalid.[43]

Conclusion: Anger and Credibility

In her assessment of the nuclear physicist and medical scientist John W. Gofman, one of the noisiest critics of the radiation safety standards adopted by the AEC, Ionna Semendeferi explores how Gofman's scientific legitimacy and credibility were undermined by the AEC and by those affiliated with or sympathetic to the AEC. Gofman ran the biomedical research division at Lawrence Livermore National Laboratory, and much of his research was funded by the AEC. But his credibility was undermined not by virtue of his close affiliation with the AEC (which he criticized relentlessly) but by AEC-affiliated administrators and scientists who attacked his emotionalism, his advocacy and his lack of 'neutrality' even as their own agency funded his research. His debate with the AEC, she notes, 'stigmatized him as a fiery nuclear critic and severely damaged his scientific credibility'. To make matters worse, she notes, historians took the AEC critique as their own:

> Existing historical accounts describe Gofman as a radical antinuclear scientist whose influence depended on scant, if any, scientific arguments, acknowledging, however, that he contributed to many public policy changes. These accounts, while valuable, are highly critical of Gofman and present views similar to those held within the AEC at the time.[44]

Thus she suggests that historians have themselves been affected by the narratives of AEC officials and scientists who branded some critics as unscientific or (of particular interest to me) *emotional* when they raised questions about radiation safety.

Note that Muller was personally despised by AEC Commissioner Willard F. Libby – the oral history with Elof Axel Carlson is almost shocking in its hostility[45] – and that Gofman was publicly called 'an opera star' by AEC Commissioner James T. Ramey in 1970.[46] Apparently concern about radiation risk was somehow feminine and melodramatic. But this fight was highly emotional on all sides, both publicly and privately – so one possible question might be: Which emotions were understood by those involved to call into question legitimacy and credibility? And which emotions could, in this network of social performance, be expressed?

From another perspective, Scott Kirsch has looked at the work of an AEC insider, the mathematician Harold Knapp, who like Gofman questioned AEC standards for radiation protection. Knapp worked for the Division of Biology and Medicine on questions of fallout, and his study in 1962 suggested that short-living radioiodine, rather than long-living nuclides such as radiostrontium, posed the greatest hazard from nuclear test fallout, and that children raised in Nevada and Utah during the 1950s had already been exposed to internal radiation doses far in excess of recommended guidelines. When Knapp sought to publish his findings in the fall of 1962, AEC officials initially determined that his report contained 'Restricted Data' and should not be published.[47]

One of those objecting to Knapp's data most loudly was the deputy director of the AEC's Division of Operational Safety, Gordon Dunning, and one of Dunning's proposed solutions involved a careful management of emotion – by the AEC:

> Let the Commission tell Dr. Knapp in a *matter-of-fact and bland* manner that the Commission interposes no objection if he, as an individual scientist, wishes to publish his paper. If Dr. Knapp can find a reputable scientific journal to accept the manuscript, we may expect letters and inquiries. We can treat these in the same *professional and unemotional* way that we have many others in the past.[48]

Emotionality, like radioactivity, was one of the things that had to be managed. It was recognized by those involved as a public and professional performance.

With a somewhat different but related agenda, John Beatty has explored the ways that disagreement among experts in contentious public debates can often be masked for the sake of public credibility – not credibility within the scientific community, but credibility in the larger world. In his close reading of the negotiations that led to the June 1956 National Academy of Sciences report on radiation risk, he elucidates the ways that participants compromised for the sake of consensus. Beatty interprets the public masking of disagreement in the final report in terms of the 'epistemological asymmetry between scientific experts and the lay public'.[49] But I would add that it also functioned to limit public awareness of the emotional dimensions of the debate.

While the geneticists obsessed about genetic effects, other scientists felt baffled by the relatively minimal attention granted to somatic effects. The Federation of American Scientists interpreted the attention to genetic effects as a kind of distraction, complaining that reporters were all referring to the low risk of genetic effects. But what about pathologic effects and cancer in people now living?[50] From this perspective, *both* Neel and Muller were facilitating an AEC strategy of distraction. Their emotional disagreement was useful, just as the artificially prolonged technical fight about tobacco and cancer was useful to the tobacco companies.[51]

Neel's prediction that studies of human heredity would, over the next thirty years, be as productive as work with flies had been, was a programmatic claim that more or less came true, and radiation risk was a critical part of the programme. When I recently reread the WHO 1957 Study Group Report, having not read it since the 1980s, I found that the Study Group had (without citing me!) outlined my 2005 book on the rise of genetic disease to medical prominence.[52] The WHO report emphasized the importance of field research with special, isolated populations like the Amish, the development of human cytogenetics, behavioural genetics and twins research, state initiatives to track genetic diseases in newborns, and the role of genetics in medical education – suggesting to my surprise that I had empirically replicated an agenda driven by radiation risk merely by looking at institutions, research, political debates and funding. The scientific study of human genetics came into being, then, with a salvage or preservationist mentality.[53] If eugenics was animated by fears about the wrong people breeding, scientific human genetics after 1945 had its own dark fears, about radiation and human devolution.

In 1960 the physicist-turned-sociologist Samuel Stewart West carried out a sociological study of the 'ideology of academic scientists'. He listed the values he found in historian of science Bernard Barber's 1952 book *Science and the Social Order.* These included emotional neutrality, faith in rationality, universalism, disinterestedness, impartiality and freedom.[54] West proposed:

> it is commonly believed that persons engaged in scientific research adhere to a set of moral values representing ideal types of behavior which facilitate the production of new knowledge. However, the many listings of these values which may be found in the literature range from intuitive to, at best, speculative.

His comments reflected Cold War tensions within the scientific community, which was simultaneously widely engaged in making weapons and theories that facilitated state violence and also in proclaiming the deep benevolence, disinterestedness and neutrality of science. Neel and Muller were right in the middle of these tensions. Their fight about flies and humans was a fight about many other things: AEC funding, emotional decorum and what it meant to be a 'physician to the gene pool' at a turning point in the history of human genetics.

So, how does the debate about radiation look if we notice the emotion? My case suggests that titrating emotional performance around radiation risk was part of establishing legitimacy and authority, or calling authority into question, and that strategic emotional display plays a little-discussed role in scientific debates. While sociologists have been keenly interested in questions about emotion as a cultural product, historians have accorded it relatively little importance, perhaps relegating it to the domain of psycho-history. Yet the point of these analyses is not to illuminate interior mental states, but to suggest that expected norms are performed in the spaces between people, that domain we commonly think of as culture. Surely it is a field of critical importance to historians of science interested in genetics in the Cold War.

16 THE STRUGGLE FOR AUTHORITY OVER ITALIAN GENETICS: THE NINTH INTERNATIONAL CONGRESS OF GENETICS IN BELLAGIO, 1948–53

Francesco Cassata

Introduction

From 24 to 31 August 1953, the Ninth International Congress of Genetics was held in Bellagio, on the banks of Lake Como in Italy.[1] Reflecting on the history of the Seventh International Congress of Genetics, Nikolai Krementsov observed:

> congresses provide a vehicle for the advancement of local agendas, particularly for the scientists of the host country. National communities routinely use such congresses to enhance their disciplines' standing and visibility in the eyes of domestic patrons, which lead to sometimes quite fierce competition among national communities for the chance to host such a congress.[2]

From this perspective, the Bellagio Congress was an expression of the developments in Italian genetics from the second half of the 1940s; from another, it triggered a further process of institutionalization.

The organization of the Bellagio Congress coincided with a period of extraordinary expansion in the activities of the three Italian professional geneticists: Adriano Buzzati-Traverso (1913–83), Claudio Barigozzi (1909–96) and Giuseppe Montalenti (1904–90).[3] In 1948 Buzzati-Traverso and Barigozzi were appointed to the newly created chairs of genetics, in Pavia and Milan respectively; Montalenti had already obtained the first chair of genetics in Italy in 1944. Formal and developmental genetics of pseudotumours in *Drosophila* and cancer cytology were the main research focus of Barigozzi's group in Milan. Before leaving for Berkeley as visiting professor of zoology in 1951, Buzzati-Traverso had trained a group of bright young collaborators, which included Luigi Luca Cavalli-Sforza, Niccolò Visconti di Modrone and Luigi Silvestri in bacterial genetics; Giovanni Magni in radiogenetics and yeast genetics; and Renzo Scossiroli in plant genetics. In Naples, Montalenti – in collaboration with the Roman haematologists Ezio Silvestroni and Ida Bianco – inaugurated a vast research programme on the genetics of microcythaemia in the early 1950s. This attracted the support of the Rockefeller Foundation Division of Medicine and Public Health (DMPH). In September 1953 Robert S. Morison, DMPH associate director, described this project as 'an opportunity for the DMPH to participate in what could become a classical experiment in the prevention of a hereditary disorder'.[4]

It was in this context of increasing internationalization that, from 1948 to 1953, the three Italian geneticists became deeply involved in the organization of the International Congress. They became the most authoritative members of the Executive Board (*Giunta esecutiva*), Barigozzi was appointed Secretary General of the Congress, and all the administrative work was carried out by the Institutes of Genetics of Milan and Pavia.

This essay analyses the organization of the Bellagio Congress as a crucial moment of scientific demarcation and discipline-building in the field of Italian genetics. It is divided into two sections, corresponding to the two different fronts that characterized the struggle for authority between Italian geneticists. First, I will examine the conflict between the Italian geneticists and the demographer and statistician Corrado Gini (1884–1965). As president of the three most important Italian institutions in the field of population policy and eugenics (the National Institute of Statistics (ISTAT) from 1926 to 1932; the Italian Society of Genetics and Eugenics (SIGE) from 1924 to 1965; and the Italian Committee for the Study of Population (CISP) from 1928 to 1965), Gini was the leading figure in Italian eugenics from 1920s to 1960s, and one of the most active proponents of *mainline* eugenics in the international arena.[5] In the case of the Bellagio Congress, Italian geneticists succeeded in shielding the scientific organization of the International Congress from Gini's influence. This ostracism increased tensions between the SIGE Sections for Eugenics and Genetics. Faced with this complex situation, the strategy of the Italian geneticists was divided: while Buzzati-Traverso and Barigozzi asked for the constitution of a new scientific association, completely separate from SIGE, Montalenti tried to reach some sort of compromise with Gini. The failure of Montalenti's moderate approach resulted in the complete disengagement of Italian geneticists from SIGE offices and activities.

Secondly, I will focus on the struggle between the Italian geneticists on the one side and the zoologist Luisa Gianferrari (1890–1977) and the physician Luigi Gedda (1902–2000) on the other. Gianferrari directed the Study Centre of Human Genetics (Centro Studi di Genetica Umana), inaugurated in December 1940, at the Institute of Biology and Zoology of the Faculty of Medicine in Milan. Gedda was president of the Italian Catholic Action from 1952 to 1959 and founder in 1948 of the anti-Communist organization Citizens' Committees (Comitati Civici). From 1953 he headed the Gregor Mendel Institute of Medical Genetics and Twin Research (Istituto di Genetica Medica e Gemellologia) in Rome. Their activity in the field they labelled as 'human' or 'medical genetics' was characterized by a craft knowledge of human heredity that was dominated by notions of constitution, predisposition and diathesis, rather than by statistical computation of Mendelian transmission ratios; furthermore, Gianferrari's and Gedda's centres had profound institutional and ideological connections with the Vatican and the Italian Catholic milieu. This 'war on two fronts' – of Italian geneticists striking against Gini's racial eugenics from one side, and Gianferrari's and Gedda's development of 'medical genetics' from the other – resulted in the constitution of the Italian Genetics Society (Associazione Italiana di Genetica, AGI) in June 1953.

The Bellagio Congress opens up a window from which to view the complex national and international interactions that characterized the activities of professional geneticists in Italy between 1948 and 1953. The organization of the Ninth International Congress enabled them to pursue two main objectives. First, in the international arena, they reinforced connections with Anglo-American scientific elites, legitimizing themselves as members of a transatlantic scientific community that shared not only a common view of 'modern' genetics, with its disciplinary consensus regarding research tools, methods, agendas, etc., but also a common liberal democratic interpretation of science and its values. Second, at the local level, they consolidated the disciplinary autonomy of genetics by constructing scientific, institutional and political boundaries that excluded SIGE eugenicists and centres of 'human' or 'medical' genetics connected with the faculties of medicine.

Genetics versus Eugenics

Founded in 1919, the Italian Society of Genetics and Eugenics (SIGE) was dominated by Corrado Gini from 1924 to 1965.[6] Most prominent among its members were demographers, statisticians, physicians and anthropologists. Despite the official name of the association, the role of biology – not to mention genetics – was marginal.

The young Italian geneticists – Barigozzi, Buzzati-Traverso and Montalenti – made their appearance at the Third Congress of SIGE, held in Bologna in September 1938. Barigozzi and Buzzati-Traverso participated in the session on general genetics, with respective contributions on cytogenetics[7] and radiation genetics.[8] Montalenti presented a paper on sex determination in the session on animal genetics.[9] The session on human genetics was dominated by the eugenic contributions of Gini and his collaborators. The proceedings of the Third Congress of SIGE were published by *Genus*, the organ of the CISP directed by Gini, with funds from the Italian National Research Council (CNR).

In 1948 Gini led the Italian delegation to the Eighth International Congress of Genetics in Stockholm. He read, as its representative, the delegation's acceptance of the invitation to host the following Congress in Italy.[10] In January 1949 Italian geneticists opposed Gini's attempts to reactivate SIGE and place the organization of the Bellagio Congress under its control. In a letter of 1 January 1949 addressed to all SIGE's members, Buzzati-Traverso and Barigozzi were explicit in their opposition. They demanded that the SIGE abandon any reference to eugenics. The designation of Italy as the seat of the next International Congress of Genetics placed SIGE in a position of responsibility with regards to the international scientific community. Therefore it could not allow them to simply maintain the status quo as it existed in Italy:

> A very serious responsibility hangs over Italian geneticists and the institution that has assumed the role of representing and coordinating them, for the obvious reasons of prestige and to demonstrate the level and dignity that these studies and their environment have reached among us. This role must not be underestimated: transactions, compromises and accommodations that might be accepted – for lack of anything better – in our own home, could be severely criticized on an international level, and must therefore be avoided.[11]

According to Buzzati-Traverso and Barigozzi, there were only two alternative solutions. First, the SIGE's structure would need to be transformed from a 'presidential' to a 'parliamentary' form, devolving the organization of the International Congress of Genetics to the president of the genetics section. The second was to allow the SIGE to maintain its 'presidential' character, but the role of president could not be held by a demographer and statistician such as Gini. It would be given 'to a professional geneticist, who, above all on an international level, can more specifically represent Italian genetics'.[12]

Therefore, just a few days away from SIGE's General Assembly, an internal fracture had occurred, as much scientific as it was ideological and political. On one side stood the statisticians and demographers gathered around Gini and the University of Rome, compromised by their past commitment to fascist eugenics. On the other were Buzzati-Traverso and Barigozzi, representing an emerging field of Italian genetics in the universities of Pavia and Milan, and wanting to eliminate any reference to Italy's fascist eugenics past.

A split, which had seemed imminent, was avoided through the mediation of Giuseppe Montalenti. His strategy was built upon the following objectives: first, to maintain the unity of SIGE under Gini's presidency; second, to give internal autonomy to the genetics section; and third, to wrest the organization of the future International Congress of Genetics from Gini's control. Although Buzzati-Traverso refused to recognize the legitimacy of the voting, SIGE's General Assembly on 15 January 1949 saw a victory for Montalenti's moderate line. Montalenti was duly elected president of the SIGE genetics section. With regards to the Bellagio Congress, he succeeded in constituting a Provisory Committee – presided over not by Gini but by Alessandro Ghigi, professor of zoology at the University of Bologna and the Italian member of the International Organizing Committee for Genetic Congresses. In November 1951 the Provisory Committee for the organization of the Congress nominated the Executive Board. The secretary general was Barigozzi, the vice-secretary was Cavalli-Sforza, and Buzzati-Traverso and Montalenti were among the permanent members.[13] The Congress was, therefore, completely under the control of the three geneticists.

However, this development only served to delay the break between Gini and the geneticists by a few months. Faced with the persistent hostility of Gini, and, in particular, his refusal to recognize the appointment of Buzzati-Traverso as secretary of the SIGE genetics section, on 30 March 1950 Montalenti resigned from his role as president.[14]

Besides the institutional conflict within SIGE, another source of tension stemmed from Gini's scientific contribution to the Bellagio Congress. In October 1952 Gini presented a paper on the 'physical assimilation of the foreign settlements in Italy'. This was based on anthropological and demographic inquiries between the 1930s and 1950s, organized by the CISP, in order to study the Albanian settlements in three isolated villages in Calabria (Carfizzi, San Nicola dall'Alto and Caraffa, August–October 1938) and the Ligurian Piedmontese settlements in two Sardinian villages (Carloforte, August 1939 and 1952; Calasetta, March–April 1940 and 1953). CISP investigations had already been the subject of Gini's papers for the Second International Congress of the Latin Eugenics Societies (Bucharest, 1939 – abandoned due to the outbreak of war), and at the Seventh and Eighth International Congresses of Genetics, held respectively in Edinburgh in 1939 and Stockholm in 1948. The main aim of CISP expeditions into foreign settlements in Italy was to shed light on the mechanisms of the 'physical assimilation' of the immigrant groups, providing data on the influences of the environment on changes in stature, pigmentation and another eighty-four anthropometric measures. According to Gini, the final results of CISP inquiries demonstrated that the near complete assimilation of Albanians in Calabria and of Ligurian and Piedmontese colonies in Sardinia was due, 'at least for a substantial part', not 'to the mingling of stocks, but to an influence, direct or indirect, of the environment'.[15] Gini's reference point for the CISP inquiries was Franz Boas's 1911 research on the changes in physical characteristics of the descendants of various European stocks that had immigrated to United States.[16] While Boas's study was intended to challenge American scientific racism, Gini adopted it to support an environmentalist form of racial eugenics.[17] During the fascist regime, CISP data had provided the theoretical foundation for Gini's celebration of fascist demographic and racial policies, which were aimed at the biological unification of the different stocks that comprised the Italian nation, while prohibiting intermixture with Jews and Africans.[18] In the post-war period, Gini adopted the same theoretical framework in order to reject the egalitarianism of UNESCO's Statements on Race of 1950–1, advocating a direct parallelism between environmental differences and racial differences. In this spirit, Gini supported the anti-UNESCO campaign by the *Mankind Quarterly*, the journal of the Anglo-American International Association for the Advancement of Ethnology and Eugenics (IAAEE).[19]

In opposing Gini's racialist eugenics, Italian geneticists pursued a threefold strategy. First, they criticized the inconsistencies of CISP investigations with reference to the methods and approaches of population genetics. They maintained, for example, that Gini's research had completely neglected such fundamental elements as blood group frequencies.[20] Second, they challenged Gini's typological concept of race, referring to its redefinition by Dobzhansky as a Mendelian population in constant flux.[21] Third, they countered the pronatalist, quantitative and racial model of fascist eugenics with a *new* form of eugenics. This was based on the reinterpretation of pathological inheritance along Mendelian and biochemical lines, and the provision of objective statements and informed advice to individuals and couples regarding their reproductive behaviour.[22]

Despite this battery of criticisms, internal diplomatic and academic considerations prevailed. While Buzzati-Traverso and Barigozzi suggested that Gini's paper be rejected, Gini's contribution on the 'physical assimilation' was finally published in the proceedings of the Bellagio Congress in accordance with Montalenti's more moderate line.

Against Gianferrari and Gedda: A Struggle for Human Genetics

The second front established by Italian geneticists during the organization of the Bellagio Congress was represented by the Centres of Human Genetics, headed in Milan by Luisa Gianferrari and in Rome by Luigi Gedda. The Milan Study Centre of Human Genetics (Centro Studi di Genetica Umana) was inaugurated in December 1940 at the Institute of Biology and Zoology of the Faculty of Medicine. Supported by the majority of local political and academic authorities, the Centre was financed by both private and public institutions. The aim of the Centre, according to article 1 of the statute, was to 'collect data on the physiological and pathological human traits, with the aim of carrying out genetic studies, also with a focus on health and demographic problems'.[23]

The first important initiative of the Milan Centre was the elaboration of a form of national genetic index of the transmission of hereditary traits. The index drew upon the archives of hospitals, surgeries, special schools, mental hospitals and many other institutions. The collection of data was entrusted to volunteers recruited from students of the Faculty of Biology and Surgery. Each volunteer was provided with data sheets by the Centre. In 1944 Gianferrari referred to 510 'student field-researchers'.[24] By this time, the Centre had gathered almost one hundred thousand index cards by sifting through a number of relevant clinics, hospitals and institutes in Milan and Lombardy. This contained over one thousand twins and approximately one thousand documented clinical pedigrees. The general index, which identified 'the branches that could be useful to study from the point of view of the hereditary transmission of several traits',[25] formed the basis for the principal studies of the Centre during the 1940s. A first research project concerned the identification of 'defective branches'. In different zones of Lombardy, the field researchers discovered 'original foci of various pathological hereditary forms', in particular dental malformations, tumours, schizophrenia and manic depression.[26] The second line of research dealt with the hereditary transmission of 'talents', starting with 'pictorial' ability.[27]

Between 1940 and 1945 the research activities of Gianferrari's Centre were perfectly in line with the demographic, eugenic and racial policies of fascist Italy, stressing in particular the dysgenic effects of consanguineous marriages in isolated Alpine rural centres.[28] After the collapse of the fascist regime, the Milan Centre abandoned the project of racial improvement, shifting its attention to 'eugenic counselling' for couples. In 1946 Gianferrari's centre provided the first 'eugenic counselling' service in Italy. In 1948 another programme of 'municipal eugenic counselling' was founded at the Milan Policlinic, again entrusted to Gianferrari's Centre.[29] The activities of the two consultancy centres were principally concerned with premarital counselling for prospective parents and counselling for maternal-foetal haematic group or blood group incompatibility. The focus of the counselling service was on mental and nervous diseases, malformations, eye diseases and haemopathy (haemophilia). Methodologically, it was based on the construction of medical pedigrees through a combination of biographic narratives and anatomical and pathological observations. Medical pedigrees constituted the family as a collective patient, comparing a set of cases that shared a single pathological entity. In Gianferrari's vision, 'eugenic counselling' was conceived as part of a more comprehensive system of preventive measures, which also included 'direct action on environmental conditions'.[30] This environmental component focused on the dimensions of mother-infant relations (including housing and feeding) and education. At the Fourth International Congress of Catholic Physicians, held in Rome in September and October 1949, Gianferrari condemned any form of compulsory eugenic intervention and instead proposed that municipalities distribute a 'sanitary booklet to inform those affected by morbid hereditary conditions or who come from defective pedigrees of the serious responsibility toward the offspring that marriage carries with it'.[31]

For the Bellagio Congress, Gianferrari proposed a paper on the 'genetics of leukaemia'. Without any reference to genes or mutations, this paper was the result of a wide genealogical and statistical survey of 278 patients admitted to hospitals in Lombardy between 1945 and 1950. Not surprisingly, the final collection of family cases did not provide any evidence concerning the pathological inheritance of leukaemia.[32] During the elaboration of the Congress's scientific programme, the Italian geneticists did not receive Gianferrari's contribution positively and tried to organize some form of opposition. At the meeting of the Executive Board on 18 February 1953, Buzzati-Traverso voted against including Gianferrari's paper on leukaemia, while Montalenti suggested an alternative topic, focused on the distribution of blood group frequencies in Italy. As in the case of Gini, Montalenti's moderate attitude finally prevailed, and Gianferrari's contribution was published in the Congress proceedings.

Besides this scientific dimension, political and academic opposition further aggravated the situation. In 1953 controversy emerged regarding the qualification exam sessions for the first Italian professorship (*libera docenza*) in human genetics. The Minister of Public Education, the Christian Democrat Antonio Segni, consulted the First Section of the High Council (Sezione I del Consiglio Superiore) of Public Education regarding the composition of the deciding committee. The High Council proposed the following names: as permanent members, Claudio Barigozzi (professor of genetics in Milan), Giuseppe Montalenti (professor of genetics in Naples) and Alfonso Giordano (professor of anatomy and pathological histology in Pavia); as substitute members, Adriano Buzzati-Traverso (professor of genetics in Pavia) and Umberto D'Ancona (professor of zoology in Padua). Without taking this recommendation into account, on 15 June 1953 Segni proposed a radical alternative: the three professors of genetics disappeared from the committee, and in their places he nominated, as permanent members, the physicians Luigi Gedda, Luisa Gianferrari and Giovanni Di Guglielmo (professor of general clinical medicine and medical therapy in Rome), and, as substitute members, Alfonso Giordano and Giovanni Dall'Acqua (professor of specialized medical pathology and clinical methodology in Bari).[33] Having petitioned in vain for the Ministry to reconsider its choice, Barigozzi, Buzzati-Traverso and Montalenti adopted the strategy of a frontal attack: the first two appealed, on 27 August, to the State Council (Consiglio di Stato),[34] while the third, in December, denounced Segni's decision directly to the President of the Italian Republic.[35] The geneticists questioned the legitimacy of the ministerial decision – the Ministry had not only ignored the recommendation of the High Council, but had also failed to give any justification for its interference. Finally, considering all sides of the controversy, the sixth session of the State Council, at its jurisdictional session on 7 April 1954, decided in favour of the geneticists and annulled Segni's decree of June 1953.

The third aspect of this struggle between geneticists and physicians pertained to the institutional organization of the discipline. In 1951 Gianferrari and Gedda inaugurated a new scientific association: the Italian Society of Medical Genetics (Società Italiana di Genetica Medica). This was headed by Carlo Foà, a fascist Jewish physiologist at the University of Milan who had immigrated to Brazil after the promulgation of the Racial Laws in 1938. In January 1952 the first issue of the international quarterly *Acta Geneticae Medicae et Gemellologiae*, the journal of the Italian Society of Medical Genetics, was published. Luigi Gedda was the editor, while Luisa Gianferrari was a member of the editorial board. In the article that opened the first issue, Gedda interpreted his approach to genetics in terms of an holistic form of constitutional medicine. According to Gedda, the three different schools of constitutional medicine – morphological, functional and neuro-endocrinal – had tried to resolve the dichotomies between 'Virchowian localism' and 'Pasteurian esogenism', but with only limited success. Only genetics could allow a synthesis between 'synchronic' (form and function in action) and 'diachronic' (individual anamnesy) studies of the phenotype and 'family stock'.[36] In Gedda's opinion, medicine had therefore reached a 'turning point' due to the decisive contributions of genetics. The focus of scientific and professional interest was shifting 'from the recognition of the imprint of illness on the phenotype and from the knowledge of esogenic moments of illness' to the 'endogenic moments, that is, to constitution'.

On 6 and 7 September 1953, just a week after the Bellagio Congress, the Italian Society of Medical Genetics organized the First International Symposium of Medical Genetics (Primum Symposium Internationale Geneticae Medicae) held in Rome, under the auspices of Pope Pius XII. The Symposium coincided with the inauguration of the Gregor Mendel Institute of Medical Genetics and Twin Research, founded in Rome with headquarters in Piazza Galeno, and directed by Gedda.[37] The intensity of the conflict between the professional geneticists and the Gedda-Gianferrari group is reflected well by these few indignant lines written by Buzzati-Traverso to Montalenti in February 1953:

> And what do you think of those S.O.B.s (if you don't know what it means, ask the nearest American) Gedda and Gianferrari, who are putting together a symposium of medical genetics, without saying even one word to the organisers of the congress? With this, they also make us look stupid, regarding those who would have been invited, who will conclude that usually in Italy, we gently lead each other to the gallows.[38]

At the inaugural ceremony of the Gregor Mendel Institute, the physiologist Carlo Foà, head of the Italian Society of Medical Genetics, attacked the so-called 'pure' geneticists directly, restating the right of medicine to engage in human genetics.[39] According to Foà, only medicine could provide geneticists with that 'verification of the most subtle clinical symptoms', necessary for the investigation of human heredity.[40]

In his inauguration speech as president of the Mendel Institute, Gedda outlined his view of the problems of human heredity, emphasizing in particular the connection between medical genetics and constitutional medicine.[41] According to Gedda, the aim of medical genetics was to 'carry its help to the clinic to study, diagnose and cure the phenotype', but also to 'make the phenotype as translucent as crystal, so that we can transparently see what is happening on the level of genotype and can provide for the individual and his offspring'.[42] From here came 'the prevention of the hereditary disease of the single individual and its cure without fatalism and purely symptomatic therapy, the treatment of diathesis, eugenics at the service of the individual rights and duties of the human person, and even premarital counselling'. In Gedda's view, genetics had to become the inheritor of family medicine, allowing it to seize the 'invisible fabric that links the illness of man to the history of his stirp'. In addition, Gedda maintained the necessity of new specialized centres 'where the problem can be posed and resolved through all the means that the insurance companies, military and sport medicine and other institutions that carry out collective medical assistance, can achieve today'.[43]

In his address to the participants of the Symposium, held at the papal summer residence of Castel Gandolfo on 8 September, and published the following day in *L'Osservatore Romano* (in its original French), Pius XII confirmed Gedda's programme. Pius XII, on the one hand, gave a summary of the basic and well-established facts and concepts of genetics: cell theory, fertilization, Mendel's laws, gene theory and mutations. On the other, with regards to the connections between the theory of heredity and evolution, the Pius XII admitted evolution only as a possibility or hypothesis not yet verified. In the final part of his discourse, Pius XII dealt with the issue of eugenics. According to his view, 'the fundamental tendency of genetics and eugenics' was 'to influence the transmission of hereditary factors in order to promote what is good and eliminate what is injurious'. This, he argued, was 'irreproachable from the moral viewpoint'. Pius XII strongly condemned 'certain defensive measures in genetics and eugenics'.[44] Sterilization, the 'interdiction of marriage', the segregation of defectives and therapeutic abortion were all rejected as affronts to the dignity of the human individual, in accordance with Catholic teachings.[45]

The reply of the 'pure' geneticists to Gedda's Symposium was swift. Following Theodosius Dobzhansky, who had criticized Pius XII's anti-evolutionism in *Science*,[46] Buzzati-Traverso provided a vitriolic review, again in *Science*, of Gedda's Symposium proceedings, which he denounced as encouraging international isolation.[47] He also criticized Gedda and Foà in person, suggesting that they at least learn the correct usage of specific terminology before occupying themselves with genetics:

> Of course, no geneticist would deny the right of medical doctors to devote themselves to human genetics, and, in fact, important contributions to the science of heredity have been made by professional physicians. They, however, should at least take the trouble to learn the proper use of terms, in order not to confuse, for example, inbreeding with backcrossings (p. 13) or chromosome markers with closely linked genes (p. 448).[48]

The struggle between the geneticists Barigozzi, Buzzati-Traverso and Montalenti and the physicians Gedda and Gianferrari triggered the process of disciplinary demarcation in the field of Italian genetics. Between March and April 1953, the three geneticists discussed the issue of the constitution of an Italian Society of Genetics – genetics 'without adjectives', as they emphasized – in order to counter the 'work of proselytism' in which the Italian Society of Medical Genetics was engaged.[49]

The Italian Society of Genetics (Associazione Genetica Italiana, AGI) was finally founded in June 1953. Initially conceived in 1949–50 as a means of distinguishing genetics from Corrado Gini's eugenics, the project of a national Genetics Society was now realized as a consequence of the struggle against Gedda's and Gianferrari's ambitions in human and medical genetics.

Conclusion

The organization of the Ninth International Congress of Genetics was a catalysing event in the process of discipline-building in Italian genetics. Defining the boundaries of their own discipline in the context of the Bellagio Congress, Italian professional geneticists drew the first line of demarcation against Gini's eugenics between 1948 and 1950. Confronted with Gini's enduring attempts to monopolize Italian research on human heredity along the lines of fascist eugenics, the response of the geneticists was articulated in two ways: while Buzzati-Traverso and Barigozzi contested Gini's hegemonic endeavours directly, Montalenti committed himself to a precarious strategy of mediation that aimed at preserving the scientific autonomy of the genetics section within SIGE. Gini's authoritarian approach and his persistent objections to the anti-racist stance of UNESCO led to the internal schism of SIGE. Italian geneticists succeeded in keeping Gini away from the organization of Bellagio Congress, but they decided, for diplomatic reasons, to include him in the programme, even though his contribution was based on a 'sub-Lamarckian' interpretation of human heredity.

The second line of demarcation was established between 1951 and 1953 against the constitution of the Italian Society of Medical Genetics and the activities of the Centres of Human Genetics, headed by the zoologist Luisa Gianferrari and by the physician Luigi Gedda. The radical conflict concerning the experimental methods and clinical practices of medical genetics was instrumental in reshaping the interpretation of pathological inheritance within the new cultural, ideological and political post-war framework. On one side, Gianferrari and Gedda supported the socio-medical and familial configuration of eugenics that had been elaborated in Italy in the 1920s and 1930s in connection with fascist social and demographic policies, and characterized by concepts such as familial transmission, constitution and predisposition. On the other, Italian experimental geneticists argued for a new biological and molecular definition of pathological heredity, focusing on inherited biochemical and metabolic disorders, re-establishing pedigrees along Mendelian lines, and proposing a genetic and biochemical reframing of the disease. The differences in the field of medical genetics not only concerned theoretical and methodological problems, but also affected the issue of professional boundaries, nurturing the opposition between clinical physicians and experimental biologists. The programme of the Bellagio Congress mirrored this scientific antagonism, as it presented Gianferrari's paper on the genetics of leukaemia and Montalenti's contribution on the genetics of microcythaemia side by side.[50]

Finally, the struggle between geneticists and physicians involved ideological and political issues as well. The contribution of Pius XII at the inauguration of Gedda's Mendel Institute, the political interference in the competition for the professorship of human genetics in 1953, and the Catholic orientation of Gianferrari's and Gedda's eugenics clearly reveal the political, ideological and academic dimensions of the strategy that the Italian Catholic political milieu pursued in the field of human and medical genetics. From this point of view, in confronting Gianferrari and Gedda, Italian professional geneticists intended not only to redefine the scientific and academic boundaries of their discipline, but also to protect medical and human genetics from the interference of the Vatican and of Catholic politics.

NOTES

Gausemeier, Müller-Wille and Ramsden, 'Introduction: Human Heredity in the Twentieth Century'

1. For classic accounts covering substantial parts of the twentieth century as well, see D. J. Kevles, *In the Name of Eugenics: Genetics and the Use of Human Heredity* (Cambridge, MA: Harvard University Press, 1985) and D. B. Paul, *Controlling Human Heredity: 1865 to the Present* (Amherst, NY: Prometheus Books, 1995) for Britain and North America. For the German case, see P. Weingart, K. Bayertz and J. Kroll, *Rasse, Blut und Gene: Geschichte der Eugenik und Rassenhygiene in Deutschland* (Frankfurt: Suhrkamp, 1992); for Scandinavia, G. Broberg and N. Roll-Hansen, *Eugenics and the Welfare State* (East Lansing, MI: Michigan State University Press, 1996); for France, A. Carol, *Histoire de l'Eugénisme en France: Les Médecins et la Procréation, XIXe-XXe Siècle* (Paris: Seuil, 1995); for Latin America, N. Stepan, *The Hour of Eugenics: Race, Gender, and Nation in Latin America* (Ithaca, NY: Cornell University Press, 1991); and for Russia and the Soviet Union, N. Krementsov, 'From "Beastly Philosophy" to Medical Genetics: Eugenics in Russia and the Soviet Union', *Annals of Science*, 68:1 (2011), pp. 61–92.
2. E. F. Keller, *The Century of the Gene* (Cambridge, MA: Harvard University Press, 2000).
3. On the role of animal and plant breeding for the emergence of Mendelism, see R. C. Olby, 'Mendelism: From Hybrids and Trade to a Science', *Comptes rendus de l'Académie des Sciences, Series III, Sciences de la vie*, 323:12 (2000), pp. 1043–1051, and P. Thurtle, *The Emergence of Genetic Rationality: Space, Time, and Information in American Biological Science, 1870–1920* (Seattle, WA: University of Washington Press, 2008); on *Drosophila melanogaster*, see R. E. Kohler, *Lords of the Fly:* Drosophila *Genetics and the Experimental Life* (Chicago, IL: University of Chicago Press, 1994).
4. Quoted from Lipphardt, Chapter 4 in this volume.
5. J.-P. Gaudillière and I. Löwy, 'Introduction: Horizontal and Vertical Transmission of Disease: The Impossible Separation', in J.-P. Gaudillière and I. Löwy (eds), *Heredity and Infection: The History of Disease Transmission* (London: Routledge, 2001), pp. 1–18.
6. S. Lindee, *Moments of Truth in Genetic Medicine* (Baltimore, MD: Johns Hopkins University Press, 2005); K. Wailoo and S. Pemberton, *The Troubled Dream of Genetic Medicine* (Baltimore, MD: Johns Hopkins University Press, 2006).
7. For excellent and well-researched recent accounts along these lines, see P. Harper, *A Short History of Medical Genetics* (Oxford: Oxford University Press, 2008); and M. Keynes, A. Edwards and R. Peel (eds), *A Century of Mendelism in Human Genetics* (Boca Raton, FL: CRC Press, 2004).

8. M. Speicher, S. Antonarakis and A. G. Motulsky (eds), *Vogel and Motulsky's Human Genetics: Problems and Approaches*, 4th edn (Heidelberg: Springer, 1997), p. 16.
9. Ibid., p. 18.
10. J. Witowski and J. R. Inglis (eds), *Davenport's Dream: 21st Century Reflections on Heredity and Eugenics* (Cold Spring Harbor, NY: Cold Spring Harbor Laboratory Press, 2008).
11. A. R. Rushton, *Genetics and Medicine in the United States, 1800 to 1922* (Baltimore, MD: Johns Hopkins University Press, 1994); see also W. Bateson, *Mendel's Principles of Heredity* (Cambridge: Cambridge University Press, 1909), pp. 210–34, for an early review of the literature.
12. Speicher, Antonarakis and Motulsky (eds), *Vogel and Motulsky's Human Genetics*, p. 20.
13. J. Sapp, *Genesis: The Evolution of Biology* (Oxford: Oxford University Press, 2003), p. 158.
14. Speicher, Antonarakis and Motulsky (eds), *Vogel and Motulsky's Human Genetics*, pp. 13, 21–23.
15. K. M. Ludmerer, *Genetics and American Society: A Historical Appraisal* (Baltimore, MD: Johns Hopkins University Press, 1972).
16. P. J. Pauly, *Biologists and the Promise of American Life: From Meriwether Lewis to Alfred Kinsey* (Princeton, NJ: Princeton University Press, 2000).
17. D. A. MacKenzie, 'Eugenics in Britain', *Social Studies of Science*, 6:3/4 (1976), pp. 499–532; T. M. Porter, *The Rise of Statistical Thinking: 1820-1900* (Princeton, NJ: Princeton University Press, 1986); P. M. H. Mazumdar, 'Two Models for Human Genetics: Blood Grouping and Psychiatry in Germany Between the World Wars', *Bulletin of the History of Medicine*, 70:4 (1996), pp. 609–57.
18. W. Schneider, 'Toward the Improvement of the Human Race: The History of Eugenics in France', *Journal of Modern History*, 54:2 (1982), pp. 268–91; P. Zylberman, 'Hereditary Diseases and Environmental Factors in the "Mixed Economy" of Public Health: Rene Sand and the French Social Medicine, 1920–1934', in Gaudillière and Löwy (eds), *Heredity and Infection*, pp. 261–81.
19. Kevles, *In the Name of Eugenics*, ch. 11.
20. P. J. Weindling, *Health, Race and German Politics between National Unification and Nazism, 1870–1945* (Cambridge: Cambridge University Press, 1989).
21. A. Schwerin, *Experimentalisierung des Menschen: Der Genetiker Hans Nachtsheim und die vergleichende Erbpathologie, 1920–1945* (Göttingen: Wallstein, 2004); A. Cottebrune, *Der planbare Mensch: Die Deutsche Forschungsgemeinschaft und die menschliche Vererbungswissenschaft, 1920–1970* (Stuttgart: Steiner, 2008); S. F. Weiss, *The Nazi Symbiosis: Human Genetics and Politics in the Third Reich* (Chicago, IL: University of Chicago Press, 2010).
22. C. López Beltrán, 'In the Cradle of Heredity: French Physicians and *l'hérédité naturelle* in the Early Nineteenth Century', *Journal of the History of Biology*, 37:1 (2004), pp. 39–72; S. Müller-Wille and H.-J. Rheinberger (eds), *Heredity Produced: At the Crossroads of Biology, Politics, and Culture, 1500–1870* (Cambridge, MA: MIT Press, 2007).
23. J. C. Waller, 'Ideas of Heredity, Reproduction and Eugenics in Britain, 1800–1875', *Studies in History and Philosophy of Science Part C: Studies in History and Philosophy of Biological and Biomedical Sciences*, 32:3 (2001), pp. 457–89; see also Waller's recent *Breeding: The Human History of Heredity, Race, and Sex* (Oxford: Oxford University Press, 2012), and C. E. Rosenberg, *No Other Gods: On Science and American Social Thought*, rev. edn (Baltimore, MD: Johns Hopkins University Press, 1997), as well as S. Müller-Wille and H.-J. Rheinberger, *A Cultural History of Heredity* (Chicago, IL: University of Chicago Press, 2012), especially ch. 5.

24. C. Renwick, 'From Political Economy to Sociology: Francis Galton and the Social Scientific Origins of Eugenics', *British Journal for the History of Science*, 44 (2011), pp. 343–69.
25. A. Powell, M. O'Malley, S. Müller-Wille, J. Calvert and J. Dupré, 'Disciplinary Baptisms: A Comparison of the Naming Stories of Genetics, Molecular Biology, Genomics and Systems Biology', *History and Philosophy of the Life Sciences*, 29:1 (2007), pp. 5–32. For a review of the historiography of classical genetics, molecular genetics and genomics that takes this point on board, see S. Müller-Wille and H.-J. Rheinberger, 'Gene Concepts', in A. Plutynsky and S. Sarkar (eds.), *A Companion to the Philosophy of Biology* (Oxford: Blackwell, 2008), pp. 3–21.
26. See A. Barahona, E. Suarez-Díaz and H.-J. Rheinberger (eds), *The Hereditary Hourglass: Genetics and Epigenetics, 1868–2000* (Berlin: Max Planck Institute for the History of Science, preprint no. 392, 2010), as well as Müller-Wille and Rheinberger, *A Cultural History of Heredity*, chs 6–8, for succinct overviews and guides to the literature.
27. L. Fleck, 'The Problem of Epistemology', in R. S. Cohen and T. Schnelle (eds), *Cognition and Fact: Materials on Ludwik Fleck* (Dordrecht: D. Reidel, 1986), pp. 70–112. For a comparison of Kuhn's and Fleck's models of scientific change, see S. Müller-Wille, 'History of Science and Medicine', in M. Jackson (ed.), *The Oxford Handbook of the History of Medicine* (Oxford: Oxford University Press), pp. 469–83.
28. For the later period of the twentieth century, see M. Fortun and E. Mendelsohn (eds), *The Practices of Human Genetics* (Dordrecht: Kluwer, 1999).
29. N. G. Comfort, *The Science of Human Perfection: How Genes Became the Heart of American Medicine* (New Haven, CT: Yale University Press, 2012).

1 Gausemeier, 'Borderlands of Heredity: The Debate about Hereditary Susceptibility to Tuberculosis, 1882–1945'

1. M. Worboys, 'From Heredity to Infection: Tuberculosis, 1870–1890', in J.-P. Gaudillière and I. Löwy (eds), *Heredity and Infection: The History of Disease Transmission* (London: Routledge 2001), pp. 81–99; P. K. Wilson, 'Confronting "Hereditary" Disease: Eugenic Attempts to Eliminate Tuberculosis in Progressive Era America', *Journal of Medical Humanities*, 27 (2006), pp. 19–37.
2. A. R. Rushton, *Genetics and Medicine in the United States, 1800 to 1922* (Baltimore, MD and London: Johns Hopkins University Press, 1994); M. Keynes, A. Edwards and R. Peel (eds), *A Century of Mendelism in Human Genetics* (Boca Raton, FL: CRC Press, 2004); P. Harper, *A Short History of Medical Genetics* (Oxford: Oxford University Press, 2008).
3. Worboys, 'From Heredity to Infection', *passim*.
4. A. Riffel, *Die Erblichkeit der Schwindsucht und tuberkuloesen Prozesse nachgewesen durch zahlreiches statistisches Material und die praktische Erfahrung* (Karlsruhe: Gutsch, 1890); A. Riffel, *Schwindsucht und Krebs im Lichte vergleichend-statistisch-genealogischer Forschung* (Karlsruhe: Gutsch, 1905).
5. B. Gausemeier, 'Auf der "Brücke zwischen Natur- und Geschichtswissenschaft". Ottokar Lorenz und die Neuerfindung der Genealogie um 1900', in F. Vienne and C. Brandt (eds), *Wissensobjekt Mensch. Praktiken der Humanwissenschaften im 20. Jahrhundert* (Berlin: Kadmos, 2008), pp. 137–64.
6. F. Martius, 'Die Vererbbarkeit des constitutionellen Factors der Tuberculose', *Berliner medizinische Wochenschrift*, 38 (1901), pp. 1125–30; R. Schlüter, *Die Anlage zur Tuberkulose* (Leipzig: Deuticke, 1905).

7. G. Cornet, *Die Tuberculose* (Wien: Hölder, 1899), pp. 278–9.
8. F. Galton, *Natural Inheritance* (London: Macmillan, 1889), pp. 164–86.
9. For guides on insurance medicine, see E. Buchheim, Ärztliche Versicherungs-Diagnostik (Vienna: Hölder, 1887); G. Florschütz, *Allgemeine Lebensversicherungsmedizin* (Berlin: Mittler, 1914).
10. According to a survey of the biggest German company, *Gothaer Lebensversicherungsbank*, 23.7 per cent of its insurants who had died from TB had a parent having suffered the same fate, while the average TB mortality accounted for 11.6 per cent; see Florschütz, *Allgemeine Lebensversicherungsmedizin*, p. 54. For the statistical use of insurance material also H. Westergaard, *Die Lehre von der Mortalität und Morbilität* (Jena: Fischer, 1901), pp. 512–22.
11. F. Condrau, *Lungenheilanstalt und Patientenschicksal. Sozialgeschichte der Tuberkulose in Deutschland und England im späten 19. und frühen 20. Jahrhundert* (Göttingen: Vandenhoeck und Ruprecht, 2000), pp. 57–65.
12. K. Pearson, *A First Study of the Statistics of Pulmonary Tuberculosis* (London: Dulau, 1907).
13. Ibid., pp. 11–13.
14. W. Weinberg, 'Pathologische Vererbung und genealogische Statistik', *Deutsches Archiv für Klinische Medizin*, 78 (1903), pp. 521–40.
15. F. Prinzing, 'Die mannigfachen Beziehungen zwischen Statistik und Medizin', *Allgemeines Statistisches Archiv*, 6 (1902–4), pp. 1–22, on p. 3.
16. W. Weinberg, 'Die württembergischen Familienregister und ihre Bedeutung als Quellen für wissenschaftliche Untersuchungen', *Württembergische Jahrbücher für Statistik und Landeskunde* (1907), pp. 174–98.
17. W. Weinberg, 'Die familiäre Belastung der Tuberkulösen und ihren Beziehungen zu Infektion und Vererbung', *Beiträge zur Klinik der Tuberkulose*, 7 (1907), pp. 257–89.
18. Ibid., p. 270.
19. Pearson, *A First Study of the Statistics of Pulmonary Tuberculosis*, p. 11.
20. W. Weinberg, 'Weitere Beiträge zur Theorie der Vererbung', *Archiv für Rassen- und Gesellschaftsbiologie*, 7 (1910), pp. 35–49 and 169–73, on p. 49
21. Weinberg, 'Familiäre Belastung', pp. 266–72.
22. W. Weinberg, 'Ueber die Fruchtbarkeit der Phthisiker beiderlei Geschlechts', *Medizinische Reform*, 16 (1908), pp. 285–8 and 298–9, on p. 299.
23. F. Reiche, 'Die Bedeutung der erblichen Belastung bei der Lungenschwindsucht', *Zeitschrift für Tuberkulose und Heilstättenwesen*, 1 (1901), pp. 302–10.
24. F. Reiche, 'Die Heredität bei Phtisis pulmonum', *Beiträge zur Klinik der Tuberkulose*, 54 (1923), pp. 394–401.
25. Weinberg, 'Familiäre Belastung', p. 260.
26. A. Gottstein, *Allgemeine Epidemiologie der Tuberkulose* (Berlin: Springer, 1931), pp. 55–63.
27. V. Haecker, 'Vererbungsgeschichtliche Probleme der sozialen und Rassenhygiene', in A. Gottstein et al. (eds), *Handbuch der sozialen Hygiene und Gesundheitsfürsorge*, Vol. I (Berlin: Springer, 1925), pp. 182–255, on pp. 233–50.
28. H. Münter, 'Lungentuberkulose und Erblichkeit. Eine erbbiologische Untersuchung', *Beiträge zur Klinik der Tuberkulose*, 76 (1930), pp. 257–344; K. Diehl and O. von Verschuer, *Zwillingstuberkulose* (Jena: Fischer, 1933), pp. 35–7.

29. J. A. Mendelsohn, 'Medicine and the Making of Bodily Inequality in Twentieth-Century Europe', in J. P. Gaudillière and I. Löwy (eds), *Heredity and Infection. The History of Disease Transmission* (London: Routledge, 2001), pp. 21–79, on p. 26.
30. Florschütz, *Allgemeine Lebensversicherungsmedizin*, pp. 56–7.
31. H. W. Siemens, 'Über eine Aufgabe und Methode der Konstitutionsforschung', *Beiträge zur Klinik der Tuberkulose*, 43 (1920), pp. 327–31.
32. E. Kretschmer, *Körperbau und Charakter. Untersuchungen zum Konstitutionsproblem und zur Lehre von den Temperamenten* (Berlin: Springer, 1921).
33. F. Ickert, 'Körpertyp und Tuberkulose', *Beiträge zur Klinik der Tuberkulose*, 72 (1929), pp. 774–83.
34. W. Hagen, 'Zur Disposition für Erkrankung an Tuberkulose', *Beiträge zur Klinik der Tuberkulose*, 58 (1924), pp. 481–7.
35. E. Rüdin, *Studien über Vererbung und Entstehung geistiger Störungen. Bd. 1: Zur Vererbung und Neuentstehung der Dementia Praecox* (Berlin: Springer, 1916). For the background of the study, see M. M. Weber, *Ernst Rüdin. Eine kritische Biographie* (Berlin: Springer, 1993).
36. H. Luxenburger, 'Tuberkulose als Todesursache in den Geschwisterschaften Schizophrener, Manisch-Depressiver und der Durchschnittsbevölkerung', *Zeitschrift für die gesamte Neurologie und Psychiatrie*, 109 (1927), pp. 313–40.
37. H. W. Siemens, *Die Zwillingspathologie* (Berlin: Springer, 1924).
38. Diehl and Verschuer, *Zwillingstuberkulose*.
39. For a concise analysis of Verschuer's twin research programme, see B. Massin, 'Mengele, die Zwillingsforschung und die "Auschwitz-Dahlem Connection"', in C. Sachse (ed.), *Die Verbindung nach Auschwitz. Biowissenschaften und Menschenversuche an Kaiser-Wilhelm-Instituten* (Göttingen: Wallstein, 2003), pp. 201–54.
40. Diehl and Verschuer, *Zwillingstuberkulose*, pp. 130–6.
41. K. Turban, 'Die Vererbung des Locus minoris resistentiae bei der Lungentuberkulose', *Zeitschrift für Tuberkulose und Heilstättenwesen*, 1 (1901), pp. 30–8 and 123–9.
42. H. W. Schmuhl, *Grenzüberscheitungen. Das Kaiser-Wilhelm-Institut für Anthropologie, menschliche Erblehre und Eugenik 1927–1945* (Göttingen: Wallstein, 2005), p. 107.
43. B. Lange, 'Äußere und innere Ursachen der Infektionskrankheiten, dargestellt am Beispiel der Tuberkulose', *Die Naturwissenschaften*, 51 (1936), pp. 802–9.
44. Schmuhl, *Grenzüberschreitungen*, pp. 240–1.
45. K. Diehl and O. von Verschuer, *Der Erbeinfluß bei der Tuberkulose (Zwillingstuberkulose II)* (Jena: Fischer, 1936).
46. Ibid., p. 147.
47. Diehl and Verschuer, *Zwillingstuberkulose*, p. 457.
48. K. Diehl, 'Tierexperimentelle Erbforschung bei der Tuberkulose', *Beiträge zur Klinik der Tuberkulose*, 97 (1942), pp. 331–49.
49. For a good survey of Nazi TB policies, see K. Kelting, *Das Tuberkuloseproblem im Nationalsozialismus* (MD dissertation, Universität Kiel, 1974).
50. O. von Verschuer, 'Zwillingsforschung und Tuberkulose', *Beiträge zur Klinik der Tuberkulose*, 97 (1942), pp. 317–31.
51. Discussion statements by E. Jüngling, C. Noeggerath and H. Rietschel, in *Beiträge zur Klinik der Tuberkulose*, 97 (1942), pp. 386–7.
52. For a review of results up the 1990s, see L. J. Boothroyd, *Genetic Susceptibility to Tuberculosis* (PhD dissertation, McGill University, 1994).

2 Wilson, 'Championing a US Clinic for Human Heredity: Pre-War Concepts and Post-War Constructs'

1. P. K. Wilson, 'Eugenicist Harry Laughlin's Crusade to Classify and Control the "Socially Inadequate in Progressive Era America"', *Patterns of Prejudice*, 36 (2002), p. 53.
2. Harry H. Laughlin, 'Notes on the Growing Demand for a Clinical Service in Human Heredity', typescript in 'Report 1937–1938' folder, box C-4-3:12, p. 2, Harry H. Laughlin Papers, Pickler Memorial Library Special Collections, Truman State University (TSU), Kirksville, Missouri (hereafter Laughlin Papers, TSU).
3. Charles B. Davenport to Ludwig Hektoen, 6 October 1923, 'Hektoen letters' file, Box 51, B/D 27, Charles B. Davenport Papers, American Philosophical Society (APS), Philadelphia, Pennsylvania; and Laughlin, 'Notes on the Growing Demand for a Clinical Service in Human Heredity'.
4. Harry H. Laughlin, 'Clinical Service in Human Heredity' (1938), typescript in 'Clinic in Human Heredity – Work and Papers' folder, box D-5-5:6, p. 19, Laughlin Papers, TSU.
5. Harry H. Laughlin, 'Explanatory Notes of the Sample Clinical Cases' (1938), typescript in 'Clinic in Human Heredity' folder, box D-5-5, p. 11, Laughlin Papers, TSU.
6. Ibid., p. 13.
7. Harry H. Laughlin, 'Brief Instructions on How to Make a Eugenical Study of a Family' (1915), in 'Eugenics in National Reconstruction; Eugenics Study Instructions' folder, box D-2-5:2, Laughlin Papers, TSU.
8. H. Bruinius, *Better for All the World: The Secret History of Forced Sterilization and America's Quest for Racial Purity* (New York: Alfred A. Knopf, 2002).
9. H. H. Laughlin, 'An Account of the Work of the Eugenics Record Office', *American Breeders Magazine*, 3 (1912), pp. 119–23, on p. 121. For a more thorough review of the use of pedigree charts in human medical practice, see R. G. Resta, 'The Crane's Foot: The Rise of the Pedigree in Human Genetics', *Journal of Genetic Counseling*, 2 (1993) pp. 235–59; A. R. Rushton, *Genetics and Medicine in the United States, 1800 to 1922* (Baltimore, MD: Johns Hopkins University Press, 1994); Y. Nukaga and A. Cambrosio. 'Medical Pedigrees and the Visual Production of Family Disease in Canadian and Japanese Genetic Counseling Practices', in M. A. Elston (ed.), *The Sociology of Medical Science and Technology* (Oxford: Blackwell, 1997), pp. 29–55; and P. K. Wilson, 'Pedigree Charts as Tools to Visualize Inherited Disease in Progressive Era America', in S. Müller-Wille and H.-J. Rheinberger (eds), *A Cultural History of Heredity: Heredity in the Century of the Gene* (Berlin: Max-Plank-Institut für Wissenschaftsgeschichte, 2008), pp. 163–90.
10. George Draper outlined his overall views of basic human types in a number of publications, among the earliest being 'Man as a Complete Organism – in Health and Disease', *New York State Medical Journal*, 34 (1934), reprint pp. 1–12, as well as in 'The Common Denominator of Disease', in I. Galdston (ed.), *Medicine and Mankind* (New York: D. Appleton-Century Co., 1936), pp. 105–35. For an overview of Draper, see S. W. Tracy, 'George Draper and American Constitutional Medicine, 1916–1946: Reinventing the Sick Man', *Bulletin of the History of Medicine*, 66 (1992), pp. 53–89.
11. S. Lindee, *Moments of Truth in Genetic Medicine* (Baltimore, MD: Johns Hopkins University Press, 2005), p. 17.
12. S. W. Tracy, 'An Evolving Science of Man: The Transformation and Demise of American Constitutional Medicine, 1920–1950', in C. Lawrence and G. Weisz (eds), *Greater than the Parts: Holism in Biomedicine, 1920–1950* (New York: Oxford University Press,

1998), pp. 161–88, on p. 170. Here we see a return to the malleable or soft hereditarianism that was frequently found in nineteenth-century discourse on heredity.

13. Harry H. Laughlin to Allan Gregg, 29 June 1936, 'Committee of Human Heredity' folder, box C-2-2:5, Laughlin Papers, TSU.
14. The Pioneer Foundation, 'Notes on Getting the Work Underway', n.d., in 'Draper-Osborn-Pioneer Fund' folder, box D-2-3, Laughlin Papers, TSU. M. E. Kopp, 'The Development of Marriage Consultation Centers as a New Field of Social Medicine', *American Journal of Obstetrics and Gynecology*, 26 (1933), pp. 122–34, described the contemporary social importance of marriage consultation clinics.
15. Laughlin argued in support of the term 'Pioneer Fund', noting that although a 'colorless term, it would be perfectly appropriate if this foundation should have for its purpose the maintenance of the pioneer traditions and the perpetuation of pioneer family-stocks and the hereditary qualities – physical, spiritual, and mental – of the pioneer families of America'; Harry H. Laughlin to Mr Malcolm Donald, 24 February 1937, 'Draper-Osborn-Pioneer Fund' folder, box D-2-3, Laughlin Papers, TSU. The Pioneer Fund's current director, Harry F. Weyher, outlined this organization's somewhat controversial history in his 'Contributions to the History of Psychology: CXII. Intelligence, Behavioral Genetics, and the Pioneer Fund', *Psychological Reports*, 82 (1998), pp. 1347–74. See also M. G. Kenny, 'Toward a Racial Abyss: Eugenics, Wickliffe Draper, and the Origins of the Pioneer Fund', *Journal of the History of the Behavioral Sciences*, 38 (2002), pp. 259–83, and R. Lynn, *The Science of Human Diversity: A History of the Pioneer Fund* (Lanham, MD: University Press of America, 2001).
16. Quip from one page typed note titled 'Private Copy for Colonel W. Draper', n.d., 'Draper-Osborn-Pioneer Fund' folder, box D-2-3, Laughlin Papers, TSU.
17. T. H. Morgan to James G. Eddy, 29 January 1938, in 'Correspondence-Eddy Clinic of Human Heredity' folder, box E-2-1, Laughlin Papers, TSU.
18. Harry H. Laughlin, 'Outline of the Organization, Staff and Service, Proposed for "The Clinic of Human Heredity"' (July 1937), 'Outline of the Organization, Staff, and Service, Proposed for "The Clinic of Human Heredity"' folder, box E-2-2, Laughlin Papers, TSU.
19. Ibid.
20. Ibid.
21. John C. Merriam to James G. Eddy, 13 January 1938, in 'Correspondence-Eddy Clinic of Human Heredity' folder, box E-2-1, Laughlin Papers, TSU.
22. L. R. Dice, 'Heredity Clinics: Their Value for Public Service and for Research', *American Journal of Human Genetics*, 4 (1952), pp. 1–13, on p. 11. For a thorough review, see N. Comfort, *The Science of Human Perfection: How Genes Became the Heart of Medicine* (New Haven, CT: Yale University Press, 2010), pp. 97–129.
23. Sheldon Reed later argued that the Dight Institute 'did not really function until I came … in 1947'; Sheldon C. Reed to Frederick Osborn, 18 March 1970, 'Osborn, Frederick: History of the American Eugenics Society' folder, American Eugenics Society Papers, APS.
24. Dice, 'Heredity Clinics', pp. 9–11. Reed, Director of the Dight Institute, identified a dozen of these sites throughout the US in his *Counseling in Medical Genetics* (Philadelphia, PA: W. B. Saunders, 1955), a work written for medical practitioners. He added a few more to the list he created for Ashley Montague's popular *Human Heredity* (Cleveland OH: World Publishing Co., 1959), Appendix C, pp. 348–9.
25. S. C. Reed, 'A Short History of Genetic Counseling', *Social Biology*, 21 (1974), pp. 332–9, on p. 335. For further discussion of the growth of 'Genetic Counseling' in the United States, see E. J. Yoxen, 'Constructing Genetic Diseases', in T. Duster and K. Garrett (eds),

Cultural Perspectives on Biological Knowledge (Norwood, NJ: Ablex Publishing Company, 1984), pp. 41–62; D. C. Wertz, 'Eugenics in Alive and Well: A Survey of Genetic Professionals around the World', *Science in Context*, 11 (1998), pp. 493–510; and H. P. Kröner, 'From Eugenics to Genetic Screening: Historical Problems of Human Genetic Applications', in R. Chadwick et al. (eds), *The Ethics of Genetic Screening* (Amsterdam: Kluwer, 1999), pp. 131–45.

26. F. Osborn, 'Eugenics: Retrospect and Prospect', 26 March 1959, prepared for the 23 April 1959 American Eugenics Society Directors Meeting, typescript, p. 4, in 'Concerning Eugenics' folder, Frederick Henry Osborn Papers, MS. Coll. 24, American Eugenics Society Papers, APS.
27. Ibid., p. 5.
28. P. K. Wilson, 'Bad Habits from Bad Genes: Early 20th-Century Eugenic Attempts to Eliminate Syphilis and Associated "Defects" from the United States', *Canadian Bulletin of Medical History*, 20 (2003), pp. 11–41.
29. T. B. Turner, *Heritage of Excellence: The Johns Hopkins Medical Institutions, 1914–1947* (Baltimore, MD: Johns Hopkins University Press, 1974), p. 167.
30. M. Warren, *Johns Hopkins: Knowledge for the World: 1876–2001* (Baltimore, MD: Johns Hopkins University Press, 2000), p. 150.
31. J. E. Moore to A. M. Harvey, 9 July 1952, p. 1. 'Medicine I – Procedures & Policies' folder, Moore Clinic box. The Victor Almon McKusick Collection, Alan Mason Chesney Medical Archives of the Johns Hopkins Medical Institutions, Baltimore, Maryland.
32. E. W. Smith to all Hopkins Out-Patient Department Physicians, 2 February 1955, p. 1. 'Medicine I-Procedures & Policies' folder, Moore Clinic box. McKusick Collection, Chesney Medical Archives.
33. Ibid., p. 2.
34. A. M. Harvey, V. A. McKusick and J. D. Stobo, *Osler's Legacy: The Department of Medicine at Johns Hopkins 1889–1989* (Baltimore, MD: Johns Hopkins University Press, 1990), p. 83.
35. J. E. Moore to A. M. Harvey, 9 July 1952, p. 13. 'Medicine I-Procedures & Policies' folder, Moore Clinic box. McKusick Collection, Chesney Medical Archives.
36. Warren, *Johns Hopkins*, p. 150.
37. L. Van Dam, 'The Gene Doctor is In', *MIT's Technological Review*, 100 (1997), pp. 46–52, on p. 47. Initially, the 'clustering of abnormalities' that McKusick frequently saw in his heart patients 'intrigued him'. Soon thereafter he became 'particularly fascinated' by Marfan's syndrome patients, though eventually 'the study and management of the whole realm of inherited diseases, symptoms and predispositions became his field'; *Uniquely Johns Hopkins* (Baltimore, MD: Johns Hopkins School of Medicine, 1988), p. 14.
38. Harvey et al., *Osler's Legacy*, p. 84.
39. J. E. Moore to A.M. Harvey, 9 July 1952, p. 1. 'Medicine I-Procedures & Policies' folder, Moore Clinic box. McKusick Collection, Chesney Medical Archives.
40. Victor A. McKusick to Arno Motulsky, 18 November 1957. 'Clinic-Medical Genetics' folder, Moore Clinic box, McKusick Collection, Chesney Medical Archives.
41. The AES was incorporated in 1926 to promote popular educational programmes in eugenics. Following World War II, Frederick Osborn was elected as president of the AES. Osborn had a long-standing interest in the research aspects of eugenics, having served as a founding director of the Eugenics Research Association (ERA) at the time of its incorporation in 1928. Typical of the various attempts to explicitly distance interested parties from anything labeled 'eugenics' by the late 1930s, the ERA was renamed

the Association for Research in Human Heredity in 1938. For general historical overviews of the AES, see M. A. Bigelow, 'Brief History of the American Eugenics Society', *Eugenical News*, 31 (1946), pp. 49–51, and F. Osborn, 'History of the American Eugenics Society', *Social Biology*, 21 (1974), pp. 115–26.

42. Victor A. McKusick, 'Log Book, Medical Genetics', 1957, vol. 1. Moore Clinic box. McKusick Collection, Chesney Medical Archives. 'Record System' taped inside front cover.
43. Of these, the most common conditions studied were neurofibromatosis, polycystic kidney disease, Marfan's syndrome, tuberous sclerosis, premature coronary artery disease, Charcot–Marie–Tooth disease and Laurence–Moon–Biedl syndrome.
44. Victor A. McKusick to F. Parkes Weber, 17 January 1958, in 'W-until 1960' folder, Moore Clinic box. McKusick Collection, Chesney Medical Archives.
45. Victor A. McKusick to a North Carolina patient, 24 November 1958, in 'Patient Follow-up Correspondence' folder, Moore Clinic box. McKusick Collection, Chesney Medical Archives.
46. Victor A. McKusick to a Washington, DC patient, 23 July 1958, in 'Patient Follow-up Correspondence' folder, Moore Clinic box. McKusick Collection, Chesney Medical Archives.
47. Victor A. McKusick to a Virginia patient, 26 December 1958, in 'Patient Follow-up Correspondence' folder, Moore Clinic box. McKusick Collection, Chesney Medical Archives.
48. Victor A. McKusick to a University of Virginia physician, 26 December 1958, in 'Patient Follow-up Correspondence' folder, Moore Clinic box. McKusick Collection, Chesney Medical Archives.
49. 'Research Summary', 18 June 1959, pp. 1–2, in 'Research Summary' folder, Moore Clinic box. McKusick Collection, Chesney Medical Archives.
50. 'Research Outline', 25 September 1959, pp. 1–2, in 'Research Summary' folder, Moore Clinic box. McKusick Collection, Chesney Medical Archives.
51. Osborn, 'Eugenics: Retrospect and Prospect', pp. 3–4.

3 Ramsden, 'Remodelling the Boundaries of Normality: Lionel S. Penrose and Population Surveys of Mental Ability'

1. D. Thom and M. Jennings, 'Human Pedigree and the "Best Stock": From Eugenics to Genetics?', in T. Marteau and M. Richards (eds), *The Troubled Helix: Social and Psychological Implications of the New Human Genetics* (Cambridge: Cambridge University Press, 1996), pp. 211–34, on p. 228.
2. D. B. Paul, *The Politics of Heredity: Essays on Eugenics, Biomedicine, and the Nature-Nurture Debate* (Albany, NY: State University of New York Press, 1998), p. 141.
3. Sean Valles has also sought to focus attention on the radical and pioneering nature of Penrose's criticism of typological thinking and promotion of human diversity – 'Lionel Penrose and the Concept of Normal Variation in Human Intelligence', *Studies in History and Philosophy of Biological and Biomedical Sciences*, 43 (2012), pp. 281–9.
4. J. R. Flynn, 'The Mean IQ of Americans: Massive Gains 1932 to 1978', *Psychological Bulletin*, 95 (1984), pp. 29–51; U. Neisser (ed.), *The Rising Curve: Long-Term Gains in IQ and Related Measures* (Washington, DC: American Psychological Association, 1998).
5. In spite of the importance of such investigations as the National Survey of Health and Development and the Scottish Mental Surveys in Britain, and the Berkeley and

Harvard Growth Studies in the United States, their histories have been left to those directly engaged in them. See J. M. Tanner, *A History of the Study of Human Growth* (Cambridge: Cambridge University Press, 1981), and M. E. J. Wadsworth, *The Imprint of Time: Childhood, History, and Adult Life* (Oxford: Clarendon Press; New York: Oxford University Press, 1991).

6. For a detailed analysis of this survey and its influence, see E. Ramsden, 'A Differential Paradox: The Controversy Surrounding the 1947 Scottish Inquiry into Intelligence and Family Size', *Journal of the History of the Behavioral Sciences*, 43 (2007), pp. 109–34.
7. I. Lakatos, 'Falsification and the Methodology of Scientific Research Programmes', in I. Lakatos and A. Musgrave (eds), *Criticism and the Growth of Knowledge* (Cambridge: Cambridge University Press, 1970), pp. 91–195. See in particular P. Urbach, 'Progress and Degeneration in the I.Q. Debate (1)', *British Journal for the Philosophy of Science*, 25 (1974), pp. 99–135.
8. F. Galton, 'Regression towards Mediocrity in Hereditary Stature', *Journal of the Anthropological Institute of Great Britain and Ireland, 15 (1886), pp.* 246–63, and F. Galton, *Natural Inheritance* (London: Macmillan, 1889).
9. See discussion in A. Desrosières, *The Politics of Large Numbers: A History of Statistical Reasoning* (Cambridge, MA: Harvard University Press, 1998), and D. A. MacKenzie, *Statistics in Britain, 1865–1930: The Social Construction of Scientific Knowledge* (Edinburgh: Edinburgh University Press, 1981).
10. F. Galton, *Hereditary Genius: An Inquiry into its Laws and Consequences*, 2nd edn (London: Macmillan, 1892), p. 28.
11. Ibid., p. 321.
12. Tanner, *A History*, p. 217.
13. W. T. Porter, 'The Physical Basis of Precocity and Dullness', *Transactions of the Academy of Science of St. Louis*, 6 (1895), pp. 161–81, on p. 168.
14. H. H. Goddard, 'The *Height and Weight of Feeble-minded Children* in American Institutions', *Journal of Nervous and Mental Disease*, 39 (1912), pp. 217–35, on p. 217.
15. H. H. Goddard, *The Kallikak Family: A Study in the Heredity of Feeble-mindedness* (New York, Macmillan, 1912), p. 110–11.
16. Ibid., p. 101.
17. Mackenzie, *Statistics in Britain*, and W. B. Provine, *The Origins of Theoretical Population Genetics* (Chicago, IL: University of Chicago Press, 1971).
18. R. C. Punnett, 'Eliminating Feeblemindedness', *Journal of Heredity*, 8 (1917), pp. 464–5. For an excellent analysis of this issue, see D. B. Paul and H. G. Spencer, 'Did Eugenics Rest on an Elementary Mistake?', in J. Beatty, C. Krimbas, D. B. Paul and R. S. Singh (eds), *Thinking about Evolution: Historical, Philosophical and Political Perspectives* (Cambridge: Cambridge University Press, 2001), pp. 103–18.
19. H. S. Jennings, 'Health Progress and Race Progress: Are They Incompatible?', *Journal of Heredity*, 18 (1927), pp. 271–6, on p. 274.
20. R. A. Fisher, 'The Correlation between Relatives on the Supposition of Mendelian Inheritance', *Transactions of the Royal Society of Edinburgh*, 52 (1918), pp. 399–433.
21. P. M. H. Mazumdar, *Eugenics, Human Genetics and Human Failings: The Eugenics Society, its Sources and Critics in Britain* (London: Routledge, 1991), p. 107–10.
22. R. A. Fisher, 'The Elimination of Mental Defect', *Eugenics Review*, 16 (1924), pp. 114–16, on p. 115.
23. Ibid., p. 116.
24. Mazumdar, *Eugenics*, p. 109.

25. Fisher, 'The Correlation', p. 400.
26. Ibid.
27. Ibid., p. 424. See J. Tabery, 'R. A. Fisher, Lancelot Hogben, and the Origin(s) of Genotype-Environment Interaction', *Journal of the History of Biology*, 41 (2008), pp. 717–61.
28. Fisher, 'The Elimination', p. 116.
29. C. Burt, *Mental and Scholastic Tests* (London: London County Council, 1921); C. Burt, 'Ability and Income', *British Journal of Educational Psychology*, 13 (1943), pp. 83–98; C. Burt and M. Howard, 'The Multifactorial Theory of Inheritance and its Application to Intelligence', *British Journal of Statistical Psychology*, 8 (1956), pp. 95–131; C. Spearman, 'The Proof and Measurement of Association between Two Things', *American Journal of Psychology*, 15 (1904), pp. 72–101; C. Spearman, 'Demonstration of Formulæ for True Measurement of Correlation', *American Journal of Psychology,* 18 (1907), pp. 161–9; C. Spearman, *The Abilities of Man: Their Nature and Measurement* (London: Macmillan, 1927). In his belief that the general factor could also be used for physical form, Burt disagreed with Spearman.
30. L. S. Hearnshaw, *Cyril Burt: Psychologist* (London: Hodder and Stoughton, 1979) p. 58.
31. For excellent analyses of Boas's challenge upon which this essay draws, see Tanner, *A History*, ch. 10, and J. M. Tanner, 'Boas' Contributions to Knowledge of Human Growth and Form', in W. Goldschmidt (ed.), *The Anthropology of Franz Boas: Essays on the Centennial of his Birth* (San Francisco, CA: American Anthropological Society and Howard Chandler, 1959), pp. 76–111.
32. F. Boas, 'On Dr. William Townsend Porter's Investigation of the Growth of the School Children of St. Louis', *Science*, new ser., 1 (1895), pp. 225–30, on p. 227. See also F. Boas, 'The Growth of Children', *Science*, 19 (1892), pp. 256–7, and 20 (1892), pp. 351–2; F. Boas, 'Observations on the Growth of Children', *Science*, 72 (1930), pp. 44–8.
33. F. Boas, 'The Effects of American Environment on Immigrants and their Descendants', *Science*, 84 (1936), pp. 522–5, on p. 523.
34. F. Boas, *Changes in Bodily Form of Descendants of Immigrants* (New York: Columbia University Press, 1912), p. 5.
35. Tanner, 'Boas' Contributions', p. 93.
36. L. S. Penrose, *A Clinical and Genetic Study of 1280 Cases of Mental Defect* (London: HMSO, 1938).
37. H. Harris, 'The Development of Penrose's Ideas in Genetics and Psychiatry', *British Journal of Psychiatry*, 125 (1974), pp. 529–36, on p. 530.
38. L. S. Penrose, 'Intelligence and Birth Rate', *Occupational Psychology*, 13 (1939), pp. 110–25.
39. L. S. Penrose and J. C. Raven, 'A New Series of Perceptual Tests: Preliminary Communication', *British Journal of Medical Psychology*, 16 (1936), pp. 97–104.
40. Penrose, 'Intelligence and Birth Rate', p. 118.
41. R. A. Fisher, *The Social Selection of Human Fertility* (Oxford: Clarendon Press, 1932).
42. Ibid., p. 29.
43. R. B. Cattell, *The Fight for our National Intelligence* (London: P. S. King, 1937), and J. A. F. Roberts, 'The Negative Association between Intelligence and Fertility', *Human Biology*, 13 (1941), pp. 410–12.
44. C. M. Langford, 'The Eugenics Society and the Development of Demography in Britain: The International Population Union, the British Population Society and the Population Investigation Committee', in R. A. Peel (ed.), *Essays in the History of Eugenics* (London: Galton Institute, 1998), pp. 81–111.

45. A. M. Carr-Saunders, 'Eugenics in the Light of Population Trends', *Eugenics Review*, 27 (1935), pp. 11–20, on p. 12.
46. G. Thomson, memorandum, June 1944, p. 7, in Carr-Saunders Papers, B/3/10, London School of Economics and Political Science.
47. This was then published as an Occasional Paper by the Eugenics Society – C. Burt, *Intelligence and Fertility: The Effect of the Differential Birthrate on Inborn Mental Characteristics* (London: Eugenics Society and Hamish Hamilton Medical Books, 1946), p. 26.
48. Ibid., p. 6.
49. Scottish Council for Research in Education, *The Trend of Scottish Intelligence: A Comparison of the 1947 and 1932 Surveys of the Intelligence of Eleven-Year-Old Pupils* (London: University of London Press, 1949).
50. O. D. Duncan, 'Is the Intelligence of the General Population Declining?', *American Sociological Review*, 17 (1952), pp. 401–7, on p. 405.
51. G. Thomson, 'Preface', in Scottish Council for Research in Education, *The Trend of Scottish Intelligence*, pp. vii–xvi, on p. viii.
52. Z. Stein and M. Susser, 'Mutability of Intelligence and Epidemiology of Mild Mental Retardation', *Review of Educational Research*, 40 (1970), pp. 29–67.
53. J. W. B. Douglas, *The Home and the School: A Study of Ability and Attainment in the Primary School* (London: MacGibbon and Kee, 1964); J. W. B. Douglas and J. M. Blomfield, *Children under Five* (London: George Allen and Unwin, 1958); D. V. Glass, *Differential Fertility, Ability and Educational Objectives: Problems for Study* (Edinburgh: Trustees of the Godfrey Lecture Fund, 1961).
54. R. Laxova, 'Lionel Sharples Penrose, 1898–1972: A Personal Memoir in Celebration of the Centenary of his Birth', *Genetics*, 150 (1998), pp. 1333–40, on p. 1337.
55. D. J. Kevles, *In the Name of Eugenics: Genetics and the Uses of Human Heredity* (Cambridge, MA: Harvard University Press, 1985), p. 251.
56. A. C. Allison, 'Protection Afforded by the Sickle Cell Trait against Subtertian Malarial Infection', *British Medical Journal*, 1 (1954), pp. 290–4.
57. L. S. Penrose, 'The Galton Laboratory: Its Work and Aims', *Eugenics Review*, 41 (1949), pp. 17–27, on p. 24.
58. Ibid.
59. L. S. Penrose, 'Natural Selection in Man: Some Basic Problems', in D. F. Roberts and G. A. Harrison (eds), *Natural Selection in Human Populations* (Oxford: Pergamon, 1959), pp. 1–10. L. S. Penrose, 'A Contribution to the Study of the Genetics of Intelligence', January 1955, Penrose Papers, 65/3, University College London (UCL).
60. Penrose, 'Galton Laboratory', p. 24.
61. In his earlier statistical studies of mental defect, he had questioned the association made by eugenicists between low intelligence and high fertility – L. S. Penrose, *Mental Defect* (London: Sidgwick and Jackson, 1933).
62. L. S. Penrose, 'Evidence of Heterosis in Man', *Proceedings of the Royal Society of London, Series B, Biological Sciences*, 144 (1955), pp. 203–13.
63. Penrose, 'Intelligence and Birth Rate', p. 123.
64. L. S. Penrose, 'Genetic Influences on the Intelligence Level of the Population', *British Journal of Psychology*, 40 (1949–50), pp. 128–36, on p. 132. See also his 'Evidence of Heterosis'.
65. K. Mather, 'Review of "Outline of Human Genetics" by L. S. Penrose', *Heredity*, 14 (1960), pp. 215–16, on p. 216.

66. J. A. F. Roberts, 'Review of L. S. Penrose, "The Biology of Mental Defect"', *Eugenics Review*, 42 (1951), pp. 225–7, on p. 226.
67. C. Burt, 'The Trend of National Intelligence: Review Article', *British Journal of Sociology*, 1 (1950), pp. 154–68, on p. 167.
68. L. S. Penrose, *Problems of Intelligence and Heredity* (Edinburgh: Trustees of the Godfrey Lecture Fund, 1959), pp. 20–1.
69. Ibid., p. 14.
70. Quoted in Royal Commission on Population, *Report* (London: HMSO, 1951), p. 155.
71. L. S. Penrose, 'Contribution to Eugenics Society Symposium', January 1947, Penrose Papers, 65/4, UCL.
72. G. Thomson, *The Trend of National Intelligence* (London: Eugenics Society and Hamish Hamilton Medical Books, 1947), pp. 33–4.
73. G. M. Morant, 'Applied Physical Anthropology in Great Britain in Recent Years', *American Journal of Physical Anthropology*, 6 (1948), pp. 329–40, on pp. 333–4.
74. Penrose then suggested a model of biological equilibrium in a BBC debate with Burt on 'Intelligence', aired 18 September 1948, Penrose Papers, 53/12, UCL. See also L. S. Penrose, 'The Supposed Threat of Declining Intelligence', *American Journal of Mental Deficiency*, 53 (1948), pp. 114–18.
75. Penrose, 'Galton Laboratory', p. 25.
76. L. H. Snyder, 'Old and New Pathways in Human Genetics', in L. C. Dunn (ed.), *Genetics in the 20th Century: Essays on the Progress of Genetics during its First 50 Years* (New York: Macmillan, 1951), pp. 369–91, on p. 382.
77. Royal Commission on Population, *Memoranda Presented to the Royal Commission on Population, Volume V* (London, 1950), p. 43.
78. L. S. Penrose, 'Limitations of Eugenics', *Proceedings of the Royal Institution*, 39 (1963), pp. 506–19, on p. 513.
79. Penrose, *Problems of Intelligence and Heredity*, p. 14.
80. G. E. Hutchinson, 'Fifty Years of Man in the Zoo', *Yale Review*, 51 (1961), pp. 56–65.
81. A. H. Halsey, 'Genetics, Social Structure and Intelligence', *British Journal of Sociology*, 9 (1958), pp. 15–28; A. H. Halsey, J. Floud and C. A. Anderson (eds), *Education, Economy, and Society* (New York: Free Press, 1961).
82. Glass to Penrose, 6 March 1953, Penrose Papers, 134/8, UCL.
83. L. S. Penrose, *The Biology of Mental Defect* (London: Sidgwick and Jackson, 1949), p. 1.
84. Ibid., p. 3.
85. Mazumdar, *Eugenics*, p. 221.
86. Paul, *The Politics of Heredity*, p. 5.
87. I. Erlenmeyer-Kimling and W. Paradowski, 'Selection and Schizophrenia', *American Naturalist*, 100 (1966), pp. 651–65; H. Osmond and A. Hoffer, 'A Comprehensive Theory of Schizophrenia', *International Journal of Neuropsychiatry*, 2 (1966), pp. 302–9; G. E. Hutchinson, 'A Speculative Consideration of Certain Possible Forms of Sexual Selection in Man', *American Naturalist*, 93 (1959), pp. 81–91; J. A. W. Kirsch and J. E. Rodman, 'Selection and Sexuality: The Darwinian View of Homosexuality', in W. Paul, J. D. Weinrich, J. C. Gonsiorek and M. E. Hotvedt (eds), *Homosexuality: Social, Psychological, and Biological Issues* (Beverly Hills, CA: Sage, 1982), pp. 183–95.
88. Neisser, *The Rising Curve*; R. Lynn, *Dysgenics: Genetic Deterioration in Modern Populations* (Westport, CT: Praeger, 1996).

4 Lipphardt, 'From "Races" to "Isolates" and "Endogamous Communities": Human Genetics and the Notion of Human Diversity in the 1950s'

1. R. S. Cowan, *Heredity and Hope: The Case for Genetic Screening* (Cambridge, MA: Harvard University Press, 2008); S. Lindee, *Moments of Truth in Genetic Medicine* (Baltimore, MD: Johns Hopkins University Press, 2005); D. B. Paul, *Controlling Human Heredity: 1865 to the Present* (Atlantic Highlands, NJ: Humanities Press, 1995); D. B. Paul and R. G. Resta, 'Historical Aspects of Medical Genetics', *American Journal of Medical Genetics, Part C: Seminars in Medical Genetics*, 115:2 (2002), pp. 73–4; D. J. Kevles, *In the Name of Eugenics: Genetics and the Use of Human Heredity* (Cambridge, MA: Harvard University Press, 1985).
2. For examples, see the contributions of Bernd Gausemeier and Jenny Bangham in this volume.
3. 'Diversity', or even 'infinite diversity', has been used since early modern times to describe the complexities of human variation in general. See, for example, 'unendliche Vielfalt' in J. G. v. Herder, 'Ideas on the Philosophy of the History of Humankind', in R. Bernasconi and T. L. Lott (eds), *The Idea of Race* (Indianapolis, IN: Hackett, 2000), first published in 1784. Its German equivalents, 'Mannigfaltigkeit' and 'Vielfalt', were used by Alexander von Humboldt to denote all kinds of differences between humans in cross-continental comparison. Parallel to the dominant usage of 'race', 'human diversity' was used by some scientists in the early twentieth century in controversies on human variation and race. It became widely used by geneticists in the 1960s and 1970s; see, for example, K. Mather, *Human Diversity: The Nature and Significance of Differences Among Men* (Edinburgh: Oliver and Boyd, 1964); J. Hiernaux, 'Human Biological Diversity in Central Africa', *Man*, 1:3 (1966), pp. 287–306; R. C. Lewontin, 'The Apportionment of Human Diversity', *Evolutionary Biology*, 6 (1972), pp. 381–98.
4. Early forerunners include G. Dahlberg and S. G. W. Wahlund, *Anthropometrical Survey: Race Biology of the Swedish Lapps* (Uppsala: Almquist and Wiksell, 1941); G. Dahlberg, *Mathematische Erblichkeitsanalyse von Populationen* (Uppsala: Almqvist and Wiksell, 1943); R. A. Fisher, *The Genetical Theory of Natural Selection* (Oxford: Clarendon Press, 1930); F. Bernstein, 'Über Mendelistische Anthropologie', in H. Nachtsheim (ed.), *Verhandlungen des 5. Internationalen Kongresses für Vererbungswissenschaft, Berlin 1927* (Leipzig: Bornträger, 1928), pp. 431–8. On Wilhelm Weinberg's work, see P. M. H. Mazumdar, 'Two Models for Human Genetics: Blood Grouping and Psychiatry in Germany between the World Wars', *Bulletin of the History of Medicine*, 70:4 (1996), pp. 609–57, and Bernd Gausemeier's contribution to this volume.
5. E. Barkan, *The Retreat of Scientific Racism: Changing Concepts of Race in Britain and the United States between the World Wars* (Cambridge: Cambridge University Press, 1992); E. Barkan, 'The Politics of Race in Science: Ashley Montagu and UNESCO's Anti-Racist Declarations', in L. T. Reynolds and L. Lieberman, *Race and Other Misadventures: Essays in Honor of Ashley Montagu in His Ninetieth Year* (New York: General Hall, 1996), pp. 96–105; N. L. Stepan, *The Idea of Race in Science: Great Britain, 1800–1960* (Basingstoke: Macmillan, 1984); N. L. Stepan, 'Science and Race. Before and after the Human Genome Diversity Project', *Socialist Register* (2003), Special Issue: Fighting Identities: Race, Religion, and Ethno-Nationalism, pp. 329–46.

6. L. Gannett, 'Racism and Human Genome Diversity Research: The Ethical Limits of "Population Thinking"', *Philosophy of Science*, 68:3 (2001), pp. S479–92; J. Reardon, 'Decoding Race and Human Difference in a Genomic Age', *differences: A Journal of Feminist Cultural Studies*, 15:3 (2004), pp. 38–65; J. Reardon, *Race to the Finish: Identity and Governance in an Age of Genomics* (Princeton, NJ: Princeton University Press, 2005).
7. L. D. Sanghvi and V. R. Khanolkar, 'Data Relating to Seven Genetical Characters in Six Endogamous Groups in Bombay', *Annals of Eugenics*, 15 (1949–51), pp. 52–76, on p. 53.
8. L. Gannett and J. R. Griesemer, 'The ABO Blood Groups: Mapping the History and Geography of Genes in Homo Sapiens', in H.-J. Rheinberger and J.-P. Gaudillière (eds), *Classical Genetic Research and its Legacy: the Mapping Cultures of Twentieth-Century Genetics* (London: Routledge, 2004), pp. 119–72; J. Marks, 'The Legacy of Serological Studies in American Physical Anthropology', *History and Philosophy of the Life Sciences*, 18 (1996), pp. 345–62; J. Marks, 'Race Across the Physical–Cultural Divide in American Anthropology', in H. Kuklick (ed.), *A New History of Anthropology* (Malden, MA: Blackwell, 2008), pp. 242–58; W. H. Schneider, 'Blood Group Research in Great Britain, France and the United States between the World Wars', *Yearbook of Physical Anthropology*, 38 (1995), pp. 77–104.
9. V. Lipphardt, 'Isolates and Crosses: Human Evolution and Population Genetics in the Mid-Twentieth Century', *Current Anthropology*, 53:S5 (April 2012), pp. S69–82.
10. See, for example, M. Brattain, 'Race, Racism, and Antiracism: UNESCO and the Politics of Presenting Science to the Postwar Public', *American Historical Review*, 112:5 (2007), pp. 1386–413; Y. Gastaut, 'L'UNESCO, les "races" et le racisme', in UNESCO (ed.), *60 ans d'histoire de l'UNESCO* (Paris: UNESCO 2007), pp. 192–210; J. Gayon, 'Do Biologists Need the Expression "Human Race"? UNESCO 1950–1951', in J. Rozenberg (ed.), *Bioethical and Ethical Issues Surrounding the Trials and Code of Nuremberg* (New York: Edwin Melon Press, 2003), pp. 23–48; S. Müller-Wille, 'Was ist Rasse? Die UNESCO Erklärungen von 1950 und 1951', in P. Lutz, T. Macho, G. Staupe and H. Zirden (eds), *Der (im-)perfekte Mensch: Metamorphosen von Normalität und Abweichung* (Cologne: Böhlau, 2003), pp. 57–71; S. Müller-Wille, 'Race et appartenance ethnique: la diversité humaine et l'UNESCO déclaration sur la race (1950 et 1951)', in UNESCO (ed.), *60 ans d'histoire de l'UNESCO* (Paris: UNESCO, 2007), pp. 211–20; R. Proctor, 'Three Roots of Human Recency: Molecular Anthropology, the Refigured Acheulean, and the UNESCO Response to Auschwitz', *Current Anthropology*, 44:2 (2003), pp. 213–39; Reardon, *Race to the Finish*; P. Selcer, 'The View from Everywhere: Disciplining Diversity in Post–World War II International Science', *Journal of the History of the Behavioral Sciences*, 45:4 (2009), pp. 309–29; P. Selcer, 'Beyond the Cephalic Index: Negotiating Politics to Produce UNESCO's Scientific Statements on Race', *Current Anthropology*, 53:S5 (2012), pp. S173–84; W. Stoczkowski, 'UNESCO's Doctrine of Human Diversity: A Secular Soteriology?', *Anthropology Today*, 25:3 (2009), pp. 7–11.
11. B. Glass, 'Blood Groups in Physical Anthropology', *Science*, 123:3204 (May 1956), pp. 927–8; C. W. Rowe, 'Genetics vs. Physical Anthropology in Determining Racial Types', *Southwestern Journal of Anthropology*, 6:2 (Summer 1950), pp. 197–211; H. H. Strandskov, 'Human Genetics and Anthropology', *Science*, 100:2608 (December 1944), pp. 570–1; H. H. Strandskov and S. L. Washburn, 'Editorial: Genetics and Physical Anthropology', *American Journal of Physical Anthropology*, 9:3 (September 1951), pp. 261–4.
12. As late as 1964, a WHO report listed anthropometry under the methodology any investigator of genetic diversity of primitive populations should take to the field; however, not without an explanation why this technique was still considered to be relevant. *Research*

in Population Genetics of Primitive Groups: Report of a WHO Scientific Group, WHO Report 279 (Geneva: World Health Organization, 1964).

13. Notably, this understanding had already been expressed by Eugen Fischer in 1930: E. Fischer, *Versuch einer Genanalyse des Menschen: mit besonderer Berücksichtigung der anthropologischen Systemrassen* (Berlin: Bornträger, 1930).
14. Numerous scientific and political committees and councils were established at the time under the guiding motto of 'population'; see, for example, the 'International Union for the Scientific Investigation of Population Problems'. The term helped to adress a number of issues and problems that had hitherto been associated with race, health and eugenics.
15. G. E. Allen, *Life Science in the Twentieth Century* (New York: Wiley, 1975); G. E. Allen, *Thomas Hunt Morgan: The Man and his Science* (Princeton, NJ: Princeton University Press, 1978); P. McLaughlin and H.-J. Rheinberger, 'Darwin und das Experiment', in K. Bayertz, B. Heidtmann and H.-J. Rheinberger (eds), *Darwin und die Evolutionstheorie* (Cologne: Pahl-Rugenstein, 1982), pp. 27–43; A. v. Schwerin, *Experimentalisierung des Menschen: Der Genetiker Hans Nachtsheim und die vergleichende Erbpathologie, 1920–1945* (Göttingen: Wallstein, 2004), p. 11. Regarding the lab–field border in biology and field biologists' focus on 'natural experiments', see R. Kohler, *Landscapes and Labscapes: Exploring the Lab–Field Border in Biology* (Chicago, IL: University of Chicago Press, 2002); for an application of Darwinian evolutionary thinking onto nature in field research, see E. Cittadino, *Nature as the Laboratory: Darwinian Plant Ecology in the German Empire, 1880–1990.* (Cambridge: Cambridge University Press, 1990); B. J. Strasser, 'Collecting Nature: Practices, Styles, and Narratives', *Osiris*, 27:1 (2012), pp. 303–40.
16. T. Dobzhansky, 'Mendelian Populations and their Evolution', *American Naturalist*, 84:819 (1950), pp. 401–18, on p. 405.
17. Ibid.
18. Ibid.
19. L. C., Dunn, *Heredity and Evolution of Human Populations* (Cambridge, MA: Harvard University Press, 1959), p. 109.
20. H. H. Strandskov, 'Genetics and the Origin and Evolution of Man', *Cold Spring Harbor Symposium on Quantitative Biology*, 15: Origin and Evolution of Man (1950), pp. 1–11, on p. 2.
21. See, for example, the *Cold Spring Harbor Symposium on Quantitative Biology*, 15: Origin and Evolution of Man (1950); or the *Proceedings of the Second International Congress of Human Genetics* (Rome: Istituto Gregor Mendel, September, 1961).
22. Taku Komia, cited in M. Demerec, 'Foreword', *Cold Spring Harbor Symposia on Quantitative Biology*, 20: Population Genetics: The Nature and Causes of Genetic Variability in Populations (1955), p. v.
23. See the documents surrounding the establishment of the Institute for the Study of Human Variation at Columbia University: Institute for the Study of Human Variation, Columbia University Archives, Historical Subject Files, 1870–2012, Series I: Academics and Research, 1750s–2000s, 32/2–3; see also M. Gormley, 'Geneticist L. C. Dunn: Politics, Activism, and Community' (PhD dissertation, Oregon State University, 2006), pp. 443–68; M. Gormley, 'Scientific Discrimination and the Activist Scientist: L. C. Dunn and the Professionalization of Genetics and Human Genetics in the United States', *Journal of the History of Biology*, 42:1 (2009), pp. 33–72.
24. *Rockefeller Annual Report* (New York: Rockefeller Foundation, 1955), p. 56.
25. See the institute's unpublished bibliography: Institute for the Study of Human Variation, Bibliography, n.d., Columbia University Archives, Historical Subject Files, 1870–2012, Series I: Academics and Research, 1750s–2000s, 32/2–3. The test subjects could be

from various populations, as well as twins and chimpanzees. Members of the institute were also researching genetic diseases and genetic transmission in families.

26. L. D. Sanghvi, 'Comparison of Genetical and Morphological Methods for a Study of Biological Differences', *American Journal of Physical Anthropology*, 11:3 (1953), pp. 385–404, on p. 385.
27. See the contribution of Jenny Bangham in this volume.
28. This refers to many geneticists' usages in their published studies; only rarely would they refer to R. A. Fisher's *The Theory of Inbreeding* (Edinburgh and London: Oliver and Boyd, 1949).
29. W. C. Boyd, *Genetics and the Races of Man: An Introduction to Modern Physical Anthropology* (Boston, MA: Little, Brown, 1950), p. 120.
30. See, for example, W. J. Schull and J. V. Neel, 'The Effect of Inbreeding on Mortality in Japan', *Proceedings of the Second International Congress of Human Genetics*, 3 (Rome: Istituto Gregor Mendel, September 1961), pp. 60–70.
31. For early examples, including research endeavours of Anglo-American scientists, see Fischer's bibliography: Fischer, *Versuch einer Genanalyse des Menschen*, p. 224–34. Fischer's students pursued research in the Pacific and elsewhere: H.-W. Schmuhl, *The Kaiser Wilhelm Institute for Anthropology, Human Heredity and Eugenics, 1927–1945: Crossing Boundaries* (Boston, MA: Springer, 2008), pp. 74ff., 82–91.
32. See the contribution of Pascal Germann in this volume.
33. Sanghvi and Khanolkar, 'Data Relating to Seven Genetical Characters'.
34. See, for example, B. Glass, M. S. Sacks, E. F. Jahn and C. Hess, 'Genetic Drift in a Religious Isolate: An Analysis of the Causes of Variation in Blood Group and Other Gene Frequencies in a Small Population', *American Naturalist*, 86:828 (May–June 1952), pp. 145–59, for the Duncker; K. R. Dronamraju, 'Genetic Studies of the Andhra Pradesh Population', in E. Goldschmidt (ed.), *The Genetics of Migrant and Isolate Populations: Proceedings of a Conference on Human Population Genetics in Israel Held at the Hebrew University, Jerusalem* (Baltimore, MD: Williams and Wilkins, 1963), pp. 154–9, for the population of Andhra Pradesh, India; and V. A. McKusick, W. B. Bias, R. A. Norum and H. E. Cross, 'Blood Groups in Two Amish Demes', *Human Genetics*, 5:1 (1967), pp. 36–41, for the Amish. For McKusick's research, see also M. S. Lindee, 'Provenance and the Pedigree: Victor McKusick's Fieldwork with the Old Order Amish', in A. H. Goodman, D. Heath and M. S. Lindee, *Genetic Nature/Culture: Anthropology and Science beyond the Two-Culture Divide* (Berkeley, CA: University of California Press, 2003), pp. 41–57.
35. J. Hiernaux, 'Physical Anthropology and the Frequency of Genes with a Selective Value: The Sickle Cell Gene', *American Journal of Physical Anthropology*, 13:3 (1955), pp. 455–72; J. Hiernaux, 'Bantu Expansion: The Evidence from Physical Anthropology Confronted with Linguistic and Archaeological Evidence', *Journal of African History*, 9:4 (January 1968), pp. 505–15; J. Hiernaux, 'Physical Anthropology of the Living Populations of Sub-Saharan Africa', *Annual Review of Anthropology*, 5 (January 1976), pp. 149–68; J. Hiernaux, and A.-M. Gauthier, 'Comparaison des affinités linguistiques et biologiques de douze populations de langue bantu' [A Comparison of the Linguistic and Biological Affinities of Twelve Bantu-Speaking People], *Cahiers d'Études Africaines*, 17:66–7 (January 1977), pp. 241–54.
36. To give but one example: B. S. Kraus and C. B. White, 'Micro-Evolution in a Human Population: A Study of the Social Endogamy and Blood Type Distributions among the Western Apache', *American Anthropologist*, 54:3 (1956), pp. 433–6.

37. G. Philipps, 'The Blood Groups of Full-Blood Australian Aborigines', *Medical Journal of Australia*, 15:2 (1928), pp. 296–300, on p. 296; as one example out of a whole series of research, see B. T. Simmons, J. J. Graydon and D. C. Gajdusek, 'A Blood Group Genetical Survey in Australian Aboriginal Children of the Cape York Peninsula', *American Journal of Physical Anthropology*, 16:1 (March 1958), pp. 59–77.
38. J. K. Moor-Jankowski and H. J. Huser, 'Sero-Anthropological Investigations of the Walser and Romansh Isolates in the Swiss Alps and their Methodological Aspects', *Acta Genetica et Statistica Medica*, 6 (1956–7), pp. 527–31.
39. H. Kalmus, 'Defective Colour Vision, P.T.C. Tasting and Drepanocytosis in Samples from Fifteen Brazilian Populations', *Annals of Human Genetics*, 21:4 (June 1957), pp. 313–17.
40. B. L. Hanna, A. A. Dahlberg and H. H. Strandskov, 'A Preliminary Study of the Population History of the Pima Indians', *American Journal of Human Genetics*, 5:4 (December 1953), pp. 377–88.
41. One of the earliest population genetic studies on Indian castes as genetic isolates was Sanghvi and Khanolkar, 'Data Relating to Seven Genetical Characters'.
42. As well as populations that had 'mixed' under 'controllable conditions'. For an overview over earlier studies on isolates and on mixing, see Fischer, *Versuch einer Genanalyse des Menschen*.
43. Most importantly, S. Wright, 'The Roles of Mutation, Inbreeding, Crossbreeding and Selection in Evolution', *Proceedings of the Sixth International Congress of Genetics*, 1 (1932), pp. 356–66. See P. S. Harper, *A Short History of Medical Genetics* (Oxford: Oxford University Press, 2008); W. B. Provine, *The Origins of Theoretical Population Genetics* (Chicago, IL: University of Chicago Press, 2001). Sanghvi and Khanolkar point to Dahlberg's publications since the 1920s, particularly his from 1938, and to Dunn's publication from 1947, which suggested estimating the average size of isolates by studying the frequency of consanguineous marriages in a population: G. Dahlberg, 'On Rare Defects in Human Populations with Particular Regard to Inbreeding and Isolate Effects', *Proceeding of the Royal Society of Edinburgh*, 58 (1938), pp. 213–32; L. C. Dunn, 'The Effects of Isolates on the Frequency of a Rare Human Gene', *Proceedings of the National Academy of Sciences of the United States of America*, 33 (1947), pp. 359–63; Sanghvi and Khanolkar, 'Data Relating to Seven Genetical Characters', p. 42.
44. W. C. Boyd, 'Natural Selection and Heredity', *Proceedings of the Second International Congress of Human Genetics*, 1 (Rome: Istituto Gregor Mendel, September 1961), pp. 37–51; Fisher, *The Theory of Inbreeding*; J. Hajnal, M. Fraccaro, J. Sutter and C. A. B. Smith, 'Concepts of Random Mating and the Frequency of Consanguineous Marriages (and Discussion)', *Proceedings of the Royal Society of London. Series B, Biological Sciences*, 159:974: A Discussion on Demography (December 1963), pp. 125–77; R. C. Lewontin, 'The Effect of Compensation on Populations Subject to Natural Selection', *American Naturalist*, 87:837 (November–December 1953), pp. 375–81; S. P. H. Mandel, 'Polymorphism in Human Populations', *Proceedings of the Second International Congress of Human Genetics*, 1 (Rome: Istituto Gregor Mendel, September 1961), pp. 131–3; B. Woolf, 'Environmental Effects in Quantitative Inheritance', in E. C. R. Reeve and C. H. Waddington (eds), *Quantitative Inheritance: Papers Read at a Colloquium Held at the Institute of Animal Genetics, Edinburgh University* (London: HMSO, 1952), pp. 81–111 (with comment by K. Mather); S. Wright, 'The Genetics of Quantitative Variability', in E. C. R. Reeve and C. H. Waddington (eds), *Quantitative Inheritance: Papers Read at a Colloquium Held at the Institute of Animal Genetics, Edinburgh University* (London:

HMSO, 1952), pp. 5–41. See also a number of publications on theoretical-mathematical issues by Cavalli-Sforza, Hajnal, Bentley Glass and Gabriel Ward Lasker.

45. Sanghvi, 'Comparison of Genetical and Morphological Methods for a Study of Biological Differences'.
46. For a differentiated list of markers, see T. Dobzhansky, 'Human Diversity and Adaptation', *Cold Spring Harbor Symposium on Quantitative Biology: Origin and Evolution of Man*, 15 (1950), pp. 385–400, on p. 391.
47. See publication list of the Institute for the Study of Human Variation: Institute for the Study of Human Variation, Publication List, n.d., Columbia University Archives, Historical Subject Files, 1870–2012, Series I: Academics and Research, 1750s–2000s, 32/2–3.
48. See, for example, Leslie Clarence Dunn's publications on his study on the Jewish community of Rome; V. Lipphardt, 'The Jewish Community of Rome: An Isolated Population? Sampling Procedures and Bio-historical Narratives in Genetic Analysis in the 1950s', *BioSocieties*, 5:3 (2010), pp. 306–29.
49. T. Dobzhansky, *Mankind Evolving: The Evolution of the Human Species* (New Haven, CT: Yale University Press, 1962), p. 234.
50. Sanghvi and Khanolkar, 'Data Relating to Seven Genetical Characters', pp. 52–3.
51. Ibid., p. 58.
52. Ibid., p. 52.
53. The problem was tackled as a quantitative one by G. W. Lasker, 'Mixture and Genetic Drift in Ongoing Human Evolution', *American Anthropologist*, 54:3 (July–September 1952), pp. 433–6.
54. F. B. Livingstone, 'On the Non-Existence of Human Races', *Current Anthropology*, 3:3 (June 1962), pp. 279–81, on p. 279.
55. J. Radin, 'Life on Ice: Frozen Blood and Human Variation in a Genomic Age, 1950–2010' (PhD dissertation, University of Pennsylvania, 2012); J. Radin, 'Latent Life: Concepts and Practices of Tissue Preservation in the International Biological Program', *Social Studies of Science* (forthcoming 2013).
56. WHO, 'Research on Human Population Genetics: Report of a WHO Scientific Group', *Current Anthropology*, 11:2 (1970), pp. 225–33, on p. 233.
57. Hiernaux, 'Human Biological Diversity in Central Africa', p. 288.
58. M. J. Herskovits, 'Variability and Racial Mixture', *American Naturalist*, 61:672 (January–February 1927), pp. 68–81, on p. 76.
59. L. C. Dunn, A Genetical Study of a Jewish Community, the Old Ghetto Community of Rome, n.d., American Philosophical Society, Philadelphia, Dunn Papers, 5/32, pp. 6ff.

5 Bangham, 'Between the Transfusion Services and Blood Group Research: Human Genetics in Britain during World War II'

1. R. A. Fisher and G. L. Taylor, 'Blood Groups in Great Britain', *British Medical Journal* (hereafter *BMJ*), 4111 (1939), p. 826.
2. For the relationship between World War II and scientific research, see D. J. Kevles, *The Physicists: The History of a Scientific Community in Modern America* (New York: Knopf, 1977); A. Roland, 'Science and War', *Osiris*, 1 (1985), pp. 247–72; R. Geiger, 'Science, Universities, and National Defence, 1945–1970', *Osiris*, 7 (1993), pp. 26–48; S. de Chadarevian, *Designs for Life: Molecular Biology after World War II* (Cambridge: Cambridge

University Press, 2002), esp. ch. 2: 'World War Two and the Mobilization of British Scientists'; D. Edgerton, *Warfare State: Britain, 1920–1970* (Cambridge: Cambridge University Press, 2006). Closely related to the disciplines and contexts dealt with in my chapter, Angela Creager explores the relationship between biomedical research on blood and the infrastructures of the US Red Cross National Blood Donation service during World War II – A. Creager, '"What Blood Told Dr. Cohn": World War II, Plasma Fractionation, and the Growth of Human Blood Research', *Studies in History and Philosophy of Biological and Biomedical Sciences*, 30 (1999), pp. 377–405.

3. L. Hogben, *Principles of Evolutionary Biology* (Cape Town and Johannesburg: Juta and Co. Ltd, 1927), quoted in P. M. H. Mazumdar, *Eugenics, Human Genetics and Human Failings: The Eugenics Society, its Source and Critics in Britain* (London: Routledge, 1992), p. 155.
4. W. H. Schneider, 'Blood Transfusion between the Wars', *Journal for the History of Medicine*, 58 (2003), pp. 187–224; H. Dodsworth, 'Blood Transfusion Services in the UK', *Journal of the Royal College of Physicians of London*, 30 (1996), pp. 457–64. For a history of blood groups in the courtroom, see M. Okroi and P. Voswinkel, '"Obviously Impossible" – The Application of the Inheritance of Blood Groups as a Forensic Method. The Beginning of Paternity Tests in Germany, Europe and the USA', *International Congress Series*, 1239 (2003), pp. 711–14.
5. For example, W. H. Schneider, 'Blood Group Research in Great Britain, France and the United States between the World Wars', *Yearbook of Physical Anthropology*, 38 (1995), pp. 87–114; Drawing particular attention to the social and political deployment of blood groups, see, for example, M. Turda, 'The Nation as Object: Race, Blood, and Biopolitics in Interwar Romania', *Slavic Review*, 66 (2007), pp. 413–41; R. E. Boaz, 'The Search for "Aryan Blood": Seroanthropology in Weimar and National Socialist Germany' (PhD dissertation, Kent State University, 2009); P. M. H. Mazumdar, 'Blood and Soil: The Serology of the Aryan Racial State', *Bulletin of the History of Medicine*, 64 (1990), pp. 186–219; L. Gannett and J. R. Griesemer, 'The ABO Blood Groups: Mapping the History and Geography of Genes in Homo Sapiens', in H.-J. Rheinberger and J.-P. Gaudillière (eds), *Classical Genetic Research and its Legacy: the Mapping Cultures of Twentieth-Century Genetics* (London: Routledge, 2004), pp. 119–72.
6. For insightful accounts of 1930s human genetics in Britain, including aspirations for blood group research, see Mazumdar, *Eugenics, Human Genetics and Human Failings*, chs 3 and 4; D. Kevles, *In the Name of Eugenics: Genetics and the Uses of Human Heredity* (Cambridge, MA: Harvard University Press, 1995), chs 11, 12 and 13. For a different national context, see see P. M. H. Mazumdar, 'Two Models for Human Genetics: Blood Grouping and Psychiatry in Germany between the World Wars', *Bulletin of the History of Medicine*, 70:4 (1996), pp. 609–57.
7. The crisis also prompted a much grander project for an Emergency Medical Service (EMS) for London; see C. L. Dunn, *The Emergency Medical Services*, Vol. 1: History of the Second World War, Medical Series (London: HMSO, 1952).
8. M. Owen, 'Dame Janet Maria Vaughan, D.B.E. 18 October 1899–9 January 1993', *Biographical Memoirs of Fellows of the Royal Society*, 41 (1995), pp. 483–98; N. Whitfield, 'A Genealogy of the Gift: Blood Donation in London, 1921–1946' (PhD dissertation, University of Cambridge, 2011), ch. 2 and references therein; T. Buchanan, *Britain and the Spanish Civil War* (Cambridge: Cambridge University Press, 1997), ch. 4.
9. For the quotation, see L. W. Proger, 'Development of the Emergency Blood Transfusion Scheme', *BMJ*, 4260 (1942), pp. 252–3; For more details, see J. M. Vaughan and P. N.

Panton, 'The Civilian Blood Transfusion Service', C. L. Dunn, *The Emergency Medical Services*, Vol. 1: History of the Second World War, Medical Series (London: HMSO, 1952), pp. 334–55.

10. Vaughan and Panton, 'The Civilian Blood Transfusion Service', p. 337.
11. 'News in Brief', *Times*, 12 August 1939, sec. Col. C. For more on donor recruitment, see Whitfield, 'A Genealogy of the Gift'.
12. On the complicated history of grouping tests in relation to transfusion in different countries, see Schneider, 'Blood Transfusion between the Wars'. Until the 1930s blood groups remained just one of many considerations when choosing a donor: Whitfield, 'A Genealogy of the Gift', chs 1 and 2.
13. Janet Vaughan later recalled that 'I can always remember George Taylor ... the English authority on blood groups, saying with great solemnity: "you must also enrol girls to determine these blood groups and this should be done at once; it is not easy to procure young girls"'. J. M. Vaughan, 'Memoirs', n.d., Wellcome Library, London, Vaughan Papers (hereafter WL VP), GC/186/1.
14. 'Emergency Blood Transfusion Service Scheme: Minutes', 11 April 1939, WL VP, GC/186/1.
15. Quotations from Taylor to Landsborough Thomson, 26 September 1939, National Archives (hereafter NA), FD1/3290; and Topley to Landsborough Thomson, 8 November 1938, NA, FD1/5845. The Cambridge Pathology Department was already an important institution for the MRC. Its physiologist Alan Drury was one of the MRC's few full-time researchers and one of the earliest to be appointed as a permanent member of their external scientific staff.
16. J. Fisher Box, *R. A. Fisher: The Life of a Scientist* (New York: John Wiley and Sons, 1978), pp. 352–3.
17. Taylor to Landsborough Thomson, 15 November 1943, NA MRC, FD1/5845.
18. To the Rockefeller Foundation, Fisher stressed that his 'old group' was 'working together as an unbroken unit'. Fisher to O'Brien, 28 December 1939, Rockefeller Archives (hereafter RA), 01.0001/401A/Box 16.
19. Fisher to Miller, 4 October 1939, RA, 01.0001/401A/Box 16.
20. Fisher Box, *R. A. Fisher: The Life of a Scientist*, p. 375.
21. W. M. Fletcher, 'MRC Memorandum. Private and Confidential, for Members of the Medical Research Council only', 15 January 1932, NA, FD1/3266.
22. Fisher to O'Brien, 18 July 1934, RA, 01.0001/401A/Box 16.
23. E.g. Fisher to Copland, 13 September 1939, R. A. Fisher Digital Archive, Fisher Correspondence, Adelaide University (hereafter AU, Fisher).
24. For further reflections on investment in depot office work, see ibid.
25. 'A Blood Transfusion Depot at Work', *BMJ*, 4109 (1939), p. 730.
26. Taylor to Landsborough Thomson, 3 July 1941, NA, FD1/5845.
27. Fisher to Landsborough Thomson, 11 July 1941, NA, FD1/5845.
28. Describing their sample as 'representative of the English population', Taylor and Prior included 'Persons with Scottish, Irish and Welsh names' and 'names suggestive of a Continental origin'. They added that there were 'two obviously Jewish families'; G. Taylor and A. M. Prior, 'Blood Groups in England, I: Examination of Family and Unrelated Material', *Annals of Eugenics*, 8 (1938), p. 344.
29. Fisher to Fraser Roberts, 17 February 1940, AU, Fisher.
30. Using transfusion records for this purpose was first suggested in print by a Dr Edward Billing: E. Billing, 'Racial Origins from Blood Groupings', *BMJ*, 4108 (1939), p. 712.

Fisher and Taylor cited this letter in their appeal; Fisher and Taylor, 'Blood Groups in Great Britain'.

31. Fisher to Taylor, 15 November 1939, AU, Fisher.
32. Schneider makes this point in W. H. Schneider, 'The History of Research on Blood Group Genetics: Initial Discovery and Diffusion', *History and Philosophy of the Life Sciences*, 18:3 (1996), pp. 277–303. For more on German racial serology, see Boaz, 'The Search for "Aryan Blood"', ch. 8; Mazumdar, 'Blood and Soil'.
33. Fisher and Janet M. Vaughan, 'Surnames and Blood-Groups', *Nature*, 144:3660 (1939), pp. 1047–8.
34. Fisher refers to 'ethnographical' work to a colleague: Fisher, 'To John Fraser Roberts', 17 February 1940, AU, Fisher.
35. R. A. Fisher and G. L. Taylor, 'Scandinavian Influence in Scottish Ethnology', *Nature*, 145 (1940), pp. 590–2, on p. 592.
36. Ibid. For contemporary accounts of the Vikings in Britain, see A.W. Brøgger, *Ancient Emigrants: A History of the Norse Settlements of Scotland* (Oxford: Clarendon Press, 1929); T. D. Kendrick, *A History of the Vikings* (London: Methuen, 1930).
37. Fisher to Vaughan, 11 March 1940, AU, Fisher.
38. Fisher was not the first to suggest this; see also the textbook: L. Lattes, *Individuality of the Blood in Biology and in Clinical and Forensic Medicine*, trans. L. W. Howard Bertie (London: Oxford University Press, 1932).
39. Fisher to Taylor, 17 January 1942, AU, Fisher.
40. Fisher to Taylor, 15 November 1939, AU, Fisher.
41. Fisher to Landsborough Thomson, 23 July 1941, NA, FD1/5845.
42. In the 1930s and 1940s, neither statistics nor genetics were part of medical training curricula.
43. Fisher to Taylor, 11 November 1939, SA/BGU F.1/1/1, Wellcome Library.
44. For example, some textbooks instructed readers on interpreting agglutination reactions; see W. C. Boyd and F. Schiff, *Blood Grouping Technic: A Manual for Clinicians, Serologists, Anthropologists and Students of Legan and Military Medicine* (New York: Interscience Publishers, 1942).
45. Taylor to Drury, 29 December 1941, NA, FD1/5845.
46. R. Drummond, 'Blood Grouping in Tubes', *BMJ*, 4307 (1943), p. 118.
47. The memorandum was finally published as War Memorandum No. 9; 'The Determination of Blood Groups', *British Medical Bulletin*, 1 (1943), pp. 52–3.
48. R. A. Kekwick, 'Alan Nigel Drury. 3 November 1889–2 August 1980', *Biographical Memoirs of Fellows of the Royal Society*, 27 (1981), pp. 173–98.
49. Drury to Taylor, 18 November 1941, NA, FD1/5901.
50. J. Vaughan et al., 'Draft Majority and Minority Report of the Sub-Committee of the Blood Transfusion Research Committee', NA, FD1/5901.
51. Vaughan to Drury, 11 February 1943, NA, FD1/5901.
52. Whitby et al., 'Criticisms on Blood Group Memorandum', n.d., NA, FD1/5901.
53. Vaughan to Drury, 11 February 1943, NA, FD1/5901.
54. Fisher Box, *R. A. Fisher: The Life of a Scientist*; A. W. F. Edwards, 'R. A. Fisher's 1943 Unravelling of the Rhesus Blood-Group System', *Genetics*, 174 (2007), pp. 471–6; W. F. Bodmer, 'Early British Discoveries in Human Genetics: Contributions of R. A. Fisher and J. B. S. Haldane to the Development of Blood Groups', *American Journal of Human Genetics*, 50 (1992), pp. 671–6; P. M. H. Mazumdar, *Species and Specificity: An Interpretation of the History of Immunology* (Cambridge: Cambridge University Press, 1995);

P. Schmidt, 'Rh-Hr: Alexander Wiener's Last Campaign', *Transfusion*, 34 (1994), pp. 180–2; M. E. Reid, 'Alexander S. Wiener: The Man and his Work', *Transfusion Medicine Reviews*, 22 (2008), pp. 300–16.

55. Fisher to Taylor, 6 January 1942, AU, Fisher. For Landsteiner's career, and a rich account of research on Rhesus, see Mazumdar's *Species and Specificity*, pp. 281–378.
56. Landsteiner and Wiener were attempting to use serological reactions to produce a taxonomy of primates; for more on serological taxonomy, see B. J. Strasser, 'Laboratories, Museums, and the Comparative Perspective: Alan A. Boyden's Quest for Objectivity in Serological Taxonomy, 1924–1962', *Historical Studies in the Natural Sciences*, 40 (2010), pp. 149–82.
57. P. L. Mollison and G. L. Taylor, 'Wanted: Anti-Rh Sera', *BMJ*, 4243 (1942), pp. 561–2.
58. R. A. Fisher, 'The Rhesus Factor: A Study in Scientific Method', *American Scientist*, 35 (1947), pp. 95–103.
59. R. Race, 'An "Incomplete" Antibody in Human Serum', *Nature*, 153 (June 1944), pp. 771–2; Edwards, 'R. A. Fisher's 1943 Unravelling of the Rhesus Blood-Group System'.
60. Race declared that the choice of letters was arbitrary, but they were chosen to follow from the A and B of the ABO blood groups. For the theoretical commitments of Wiener, Fisher and Race, see Mazumdar, *Species and Specificity*, p. 350.
61. J. B. S. Haldane, 'Two New Allelomorphs for Heterostylism in *Primula*', *American Naturalist*, 67 (1933), pp. 559–60.
62. For an early account of the Rhesus story by Fisher, see Fisher, 'The Rhesus Factor: A Study in Scientific Method'.
63. L. E. H. Whitby, 'The Hazards of Transfusion', *Lancet*, 239 (16 May 1942), pp. 581–5.
64. Vaughan and Panton, 'The Civilian Blood Transfusion Service', p. 344; 'Importance of the Rh Factor', *Lancet*, 241 (8 May 1943), pp. 587–8.
65. 'A New Blood-Grouping', *Lancet*, 239 (10 January 1942), p. 50.
66. The first of which was K. E. Boorman, B. E. Dodd and P. L. Mollison, 'The Clinical Significance of the Rh Factor', *BMJ*, 4270 (1942), pp. 535–8.
67. These textbooks were largely theoretical, and blood groups were almost their only concrete examples of human inheritance, aside from sex-linked diseases. E. B. Ford, *Genetics for Medical Students* (London: Methuen and Co. Ltd, 1942); J. A. Fraser Roberts, *An Introduction to Medical Genetics* (London: Oxford University Press, 1940).
68. The varied functions of the Rhesus nomenclatures are the topic of a forthcoming paper: J. Bangham, 'Writing, Printing, Speaking: Rhesus Blood-Group Genetics and Nomenclatures in the Mid-Twentieth Century', *British Journal for the History of Science*, forthcoming.
69. J. B. S. Haldane, *New Paths in Genetics* (London: George Allen & Unwin, 1941), p. 194.
70. J. T. Saunders to Landsborough Thomson, 25 May 1945, NA, FD1/3290.

6 Germann, 'The Abandonment of Race: Researching Human Diversity in Switzerland, 1944–56'

1. See especially C. Pogliano, *L'ossessione della razza: Antropologia e genetica nel XX secolo* (Pisa: Scuola Normale Superiore, 2005). Older publications emphasize the decline of the race concept in the twentieth century. See, for example, E. Barkan, *The Retreat of Scientific Racism: Changing Concepts of Race in Britain and the United States between the World Wars* (Cambridge: Cambridge University Press, 1992); N. L. Stepan, *The Idea of Race in Science: Great Britain, 1800–1960* (London and Basingstoke: Macmillan, 1982). For the history

of human diversity research in the twentieth century, see the project 'Twentieth Century Histories of Knowledge about Human Variation' by Veronika Lipphardt, Susanne Bauer, Alexandra Widmer and Staffan Müller-Wille, at http://www.mpiwg-berlin.mpg.de/de/forschung/projects/NWGLipphardt [accessed 12 May 2012].

2. For this perspective, see, for example, J. Marks, 'The Two 20th-Century Crises of Racial Anthropology', in M. A. Little and K. A. R. Kennedy (eds), *Histories of American Physical Anthropology in the Twentieth Century* (Lanham: Lexington Books, 2010), pp. 187–206; S. Kühl, *Die Internationale der Rassisten: Aufstieg und Niedergang der internationalen Bewegung für Eugenik und Rassenhygiene im 20. Jahrhundert* (Frankfurt: Campus, 1997); P. Weingart, K. Bayertz and J. Kroll, *Rasse, Blut und Gene: Geschichte der Eugenik und Rassenhygiene in Deutschland* (Frankfurt: Suhrkamp, 1988).
3. The inner developments of science are emphasized in P. L. Farber, *Mixing Races: From Scientific Racism to Modern Evolutionary Ideas* (Baltimore, MD: John Hopkins University Press, 2011); P. L. Farber, 'Race-Mixing and Science in the United States', *Endeavour*, 27:4 (2003), pp. 166–70; P. S. Harper, *A Short History of Medical Genetics* (New York: Oxford University Press, 2008), especially pp. 213ff.
4. J. Reardon, *Race to the Finish: Identity and Governance in an Age of Genomics* (Princeton, NJ and Oxford: Princeton University Press, 2005), pp. 6–10. A similar point was made earlier by Donald MacKenzie and Ruth Schwartz Cowan in their studies of the English biometricians: D. A. MacKenzie, *Statistics in Britain, 1865–1930: The Social Construction of Scientific Knowledge* (Edinburgh: Edinburgh University Press, 1981), especially pp. 120–52; R. S. Cowan, 'Nature and Nurture: The Interplay of Biology and Politics in the Work of Francis Galton', *Studies in the History of Biology*, 1 (1977), pp. 133–208.
5. S. Müller-Wille, 'Was ist Rasse? Die UNESCO Erklärung von 1950 und 1951', in P. Lutz, T. Macho and G. Staupe (eds), *Der (im-)perfekte Mensch : Metamorphosen von Normalität und Abweichung* (Köln: Böhlau, 2003), pp. 79–93.
6. V. Roelcke, 'Auf der Suche nach der Politik in der Wissensproduktion: Plädoyer für eine historisch-politische Epistemologie', *Berichte zur Wissenschaftsgeschichte*, 33 (2010), pp. 176–92.
7. M. Brittain, 'Race, Racism, and Antiracism: UNESCO and the Politics of Presenting Science to the Postwar Public', *American Historical Review*, 112:5 (December 2007), pp. 1368–413; J. P. Jackson and N. M. Weidman, *Race, Racism, and Science: Social Impact and Interaction* (New Brunswick, NJ: Rutgers University Press, 2005); S. Müller-Wille, 'Claude Lévi-Strauss on Race, History and Genetics', *BioSocieties*, 5:3 (2010), pp. 330–47; Kühl, *Die Internationale der Rassisten*; I. Hannaford, *Race: The History of an Idea in the West* (Washington, DC: Woodrow Wilson Center Press, 1996); Barkan, *Retreat*; Weingart et al., *Rasse, Blut und Gene*; Stepan, *The Idea of Race*.
8. O. Schlaginhaufen, *Anthropologia Helvetica. Die Anthropologie der Eidgenossenschaft*, Vols 1 and 2 (Zurich: Orell Füssli, 1946). Two further volumes were not published until 1959: O. Schlaginhaufen, *Anthropologia Helvetica II: Die Antropologie der Kantone und der natürlichen Landschaften*, Vols 1 and 2 (Zurich: Orell Füssli, 1959). On Otto Schlaginhaufen, see especially C. Keller, *Der Schädelvermesser. Otto Schlaginhaufen – Anthropologe und Rassenhyigieniker. Eine biographische Reportage* (Zurich: Limmat Verlag, 1995); H.-K. Schmutz, 'Homo alpinus oder die vermessene Nation', in W. Egli and I. Tomkowiak (eds), *Berge* (Zurich: Chronos, 2011), pp. 125–38; E. Keller, 'Das Herauskristallisieren der Rasse: Vom langsamen Verschwinden eines Phantoms am Anthropologischen Institut in Zurich', *Historische Anthropologie*, 14:1 (2006), pp. 49–67.

9. S. Rosin, 'Die Verteilung der AB0-Blutgruppen in der Schweiz', in *Archiv der Julius Klaus-Stiftung für Vererbungsforschung, Sozialanthropologie und Rassenhygiene*, 31:1–2 (1956), pp. 17–127.
10. Ibid., p. 121; see also p. 105.
11. Ibid., p. 121.
12. The reconstruction of the project rests upon R. Salber, *Über Fehlerquellen bei Massenblutgruppenbestimmungen* (Uster: Buchdruckerei Eugen Weilenmann, 1951), pp. 28–35, and Rosin, 'Verteilung der AB0-Blutgruppen', pp. 19–25; further it is based on the following archive material: Protokolle des Kuratoriums der Julius Klaus-Stiftung, Archive of the Anthropological Institute at the University of Zurich; Blutspendedienst SRK, 1944–50, Swiss Federal Archives, J2.15 1969/7_12.
13. W. Gautschi, *General Henri Guisan: Commander-in-Chief of the Swiss Army in World War II*, trans. K. Vonlanthen (Rockville Center, NY: Front Street Press, 2003).
14. R. Schütz, 'Das Vorkommen der Blutgruppen in der Schweiz an Hand von 33 964 Bestimmungen nach Bürgerort eingetragen', *Archiv der Julius Klaus-Stiftung für Vererbungsforschung, Sozialanthropologie und Rassenhygiene*, 21 (1946), p. 207–29, on p. 227.
15. E. Hadorn, 'Zur Verteilung der Blutgruppen in der Schweiz', *Neue Zürcher Zeitung*, 6 December 1957, p. 6.
16. S. Rosin, 'Die Bedeutung der Blutgruppen für die Humangenetik', *Jahresbericht der Schweizerischen Gesellschaft für Vererbungsforschung*, 17 (1957), pp. 440–52, on p. 441.
17. H. R. Schinz, U. Cocchi and J. Neuhaus, 'Die Vererbung des Krebses beim Menschen', *Archiv der Julius Klaus-Stiftung für Vererbungsforschung, Sozialanthropologie und Rassenhygiene*, 23 (1948), pp. 1–233; H. R. Schinz, S. Rosin and A. Senti, 'Die neueste Entwicklung der Krebssterblichkeit in Zurich', special print from *Zürcher Statistische Nachrichten*, 3 (1945).
18. J. Eugster, 'Zur Erblichkeitsfrage der endemischen Struma: Genetische Untersuchungen über die Ursachen des Kropfes, Teil 1', *Archiv der Julius Klaus-Stiftung für Vererbungsforschung, Sozialanthropologie und Rassenhygiene*, 9:3–4 (1934), pp. 275–365; J. Eugster, 'Zur Erblichkeitsfrage des endemischen Kretinismus: Untersuchungen an 204 Kretinen und deren Blutsverwandten', *Archiv der Julius Klaus-Stiftung für Vererbungsforschung, Sozialanthropologie und Rassenhygiene*, 13 (1938), pp. 383–494.
19. For the German Society for Blood Group Research, see M. Spörri, *Reines und gemischtes Blut: Zur Kulturgeschichte der Blutgruppenforschung, 1900–1933* (Bielefeld: Transcript, 2013); R. E. Boaz, *In Search of 'Aryan Blood': Serology in Interwar and National Socialist Germany* (Budapest: Central European University Press, 2012); K. Geisenhainer, *'Rasse ist Schicksal': Otto Reche (1879 – 1966): Ein Leben als Anthropologe und Völkerkundler* (Leipzig: Evangelische Verlagsanstalt, 2002); P. M. H. Mazumdar, 'Blood and Soil: The Serology of the Aryan Racial State', *Bulletin of the History of Medicine*, 64 (1990), pp. 187–219.
20. Spörri, *Reines und gemischtes Blut*; Mazumdar, 'Blood and Soil'.
21. Schütz, 'Das Vorkommen'.
22. Ibid., pp. 225ff.
23. The blood group research of the Walser population was booming in the 1950s. See especially W. Knoll, 'Blutgruppenbestimmungen bei den Walsern im Rheinwald und oberen Avers', *Bulletin der Schweizerischen Gesellschaft für Anthropologie und Ethnologie*, 26 (1950), pp. 35–55; J. K. Moor-Jankowski, 'La prépondérance du goupe sanguin 0 et du facteur rhésus négativ chez les Walser de suisse', *Journal de génétique humaine*, 3 (1954), pp. 25–70; J. K. Moor-Jankowski and H. J. Huser, 'Sero-anthropological Investigations in the Walser and Romansh Isolates in the Swiss Alps and their Methodological Aspects',

Proceedings of the First International Congress of Human Genetics, Copenhagen (August 1956), pp. 527–31; E. W. Ikin, A. E. Mourant, A. C. Kopec, J. K. Moor-Jankowski and H. J. Huser: 'The Blood Groups of the Western Walsers', *Vox Sanguinis*, 2 (1957), pp. 159–74; J. K. Moor-Jankowski and H. J. Huser, 'Research on Alpine Isolates in Switzerland', *Eugenics Quarterly*, 6 (1959), pp. 14–22.

24. For this criticism, see Rosin, 'Verteilung der AB0-Blutgruppen', p. 102; J. K. Moor-Jankowski and Hans Jürg Huser, who were the leading geneticists in the Walser research, stated that Schütz's oberservation was numerically too small to be significant; Moor-Jankowski and Huser, 'Research on Alpine Isolates', p. 16.
25. For more on Siegfried Rosin's biographical background, see P. Tschumi, 'Siegfried Rosin 1913–1976', *Verhandlungen der Schweizerischen Naturforschenden Gesellschaft*, 156 (1976), pp. 127–9; A. Linder, 'Nachruf: Siegfried Rosin', *ROeS-Nachrichten* (1976), pp. 6ff.
26. 'Der Wert der Arbeit liegt ... in der modellhaften Durcharbeitung eines für die ganze Welt einzigartigen Materials'. Rosin cited in 'Das A und O des Schweizerblutes', *Die Woche: Schweizerische Illustrierte Zeitschrift*, 18–24 November 1957, p. 6; see also N. Stettler, *Natur erforschen. Perspektiven einer Kulturgeschichte der Biowissenschaften an Schweizer Universitäten 1945–1975* (Zurich: Chronos, 2002), p. 59.
27. In Switzerland the Julius Klaus-Foundation, which was founded in 1921, played a crucial role in funding eugenic, racial and genetic research in the first half of the twentieth century. See H.-K. Schmutz, 'Schokolade und Messzirkel – Zur Steuerung rassenhygienischer Forschungsprojekte an der Universität Zurich in den zwanziger und dreissiger Jahren: die Tätigkeit der Julius Klaus-Stiftung für Vererbungsforschung, Sozialanthropologie und Rassenhygiene', in E. Höxtermann, J. Kaasch and M. Kaasch (eds), *Berichte zur Geschichte und Theorie der Ökologie und weitere Beiträge zur 9. Jahrestagung der DGGTB in Neuburg a. d. Donau 2000* (Berlin: VWB, 2001), pp. 305–17. See also Keller, *Schädelvermesser.*
28. Protokolle des Kuratoriums der Julius Klaus-Stiftung, Archive of the Anthropological Institute at the University of Zurich.
29. See, for example, A. Hässig, 'Ergebnisse und Ausblick der Blutgruppenserologie', in Schweizerisches Rotes Kreuz (ed.), *Der Blutspendedienst des Schweizerischen Roten Kreuzes* (Zurich: Schulthess, 1953), pp. 13–18, on p. 17.
30. Remund to Eugster, 21 April 1950, Swiss Federal Archives, J2.15 1969/7_12, Blutspendedienst SRK, 1944–50.
31. Eugster to Remund, 20 March 1950, Swiss Federal Archives, J2.15 1969/7_12, Blutspendedienst SRK, 1944–50.
32. Schweizerischer Nationalfonds zur Förderung der wissenschaftlichen Forschung (ed.), *Jahresbericht* (Bern: Schweizerischer Nationalfonds 1953); on the history of research funding in Switzerland, see F. Joye-Cagnard, *La construction de la politique de la science en Suisse : enjeux scientifiques, stratégiques et politiques (1944–1974)* (Neuchâtel: Editions Alphil, 2010); A. Fleury and J. Frédéric, *Die Anfänge der Forschungspolitik in der Schweiz: Gründungsgeschichte des Schweizerischen Nationalfonds zur Förderung der wissenschaftlichen Forschung, 1934–1952* (Baden: Hier und Jetzt, 2002).
33. Schweizerischer Nationalfonds zur Förderung der wissenschaftlichen Forschung (ed.): *Jahresbericht* (Bern: Schweizerischer Nationalfonds, 1955), p. 29.
34. Marcel Benoist Stiftung, Preisträger 1956 Siegfried Rosin, at http://www.marcel-benoist.ch/index.php?option=com_content&task=view&id=85&Itemid=55 [accessed 1 July 2011]. On the history of the Marcel Benoist Prize, see M. Stuber and S. Kraut, *Der*

Marcel-Benoist-Preis 1920–1995: Die Geschichte des eidgenössischen Wissenschaftspreises (Bern: Fondation Marcel Benoist, 1995).

35. 'Das A und O des Schweizerblutes', pp. 6ff.
36. Hadorn, 'Zur Verteilung der Blutgruppen in der Schweiz'.
37. For A. E. Mourant and blood group research in England, see the contribution of Jenny Bangham in this volume.
38. A. Manuila, 'Recherches sérologiques et anthropologiques chez les populations de la Roumanie, etc.', *Archiv der Julius Klaus-Stiftung für Vererbungsforschung, Sozialanthropologie und Rassenhygiene*, 32:3–4 (1957), pp. 219–357.
39. On Ioannis Koumaris and racial anthropology in Greece, see S. Trubeta, 'Anthropological Discourse and Eugenics in Interwar Greece', in M. Turda and P. Weindling (eds), *Blood and Homeland: Eugenics and Racial Nationalism in Central and Southeast Europe, 1900–1940* (Budapest: Central European University Press, 2007), pp. 123–42; see also C. Promitzer, 'The Body of the Other: Racial Science and Ethnic Minorities in the Balkans', in S. Trubeta and C. Voss (eds), *Minorities in Greece: Historical Issues and New Perspectives* (Munich: Slavica Verlag, Dr Anton Kovac, 2003), pp. 27–40.
40. J. G. Koumaris, 'Les groupes sanguins et l'hellénisme', *Archiv der Julius Klaus-Stiftung für Vererbungsforschung, Sozialanthropologie und Rassenhygiene*, 33:1–2 (1958), pp. 81.
41. See, for example, the chapter on Switzerland in M.-R. Sauter, *Les races de l'Europe* (Paris: Payot, 1952), pp. 274ff.
42. See, for example, A. Schmid, *Die Entwicklung des Verhältnisses zwischen Deutsch und Welsch in der Schweiz seit Ausbruch des Krieges* (Basel: Finckh 1917). See also P. Du Bois, 'Mythe et réalité du fossé pendant la Première Guerre Mondiale', in P. Dubois (ed.), *Union et Division des Suisses: les Relations entre Alémaniques, Romands et Tessinois aux XIXe et XXe siècles* (Lausanne: Editions de l'Aire, 1983), pp. 65–91.
43. See especially R. Wecker, 'Eugenik – Individueller Ausschluss und nationaler Konsens', in S. Guex, B. Studer and B. Degen (ed.), *Krisen und Stabilisierung. Die Schweiz in der Zwischenkriegszeit* (Zurich: Chronos, 1998), pp. 167–79; V. Mottier, 'Narratives of National Identity: Sexuality, Race and the Swiss "Dream of Order"', *Swiss Journal of Sociology*, 26:3 (2000), pp. 533–56; P. Kury, *Über Fremde reden: Überfremdungsdiskurs und Ausgrenzung in der Schweiz 1900–1945* (Zurich: Chronos, 2003).
44. Joseph Kälin, cited in Fleury and Frédéric, *Die Anfänge der Forschungspolitik*, p. 180.
45. 'Marcel Benoist Foundation: Preisträger 1956: Siegfried Rosin', at http://www.marcelbenoist.ch/index.php?option=com_content&task=view&id=85&Itemid=55 [accessed 1 July 2011].
46. L. Gannett and J. R. Griesemer, 'The ABO Blood Groups: Mapping the History and Geography of Genes in Homo Sapiens', in H.-J. Rheinberger and J.-P. Gaudillière (eds), *Classical Genetic Research and its Legacy: the Mapping Cultures of Twentieth-Century Genetics* (London: Routledge, 2004), pp. 119–72, especially pp. 128–39.
47. See B. Studer, G. Arlettaz, R. Argast and A. Gidkov, *Das Schweizer Bürgerrecht: Erwerb, Verlust, Entzug von 1848 bis zur Gegenwart* (Zurich: Verlag Neue Zürcher Zeitung, 2008); R. Argast, *Staatsbürgerschaft und Nation: Ausschliessung und Integration in der Schweiz 1848–1933* (Göttingen: Vandenhoeck & Ruprecht, 2007); G. P. Marchal, 'National Historiography and National Identity: Switzerland in Comparative Perspective', in S. Berger and C. Lorenz (eds), *The Contested Nation. Ethnicity, Class, Religion and Gender in National Histories* (New York: Palgrave Macmilian, 2008).
48. Schütz, 'Vorkommen', pp. 207ff; Schlaginhaufen, *Anthropologia Helvetica*, Vol. 1, pp. 49ff.
49. Schütz, 'Vorkommen', p. 207.

50. Tellingly, Siegfried Rosin considered all naturalized foreigners 'genetic strangers'. Therefore he regarded it as a problem that it was not possible to exclude naturalized citizens from data pool. Rosin, 'Verteilung der AB0-Blutgruppen', p. 29.
51. Rosin, 'Verteilung der AB0-Blutgruppen', p. 52.
52. Ibid., pp. 51ff.
53. Ibid., p. 22.
54. For more on this shift, see the contribution of Veronika Lipphardt in this volume.
55. R. H. Post, 'Review of "S. Rosin, Die Verteilung der AB0-Blutgruppen in der Schweiz"', *American Journal of Human Genetics*, 10:2 (June 1958), pp. 230ff, on p. 231.
56. E. Hanhart, 'Principal Results of 30 Years-Studies in Swiss and Foreign Isolates', *Caryologia: International Journal of Cytology, Cytosystematics and Cytogenetics*, vol. suppl. (1954), pp. 925–7, on p. 925.
57. See especially H. J. Huser, J. K. Moor-Jankowski and S. Rosin, 'Genetische Untersuchungen der sero-anthropologischen Zusammenhänge in zwei Walsertälern', *Jahresbericht der Schweizerischen Gesellschaft für Vererbungsforschung*, 14 (1954), pp. 298–304; Rosin, 'Die Bedeutung der Blutgruppen', pp. 440–52.
58. See, for example, Rosin, 'Die Bedeutung der Blutgruppen', especially p. 447.
59. L. C. Dunn and T. Dobzhansky, *Heredity, Race and Society* (New York: Mentor, 1946), p. 108.
60. Moor-Jankowski summed up all these results in 'La prépondérance du goupe sanguin 0'.
61. On the term 'biohistorical narrative', see V. Lipphardt and J. Niewöhner, 'Producing Difference in an Age of Biosociality. Biohistorical Narratives, Standardisation and Resistance as Translations', *Science, Technology & Innovation Studies*, 3:1 (2007), pp. 45–65.
62. See, for example, P. Gysi, 'Erbbiologische Bestandesaufnahme einer abgelegenen Bündner Walsergemeinde', *Archiv der Julius Klaus-Stiftung für Vererbungsforschung, Sozialanthropologie und Rassenhygiene*, 26 (1951), pp. 97–127, on pp. 98–105.
63. Rosin, 'Verteilung der AB0-Blutgruppen', pp. 106–8.
64. Ibid., pp. 105–8.
65. See, for example, N. E. Morton, N. Yasuda, C. Miki and S. Yee, 'Population Structure of the ABO Blood Groups in Switzerland', *American Journal of Human Genetics*, 20:5 (September 1968), pp. 420–9.

7 Suárez-Diaz and Barahona, 'Post-War and Post-Revolution: Medical Genetics and Social Anthropology in Mexico, 1945–70'

1. G. Basalla, 'The Spread of Western Science', *Science*, 156 (1967), pp. 611–22. For a more recent example, see T. F. Glick, M. A. Puig-Samper and R. Ruiz, *El Darwinismo en España e Iberoamérica* (Madrid: CSIC, 1999).
2. F. H. Cardoso and E. Faletto, *Dependency and Development in Latin America* (Berkeley, CA: University of California Press, 1979).
3. S. Subrahmanyam, 'Connected Histories: Notes towards a Reconfiguration of Early Modern Eurasia', *Modern Asian Studies*, 31 (1997), pp. 735–62, on p. 745.
4. Although this is not the subject of the present essay, we must further emphasize the role of local elites in transnational collaboration. Further examples of elites as active agents are as follows: Moisés Saénz (1888–1941) studied in Paris, and then travelled to New York, where he gained a PhD in philosophy at Columbia University. Saénz met John Dewey, whose influence on the development of secondary schools was decisive in 1925.

He is also known for his long-standing concern for indigenous populations in Mexico (*indigenismo*), becoming the first director of the Inter-American Institute for Indigenous Affairs. Moreover, Gamio (1883–1960) was considered by Franz Boas to be one of his best students; he is recognized in Mexico as a fierce promoter of cultural anthropology.

5. T. Blanchette, 'La antropología aplicada y la administración indígena en Estados Unidos: 1934–1945', *Desacatos*, 33 (2010), pp. 33–52, on p. 44.
6. The spectre of war was already apparent, and as many scholars have recognized, US diplomacy towards Latin America centred on cutting its relations with Europe, in particular Germany. In the domestic sphere, the Indian Reorganization Act (IRA) was passed by the United States Congress in 1934 at the urging of Collier. The IRA is considered to be a very influential piece of legislation, as it reversed previous federal policies towards indigenous peoples in the United States. The new law recognized a degree of self-determination and the commitment of the federal government to alleviating the economic and social inequalities affecting its indigenous populations. During the 1930s this was followed by explicit policies of employment and welfare for these communities (known as the Indian New Deal).
7. See, for instance, S. Lindee, *Moments of Truth in Genetic Medicine* (Baltimore, MD: Johns Hopkins University Press, 2005); N. Comfort, *The Science of Human Perfection: How Genes Became the Heart of American Medicine* (New Haven, CT: Yale University Press, 2012).
8. M. Gamio, *Forjando Patria* (Mexico City: Porrúa Editores, 1916); M. Gamio, *La poblacion del valle de Teotihuacan* (Mexico City: Instituto Nacional Indigenista, 1979). On the 'modernizing nationalism' of Gamio, see D. A. Brading and M. Urquidi, 'Manuel Gamio y el indigenismo oficial en México', *Revista Mexicana de Sociología*, 51 (1989), pp. 267–84.
9. The history of cultural anthropology in Mexico is not the subject of this essay. However, it is important to note the influential work of Morris Swadesh, student of Edward Sapir, in Mexico. Swadesh first arrived in Mexico in the 1930s, attracted by the nationalist policies of Lázaro Cárdenas (see main text, p. 104). He finally settled in Mexico in 1956, having been blacklisted as a communist in the United States in 1949. As this essay shows (see main text, p. 109), his linguistic classification of Mexican indigenous groups was adopted in the research of Rubén Lisker. See M. Swadesh, *The Origin and Diversification of Language* (Chicago, IL: Aldine Atherton, 1971). On the changing attitudes towards the indigenous cultures in Mexican nationalism, see D. A. Brading, *The Origins of Mexican Nationalism* (Cambridge: Cambridge Centre for Latin American Studies, 1985).
10. Alfonso Caso Andrade (1896–1970) was a lawyer, philosopher and archaeologist who had been in charge of the Monte Albán archaeological site in southern Oaxaca since the mid-1920s. He made important contributions to the archaeology and chronology of pre-Columbian cultures. As a result of his interaction with the living indigenous populations, he became a cultural anthropologist and, like Gamio before him, was largely influenced by the culturalism of Franz Boas. Caso was instrumental in the use of linguistic differences (as opposed to racial and anatomical criteria) as a criterion for studying the diversity of human populations in Mexico.
11. In 1952 Caso was awarded the prestigious Viking Fund Medal (today the Wenner Gren Foundation). From the 1930s until his death in 1970, he was instrumental in the consolidation of close connections between Mexican anthropologists and archaeologists with the Carnegie and Rockefeller Foundations and with the Viking Fund of New York.

12. E. Zolla-Marques, 'Estado, Antropología e Indígenas en el México Posrevolucionario' (unpublished thesis, UNAM, 2004), pp. 34.
13. 'Para nuestros pueblos de America la antropología no es algo puramente teórico ni de una aplicación mediata; es una disciplina que está encajada en nuestro corazón y en nuestra vida'. Alfonso Caso, 'Discurso de ingreso a El Colegio Nacional', 15 May 1943, Alfonso Caso Archive, Instituto de Investigaciones Antropólogicas, UNAM, México City.
14. As far as we can tell, the Centres' mediation was extremely effective in implementing the 'incorporation' of the indigenous communities into the city projects. Lewis maintains that the Coordinating Centres were even more effective in raising a self-reflective attitude, which, paradoxically, fed into the Mexican guerrilla movements in the 1970s. See S. E. Lewis, 'The Tragedy of Success: Mexico's National Indigenist Institute (INI) in Highland Chiapas', paper presented at the American Historical Association Conference, San Diego, January 2009; and M. Rankin, 'Each One, Teach One: Education and Literacy in Mexico during World War II', paper presented at the American Historical Association Conference, San Diego, January 2009.
15. See J. Marks, 'The Legacy of Serological Studies in American Physical Anthropology', *History and Philosophy of the Life Sciences*, 18 (1996), pp. 345–62; L. Gannett and J. Griesemer, 'Classical Genetics and the Geography of Genes', in H.-J. Rheinberger and J.-P. Gaudillière (eds), *Classical Genetic Research and its Legacy: the Mapping Cultures of Twentieth-Century Genetics* (New York: Routledge, 2004), pp. 57–87.
16. A. Solórzano, 'La influencia de la Fundación Rockefeller en la conformación de la profesión médica mexicana, 1921–1949', *Revista Mexicana de Sociología*, 58 (1996), pp. 173–203.
17. See A. Barahona, 'Medical Genetics in Mexico. Circulation of Knowledge and the Development of Cytogenetics' (Mexico City: UNAM, forthcoming).
18. M. Salazar-Mallén and R. Hernández de la Portilla, 'Existencia del aglutinógeno Rh en los hematíes de 250 individuos Mexicanos', *Revista de la Sociedad Mexicana de Historia Natural*, 5 (1944), pp. 183–5.
19. A. S. Wiener, J. P. Zepeda, E. B. Sonn and H. R. Polivka, 'Individual Blood Differences in Mexican Indians with Special Reference to HR Blood Types and HR Factors', *Journal of Experimental Medicine*, 81 (1945), pp. 559–67. See also A. Mourant, *The Distribution of the Human Blood Groups* (Oxford: Blackwell, 1954), in particular ch. XIII on 'The Aborigines of America'.
20. Salazar-Mallén and Hernández de la Portilla, 'Existencia del aglutinógeno Rh'; M. Salazar-Mallén, 'El aglutinógeno Lewis en la sangre de los mexicanos', *Bol. Inst. Med. Bio.*, 7 (1949), pp. 25–30; C. Arteaga, M. Salazar-Mallén, E. Ugalde E. and A. Vélez-Orozco, 'Blood Agglutinogens of Mexicans', *Ann. Eugen*, 16 (1952), pp. 351–5.
21. A. Barahona, *Historia de la genética humana en México 1879–1970* (Mexico City: UNAM, 2009).
22. After World War II, Ruth Sanger moved from Sydney to London and worked for Dr Race, her future husband, and co-wrote *Blood Groups in Man*, a reference book, for nearly thirty years. See R. Sanger and R. R. Race, 'The Combination of Blood Groups in a Sample of 250 People', *Ann. Eugen.*, 15 (1949), pp. 77–90. See also R. R. Race and R. Sanger, *Blood Groups in Man*, 5th edn (Oxford: Blackwell Scientific, 1968).
23. Both Grajales (Director of the Army School at the time) and Corona del Rosal (a Mexican senator) are infamous for their later participation in the repressive actions of the Mexican government against the student movement in Mexico in 1968. See Arteaga et al., 'Blood Agglutinogens of Mexicans', p. 354.

24. Letters sent to de Garay (1 February 1963) and Agustín Romero Delgado (2 February 1963), and letter from de Garay to Caso (3 March 1963); Alfonso Caso Archive, Instituto de Investigaciones Antropólogicas, UNAM, México. See also V. Tiburcio, A. Romero and A. L. de Garay, 'Gene Frequencies and Racial Intermixture in a Mestizo Population from Mexico City', *Annals of Human Biology*, 5 (1978), pp. 131–8; and H. Kalmus, A. L. de Garay, U. Rodarte and L. Cobo, 'The Frequency of PTC Tasting, Hard Ear Was, Colour Blindness and Other Genetical Characters in Urban and Rural Mexican Populations', *Human Biology*, 36 (1964), pp. 134–45.
25. A. Basave, *México Mestizo. Análisis del nacionalismo mexicano en torno a la mestizofilia de Andrés Molina Enríquez* (Mexico City: Fondo de Cultura Económica, 2002); P. Wade, 'Racial Identity and Nationalism: A Theoretical View from Latin America', *Ethnic and Racial Studies*, 24 (2001), pp. 845–65.
26. A. Karl, 'Estudio electroforético de la hemoglobina de los indígenas mazatecos de la cuenca del Papaloapan', *Ciencia*, 17 (1957), pp. 85–6.
27. Another further reason for our focus on Lisker is his enduring influence in the education of human geneticists in Mexico, some of whom now form part of INMEGEN. For a more detailed account of Lisker's research, see E. Suárez-Díaz, 'Indigenous Populations in Mexico: Medical Anthropology in the Work of Rubén Lisker in the 1960s', *Studies in History and Philosophy of Biological and Biomedical Sciences* (forthcoming).
28. C. Dreyfuss, 'A Genetics Pioneer Sees a Bright Future, Cautiously. A Conversation with Arno Motulsky', *New York Times*, 29 April 2008, p. 8.
29. Barahona, *Historia de la genética humana en México*.
30. Ibid., p. 103.
31. R. Lisker, A. Loría, J. González-Llaven, S. Guttman and G. Ruiz-Reyes, 'Note préliminaire sur la fréquence des hemoglobines anormales et de la déficience en gluxose-6-phosphate déhydrogénase dans la population Mexicaine', *Rev. Franc. d'Etud. Clin. Biol.*, 1 (1962), pp. 76–8.
32. See the section 'Indigenous Policies and Health Services' in the main text, pp. 103–5, and p. 257 n. 9. For an extended description of the sampling design, see Lisker et al., 'Note préliminaire'; and for a detailed account of the relation between Lisker's research and Swadesh's method, see also Suárez-Díaz, 'Indigenous Populations in Mexico'.
33. M. Cueto, *Cold War, Deadly Fevers: Malaria Eradication in Mexico 1955–1975* (Baltimore, MD: Johns Hopkins University Press, 2007).
34. Lisker et al., 'Note préliminaire'.
35. R. Lisker, A. Loría and S. Córdova, 'Studies on Several Hematological Traits of the Mexican Population. VIII. Hemoglobin S, Glucose-6-Phospate Dehydrogenase Deficiency and Other Characteristics in a Malarial Region', *Amer. J. Human. Genet.*, 17 (1965), pp. 179–87.
36. R. Lisker, A. Loría, S. Ibarra and L. Sánchez-Medal, 'Características genéticas hematológicas de la población Mexicana. VII. Estudio en la Costa Chica', *Salud Pública Méx.*, 7 (1965), pp. 45–50; and R. Lisker, G. Zárate and A. Loría, 'Studies on Several Genetic Hematological Traits of Mexicans. IX: Abnormal Hemoglobins and Erythrocyte Glucos-6-Phospate Dehydrogenase Deficiency in Several Indian Tribes', *Blood*, 27 (1966), pp. 824–30.
37. See Suárez-Díaz, 'Indigenous Populations in Mexico' for more details on Lisker.
38. L. Melartin, B. Blumberg and R. Lisker, 'Albumin Mexico, a New Variant of Serum Albumin', *Nature*, 215 (1967), pp. 1288–9.
39. Lisker, Zárate and Loría, 'Studies on Several Genetic Hematological Traits of Mexicans'.
40. Mourant, *The Distribution of the Human Blood Groups*.

8 Schwerin, 'From Agriculture to Genomics: The Animal Side of Human Genetics and the Organization of Model Organisms in the Longue Durée'

1. For a short history of experimental organisms and its literature, see R. A. Ankeny and S. Leonelli, 'What's So Special About Model Organisms?', *Studies in History and Philosophy of Science*, 42 (2011), pp. 313–23, on pp. 314–15.
2. R. A. Ankeny, 'Model Organisms as Models: Understanding the "Lingua Franca" of the Human Genome Project', *Philosophy of Science*, 68 suppl. (2001), pp. S250–S61, on p. S252, fn.
3. C. A. Logan, 'Before There Were Standards: The Role of Test Animals in the Production of Empirical Generality in Physiology', *Journal of the History of Biology*, 35 (2002), pp. 329–63, on pp. 349–50.
4. A prominent example is the controversy over the dysgenic effects of radiological treatment in Germany; A. v. Schwerin, *Experimentalisierung des Menschen: Der Genetiker Hans Nachtsheim und die vergleichende Erbpathologie, 1920–1945* (Göttingen: Wallstein, 2004), pp. 119–35.
5. Schwerin, *Experimentalisierung*, p. 226 (also pp. 223–8); H.-J. Rheinberger, 'Reflections sur les organismes modèles dans la recherche biologique aux XXe siècle', in G. Gachelin (ed.), *Les organismes modèles dans la recherche médicale* (Paris: Presses Universitaires de France), pp. 45–52, on p. 51.
6. B. T. Clause, 'The Wistar Rat as a Right Choice: Establishing Mammalian Standards and the Ideal of a Standardized Mammal', *Journal of the History of* Biology, 26 (1993), pp. 329–49; K. R. Rader, '"The Mouse People": Murine Genetics Work at the Bussey Institution, 1909–1936', *Journal of the History of* Biology, 31 (1998), pp. 327–54; I. Löwy and J.-P. Gaudillière, 'Disciplining Cancer: Mice and the Practice of Genetic Purity', in J.-P. Gaudillière and I. Löwy (eds), *The Invisible Industrialist: Manufactures and the Production of Scientific Knowledge* (Hampshire and London: Macmillan Press Ltd, 1998), pp. 209–49; J.-P. Gaudillière, 'Circulating Mice and Viruses: The Jackson Memorial Laboratory, the National Cancer Institute, and the Genetics of Breast Cancer, 1930–1945', in M. Fortun and E. Mendelsohn (eds), *The Practices of Human Genetics* (Dordrecht: Kluwer, 1999), pp. 89–124; J.-P. Gaudillière, 'Making Heredity in Mice and Men: The Production and Uses of Animal Models in Postwar Human Genetics', in I. Löwy and J.-P. Gaudillière (eds), *Heredity and Infection: A History of Disease Transmission* (Amsterdam: Harwood, 2001), pp. 181–202; K. R. Rader, *Making Mice: Standardizing Animals for American Biomedical Research, 1900–1955* (Princeton, NJ: Princeton University Press, 2004); Schwerin, *Experimentalisierung*, pp. 136–77; G. Moser, *Deutsche Forschungsgemeinschaft und Krebsforschung, 1920–1970* (Stuttgart: Steiner, 2011), pp. 156–86.
7. Löwy and Gaudillière, 'Disciplining Cancer'; Rader, *Making Mice*; Schwerin, *Experimentalisierung*, pp. 161–8.
8. L. Campos and A. v. Schwerin, 'Transatlantic Mutants: Evolution, Epistemics, and the Engineering of Variation, 1903–1930', in C. Brandt and S. Müller-Wille (eds), *Heredity Explored: Between Public Domain and Experimental Science, 1850–1930* (Harvard, MA: MIT Press, forthcoming).
9. On Nachtsheim's experimental research, see Schwerin, *Experimentalisierung*, pp. 35–118 and 178–228.
10. For this French-German history, see also T. Hoquet, 'Non-Evolutionary Mutants? A Note on the Castorrex Rabbit', in L. Campos and A. v. Schwerin (eds), *Making Muta-*

tions: Objects, Practices, Contexts. Cultural History of Heredity Workshop at the Max Planck Institute for the History of Science, Berlin, 13–15 January 2009, Preprint series 393 (Berlin: Max Planck Institute for the History of Science, 2010), pp. 85–107.

11. For an analysis of this research programme, see Schwerin, *Experimentalisierung*, pp. 217–28.
12. H. Nachtsheim and H. Gürich, 'Erbleiden des Kaninchenauges. 1. Erbliche Nahtbändchentrübung der Linse mit nachfolgendem Kernstar', *Zeitschrift für menschliche Vererbungs- und Konstitutionslehre*, 23 (1939), pp. 463–83, on p. 465.
13. Also, see Schwerin, *Experimentalisierung*, pp. 212–16.
14. Kühn to DFG, 28 November 1935, Bundesarchiv Koblenz, R 73, 15057. For the connection of organization, standardization and production of difference, see Schwerin, *Experimentalisierung*, pp. 172–4.
15. Schwerin, *Experimentalisierung*, pp. 229–76; H.-W. Schmuhl, *Grenzüberschreitungen. Das Kaiser-Wilhelm-Institut für Anthropologie, menschliche Erblehre und Eugenik 1927–1945* (Göttingen: Wallstein, 2005), pp. 313–50. In addition, comparative genetics came right at hand with a methodological crisis of human genetics in the 1930; Schwerin, *Experimentalisierung*, pp. 237–42 and 259. For the crisis of twin research, see Schmuhl, *Grenzüberschreitungen*, pp. 258–63.
16. C. Sachse, 'Ein "Als Neugründung zu deutender Beschluß…": Vom Kaiser-Wilhelm-Institut für Anthropologie, menschliche Erblehre und Eugenik zum Max-Planck-Institut für Molekulare Genetik', *Medizinhistorisches Journal*, 46 (2011), pp. 24–50.
17. U. Ehling, *Von Zehdenick nach Oak Ridge: Erinnerungen eines Genetikers. Erster Teil: 1948–1968* (Berlin: Ehlingsche Verlags- und Vertriebsgesellschaft, 2003).
18. Ibid., p. 22.
19. U. Ehling, 'Untersuchungen zur kausalen Genese erblicher Katarakte beim Kaninchen', *Zeitschrift für menschliche Vererbungs- und Konstitutionslehre*, 34 (1957), pp. 77–104, on p. 78.
20. A. N. H. Creager, 'Tracing the Politics of Changing Postwar Research Practices: The Export of "American" Radioisotopes to European Biologists', *Studies in History and Philosophy of Biological and Biomedical Sciences*, 33 (2002), pp. 367–88.
21. Ehling, *Zehdenik nach Oak Ridge*, p. 25; for the Harwell school, see N. Herran, 'Spreading Nucleonics: The Isotope School at the Atomic Energy Research Establishment, 1951–67', *British Journal for the History of Science*, 39 (2006), pp. 569–86.
22. Rader, *Making Mice*, pp. 235–42.
23. A. M. Weinberg, *Reflections on Big Science* (Cambridge, MA and London: MIT Press, 1967), p. 107.
24. For the SLT, see Rader, *Making Mice*, pp. 242–6; Weinberg, *Reflections*, p. 101.
25. H. P. Kröner, 'Förderung der Genetik und Humangenetik in der Bundesrepublik durch das Ministerium für Atomfragen in den fünfziger Jahren', in K. Weisemann, H.-P. Kröner and R. Toellner (eds), *Wissenschaft und Politik – Genetik und Humangenetik in der DDR (1949–1989)* (Münster: LIT Verlag, 1997), pp. 69–82, on pp. 39–40.
26. Ehling, *Zehdenik nach Oak Ridge*, p. 35 (trans. A. von Schwerin).
27. The Russells collected mutants from time to time for research and informal distribution. In comparison, the Jackson Laboratory was reluctant in this respect; see Gaudillière, 'Making Heredity', p. 160.
28. Ehling, *Zehdenik nach Oak Ridge*, pp. 35–6.
29. Kröner, 'Förderung'; A. v. Schwerin, 'Humangenetik im Atomzeitalter: Von der Mutationsforschung zum Erbregister', in A. Cottebrune and W. Eckart (eds), *Das Hei-*

delberger Institut für Humangenetik: Vorgeschichte und Ausbau (1962–2012); Festschrift zum 50jährigen Jubiläum (Heidelberg: C. R. Bartram, 2012), pp. 82–105.

30. Kaplan to Buzzati-Traverso, 28 May 1963, American Philosophical Society, Library (APS), B H717, box 4, fol. 2.
31. Ehling, *Zehdenik nach Oak Ridge*, p. 61.
32. C. Reuter-Boysen, *Von der Strahlen- zur Umweltforschung. Geschichte der GSF 1957–1972* (Frankfurt and New York: Campus Verlag, 1992), p. 138.
33. Ehling, *Zehdenik nach Oak Ridge*, pp. 62 and 66–77.
34. Gesellschaft für Strahlen- und Umweltforschung mbH München (ed.), *Jahresbericht 1973. Kurzfassung* (Munich: Südd. Verlag GmbH, 1974), p. 41.
35. S. Frickel, *Chemical Consequences: Environmental Mutagens, Scientist Activism, and the Rise of Genetic Toxicology* (New Brunswick, NJ and London: Rutgers University Press, 2004), pp. 73–7.
36. U. Ehling, *Die Müchner Jahre: Erinnerungen eines Genetikers. Zweiter Teil: 1968–1993* (Berlin: Ehlingsche Verlags- und Vertriebsgesellschaft, 2006), p. 9; see also Frickel, *Chemical Consequences*, p. 67.
37. A. v. Schwerin, 'The Hollaender Legacy. Mutagens and a New Problematisation of the Consumer Society, 1954–1970', in S. Boudia and N. Jas (eds), *Carcinogens, Mutagens, Reproductive Toxicants: The Politics of Limit Values and Low Doses in the Twentieth and Twenty-First Centuries (Book of Papers of an International Conference, Strasbourg, 29–31 March 2010)*, pp. 109–20, on p. 119, at http://pharmgesch-bs.de/fileadmin/pharmgesch/Dokumente/Schwerin_2010_Hollaender_Legacy.pdf; for the USA, see Frickel, *Chemical Consequences*, p. 58.
38. A. v. Schwerin, 'Mutagene Umweltstoffe: Gunter Röhrborn und die neue eugenische Bedrohung', in A. Cottebrune and W. Eckart (eds), *Das Heidelberger Institut für Humangenetik: Vorgeschichte und Ausbau (1962–2012); Festschrift zum 50jährigen Jubiläum* (Heidelberg: C. R. Bartram, 2012), pp. 106–129.
39. U. Ehling (ed.), *Methodik der Mutagenitätsprüfung I*, GSF-Bericht B 564 (Munich: GSF, 1975), p. 3.
40. A. Creager, 'The Political Life of Mutagens: A History of the Ames Test', in L. Campos and A. v. Schwerin (eds), *Making Mutations: Objects, Practices, Contexts. Cultural History of Heredity Workshop at the Max Planck Institute for the History of Science, Berlin, 13–15 January 2009*, Preprint series 393 (Berlin: Max Planck Institute for the History of Science, 2010), pp. 285–306.
41. U. H. Ehling and A. Neuhäuser, 'Procarbazine-Induced Specific-Locus Mutations in Male Mice', *Mutation Research*, 59 (1979), pp. 245–56.
42. U. Ehling, 'The Multiple Loci Method', in G. Röhrborn and F. Vogel (eds), *Chemical Mutagenesis in Mammals and Man* (Heidelberg and New York: Springer-Verlag, 1970), pp. 156–61, on pp. 159–60.
43. Ibid., p. 159.
44. U. H. Ehling, 'Mutagenicity Testing and Risk Estimation with Mammals', *Mutation Research/Fundamental and Molecular Mechanisms of Mutagenesis*, 41 (1976), pp. 113–22, on pp. 119–20.
45. U. Ehling, 'Evaluation of Presumed Dominant Skeletal Mutations', in G. Röhrborn and F. Vogel (eds), *Chemical Mutagenesis in Mammals and Man* (Heidelberg and New York: Springer-Verlag, 1970), pp. 162–6, on p. 165.
46. Ehling, *Müchner Jahre*, p. 95.
47. U. H. Ehling, 'Induction of Gene Mutations in Germ Cells of the Mouse', *Archives of Toxicology*, 46 (1980), pp. 123–38, on pp. 125–6; J. Kratochvilova and U. H. Ehling,

'Dominant Cataract Mutations Induced by Gamma-Irradiation of Male Mice', *Mutation Research*, 63 (1979), pp. 221–3, on p. 221.

48. UNSCEAR (ed.), *Ionizing Radiation: Sources and Biological Effects. United Nations Scientific Committee on the Effects of Atomic Radiation, 1982 Report to the General Assembly, with Annexes* (New York: United Nations, 1982), p. 478.
49. For the citation, see Ehling, 'Mutagenicity Testing', p. 120.
50. J. Favor, 'A Comparison of the Dominant Cataract and Recessive Specific-Locus Mutation Rates Induced by Treatment of Male Mice with Ethylnitrosourea', *Mutation Research*, 110 (1983), pp. 367–82, on p. 368.
51. Ehling, *Zehdenik nach Oak Ridge*, p. 62.
52. W. L. Russell, E. M. Kelly, P. R. Hunsicker, J. W. Bangham, S. C. Maddux, and E. L. Phipps, 'Specific-Locus Test Shows Ethylnitrosourea to Be the Most Potent Mutagen in the Mouse', *Proceedings of the National Academy of Sciences of the United States of America*, 76 (1979), pp. 5818–19.
53. U. Ehling, 'Induction of Dominant Lethal Mutations in Mice by Ethylnitrosourea (ENU)', Progress Report, January–October 1980, EC Contract No. 136-77-1 ENV D, Ehling Family Archive.
54. Favor in personal communication, see M. Hrabě de Angelis and R. Balling, 'Large Scale ENU Screens in the Mouse: Genetics Meets Genomics', *Mutation Research*, 400 (1998), pp. 25–32, on p. 28.
55. Rudi Balling, Curriculum Vitae, Congress Secretariat of the XX International Congress of Genetics, Berlin, 2008, CD Press information.
56. Hrabě de Angelis and Balling, 'Large Scale ENU Screens', p. 28.
57. Ibid., pp. 27–8; for the protocol, see J. Favor, 'The Frequency of Dominant Cataract and Recessive Specific-Locus Mutations in Mice Derived from 80 or 160 mg Ethylnitrosourea per kg Body Weight Treated Spermatogonia', *Mutation Research*, 162 (1986), pp. 69–80.
58. Hrabě de Angelis and Balling, 'Large Scale ENU Screens', p. 29.
59. Hrabě de Angelis et al., 'Genome-Wide, Large-Scale Production of Mutant Mice by ENU Mutagenesis', *Nature Genetics*, 25 (2000), pp. 444–7, on p. 444.
60. Hrabě de Angelis and Balling, 'Large Scale ENU Screens', p. 26.
61. For the distinction of supplements and surrogates in detail, see Schwerin, *Experimentalisierung*, pp. 223–8; for the citation, see Ehling, 'Mutagenicity Testing', p. 120.
62. For this expression, see S. P. Cordes, 'N-Ethyl-N-Nitrosourea Mutagenesis: Boarding the Mouse Mutant Express', *Microbiology and Molecular Biology Reviews*, 69 (2005), pp. 426–39.
63. For this transformation, see also M. Morange, 'The Transformation of Molecular Biology on Contact with Higher Organisms, 1960–1980: From a Molecular Description to a Molecular Explanation', *History & Philosophy of the Life Sciences*, 19 (1997), pp. 369–93.
64. Cordes, 'N-Ethyl-N-Nitrosourea Mutagenesis', p. 427.

9 Santesmases, 'Cereals, Chromosomes and Colchicine: Crop Varieties at the Estación Experimental Aula Dei and Human Cytogenetics, 1948–58'

1. J.-P. Gaudillière, 'The Farm and the Clinic: An Inquiry into the Making of our Biotechnological Modernity', *Studies in History and Philosophy of Biological and Biomedical Sciences*, 38 (2007), pp. 521–9. On the improvement of crop varieties and its impact

in Spain, see J. Pujol Andreu, 'Agricultura y crecimiento económico: las innovaciones biológicas en la cerealicultura europea 1820–1940', *Revista de Historia Industrial*, 21 (2002), pp. 63–88; L. Camprubí, 'One Grain, One Nation: Rice Genetics and the Corporate State in Early Francoist Spain (1939–1952)', *Historical Studies in the Natural Sciences*, 40 (2010), pp. 499–531. The situation in Great Britain during the same period is described in P. Palladino, *Plants, Patients, and Historians: (Re)membering in the Age of Genetic Engineering* (New Brunswick, NJ: Rutgers University Press 2002); and P. Palladino, 'Science, Technology and the Economy: Plant Breeding in Great Britain 1920–1970', *Economic History Review*, 49 (1996), pp. 116–36. On the USA, see A. L. Olmstead and P. W. Rhode, *Creating Abundance: Biological Innovation and American Agricultural Development* (New York: Cambridge University Press, 2008).

2. M. Kottler, 'From 48 to 46: Cytological Technique, Preconception and the Counting of the Human Chromosomes', *Bulletin of the History of Medicine*, 48 (1974), pp. 465–502. A. Martin, 'Can't Anybody Count? Counting as an Epistemic Theme in the History of Human Chromosomes', *Social Studies of Science*, 34 (2004), pp. 923–48.
3. For earlier work on genetics in Spain, see S. Pinar, 'The Emergence of Modern Genetics in Spain and the Effecs of the Spanish Civil War (1936–1939) on its Development', *Journal of the History of Biology*, 35 (2002), pp. 111–48; I. Delgado Echeverría, *El descubrimiento de los cromosomas sexuales: un hito en la historia de la biología* (Madrid: CSIC, 2007), ch. 10.
4. H. A. Curry, 'Making Marigolds: Colchicine, Mutation Breeding, and Ornamental Agriculture', in L. Campos and A. von Schwerin (eds), *Making Mutations: Objects, Practices and Contexts*, Preprint 393 (Berlin: Max Planck Institute for the History of Science, 2010), pp. 259–83; H. A. Curry, 'Accelerating Evolution, Engineering Life: American Agriculture and Technologies of Genetic Modification, 1925–1960' (PhD dissertation, Yale University, 2012), ch. 4; J. Goodman, 'Plants, Cells and Bodies: The Molecular Biography of Colchicine, 1930–1975', in S. de Chadarevian and H. Kamminga (eds), *Molecularizing Biology and Medicine: New Practices and Alliances, 1910s–1970s* (Amsterdam: Harwood, 1998), pp. 17–46.
5. H. Dermen, 'Colchicine, Polyploidy and Technique', *Botanical Review*, 6 (1940), pp. 599–635, on p. 606.
6. J. V. Cook and J. D. Loudon, 'Colchicine', in R. H. F. Manske (ed.), *The Alkaloids. Chemistry and Physiology, Vol. II* (New York: Academic Press, 1952) pp. *261–329, on p.* 297.
7. The quote I am using here is on p. 6 of T. C. Hsu, *Human and Mammalian Cytogenetics: An Historical Perspective* (New York and Heidelberg: Springer Verlag, 1979), although the whole book is greatly inspiring for a historian of biological practices.
8. S. Lindee, *Moments of Truth in Genetic Medicine* (Baltimore, MD: Johns Hopkins University Press, 2006), and for a wider and longer account, D. Kevles, *In the Name of Eugenics: Genetics and the Uses of Human Heredity* (Berkeley, CA: University of California Press, 1985).
9. Joe Hin Tjio, Curriculum Vitae, preserved at the NIH Archives in Bethesda, Maryland.
10. Interview with E. Sánchez-Monge, Madrid, 4 December 2007.
11. See Sanchez-Monge's curriculum vitae, sent to the Rockefeller Foundation in 1958; Rockefeller Archive Center, Rockefeller Foundation, Record Group 1.2; Series 795, box 1 folder 4. Corn Improvement 1958–1961, 1963; Folder 5 (University of Madrid – Agricultural Library 1960–1).
12. See the report published by a Spanish visitor, A. Vázquez, *Estación de Ensayos de Semillas de Svalof, Ceres Hispánica* (Madrid: Estación de Ensayos de Semillas, 1919), pp. 51–78.

13. S. Müller-Wille, 'Hybrids, Pure Cultures and Pure Lines: From Nineteenth Century Biology to Twentieth Century Genetics', *Studies in History and Philosophy of Biological and Biomedical Sciences*, 38 (2007), pp. 796–806; S. Müller-Wille and C. Bonneuil, 'Trials and Registers: The Archives of Svaloev Weibull and Vilmorin Companies', *Mendel Newsletter*, 16 (2007), pp. 16–21.
14. Vázquez, *Estación de Ensayos*, pp. 51–2.
15. Müller-Wille, 'Hybrids, Pure Cultures'.
16. On Svalöf and its cytogenetic programme, see A. Tunlid, Ärftlighetsforskningens gränser: Individer och institutioner i framväxten av svensk genetik, Ugglan: Minerva-serien, Vol. 11 (Lund: Lund University, 2004), in Swedish with an abstract in English. See also S. Ellerström and A. Hagberg, 'The Cytogenetics Department of the Swedish Seed Association 1931–1961', *Sveriges Utsädesfören Tidskrift*, 72 (1962), pp. 192–209.
17. Tjio CV, NIH Archives; J. H. Tjio, 'The Somatic Chromosomes of Some Tropical Plants', *Hereditas*, 34 (1948), pp. 135–46; J. H. Tjio, 'Notes on Nucleolar Conditions of Ceiba Pentandra', *Hereditas*, 34 (1948), pp. 204–8; A. Levan and J. H. Tjio, 'Induction of Chromosome Fragmentation by Phenols', *Hereditas*, 34 (1948), pp. 453–84.
18. Sánchez-Monge interview, Madrid, 4 December 2007; the results of this research were published in E. Sánchez-Monge and J. MacKey, 'On the Origin of Subcompactoids in Triticum Vulgare', *Hereditas*, 34 (1948), pp. 321–37.
19. E. Akerberg and W. M. Myers, *Recent Plant Breeding Research: Svalöf 1946–1961* (New York: Wiley, 1963), p. 85, fig. 5.
20. On cereals in the history of the Aragón region in historical perspective, see V. Pinilla, *Entre la inercia y el cambio. El sector agrario aragonés, 1850–1935* (Madrid: Ministerio de Agricultura, Pesca y Alimentación, 1995), pp. 283–392.
21. 'La Estación Experimental Aula Dei hasta su 50 aniversario', Archive of the Estación, n.d. See also CSIC 1950 (Memoria 1948), p. 219.
22. From Ramón Esteruelas to the President of the CSIC, 4 February 1948 (carbon copy). Carpeta 'Nombramientos Consejo', and from José María Albareda, secretary general of the CSIC, to Joe Hin Tjio, 10 March 1948. Both letters are preserved at Registro Joe Hin Tjio, Archivo de la Estación Experimental Aula Dei, Zaragoza (hereafter Archivo Tjio at the Estación Experimental Aula Dei).
23. Tjio and Levan published their first paper together in 1948, and maintained their collaboration through publications until 1956. See Tjio CV, NIH Archives, and Archivo Tjio at the Estación Experimental Aula Dei.
24. See A. Levan, 'The Effect of Colchicine on Root Mitosis in Allium', *Hereditas*, 24 (1938), pp. 471–82.
25. See, for example, ibid. The original paper is A. F. Blakeslee and A. G. Avery, 'Methods of Inducing Doubling of Chromosomes in Plants by Treatment of Colchicine', *Journal of Heredity*, 28 (1927), pp. 393–411. On Blakeslee, see B. A. Kimmelman, 'Mr Blakeslee Built his Dreamhouse: Agricultural Institutions, Genetics and Careers', *Journal of the History of Biology*, 39 (2006), pp. 241–80; L. Campos, 'Genetics without Genes: Blakeslee, Datura and "Chromosomal Mutations"', in *A Cultural History of Heredity IV: Heredity in the Century of the Gene*, Preprint 343 (Berlin: Max Planck Institute for the History of Science, 2008), pp. 243–57. On the origins of polyploidy, M. Richmond, 'Women in Mutation Studies: The Role of Gender in the Methods, Practices and Results of Early Twentieth Century Genetics', in L. Campos and A. von Schwerin (eds), *Making Mutations: Objects, Practices and Contexts*, Preprint 393 (Berlin: Max Planck Institute for the History of Science, 2010), pp. 11–47.

26. Levan, 'The Effect of Colchicine'. See also O. J. Eigsti and P. Dustin, Jr, *Colchicine in Agriculture, Medicine, Biology and Chemistry* (Ames, IO: Iowa State College Press, 1955), p. 21: 'Doctors B. R. Nebel and M. L. Ruttle began research in April, 1937, and concluded important experiments that year clearly demonstrating that colchicine acted upon mitosis'.
27. A. Hagberg and J. H. Tjio, 'Cytological Localisation of the Translocation Point for the Barley Mutant Erectoides', *Hereditas*, 36 (1950), pp. 487–91; J. H. Tjio, 'Chromosome Fragmentation in Pyrogallol', *Anales de la Estación Experimental Aula Dei*, 2 (1951), pp. 187–94.
28. E. Sánchez-Monge, 'Studies on 42-Chromosome Triticale', *Anales de la Estación Experimental Aula Dei*, 4 (1956), pp. 191–207; E. Sánchez-Monge, 'Hexaploid Triticale', *Proceedings of the First International Wheat Genetics Symposium* (1958), pp. 181–94.
29. On the wheat black market after the Spanish War, see C. Barciela, 'Crecimiento y cambio en la agricultura española desde la Guerra Civil', in J. A. Nadal, A. Carreras and C. Sudriá (eds), *La economía española en el siglo XX. Una perspectiva histórica* (Barcelona: Ariel, 1987), pp. 258–79.
30. I have stressed elsewhere this contradiction between the rhetoric of the regime and the practices within industry; for the case of industrial penicillin production, see M. J. Santesmases, 'Distributing Penicillin: The Clinic, the Hero and Industrial Production in Spain, 1943–1952', in V. Quirke and J. Slinn (eds) *Perspectives on Twentieth Century Pharmaceuticals* (Oxford: Peter Lang, 2010), pp. 91–117. The historiography of economics shows these contradictions; see, for example, F. Guirao, *Spain and the Reconstruction of Western Europe 1945–57* (London: MacMillan, 1998).
31. E. Sánchez-Monge and J. H. Tjio, 'Note on 42 Chromosome Triticale', *Atti del IX Congresso Internazionale di Genetica, Caryologia*, suppl. (1954), p. 748.
32. G. D. H. Bell, 'Investigations in the Triticinae I. Colchicine Techniques for Chromosome Doubling in Interspecific and Intergeneric Hybridization', *Journal of Agricultural Science*, 40 (1959), pp. 9–18.
33. See Sánchez-Monge and Tjio, 'Note on 42 Chromosome Triticale'. Tjio was mentioned in the Acknowledgements in Sánchez-Monge, 'Hexaploid Triticale'. A caption of tetraploid rye grains obtained by Tjio was reproduced in Sánchez-Monge's earliest book on plant breeding: E. Sánchez-Monge, *Fitogenética, Mejora de Plantas* (Barcelona: Salvat 1955), p. 127.
34. Sánchez-Monge, *Fitogenética, Mejora de Plantas*, p. 32.
35. Sánchez-Monge, 'Hexaploid Triticale'.
36. See the discussion in ibid., pp. 193–4.
37. See Pinar, 'Emergence of Modern Genetics in Spain', p. 139, and also Sánchez-Monge's personal reconstruction in E. Sánchez-Monge, 'Triticale', *Anales de la Estación Experimental Aula Dei*, 21 (1995), pp. 159–63.
38. Tjio-Esteruelas correspondence, 1948–58, Archivo Tjio at the Estación Experimental Aula Dei. Sometimes Tjio delayed his return, but Esteruelas never complained; on the contrary, he supported Tjio's decisions every time a delay was requested or suggested to him by Tjio.
39. Tjio CV, NIH Archives; Tjio, 'Somatic Chromosomes'; Levan and Tjio, 'Induction of Chromosome Fragmentation by Phenols'.
40. J. H. Tjio and A. Levan, 'Some Experiences with Acetic Orcein in Animal Chromosomes', *Anales de la Estación Experimental Aula Dei*, 3 (1954), pp. 224–8.
41. A. Levan, 'The Background to the Determination of the Human Chromosome Number', *American Journal of Obstetrics and Gynecology*, 130 (1978), pp. 725–6.

42. On the subject of counting human chromosomes, see Kottler, 'From 48 to 46'; and Martin, 'Can't Anybody Count?'
43. Hsu, *Human and Mammalian Cytogenetics*, p. 18.
44. For the case of the Barr body, see F. A. Miller, '"Your True and Proper Gender": The Barr Body as a Good Enough Science of Sex', *Studies in History and Philosophy of Biological and Biomedical Sciences*, 37 (2006), pp. 459–83.
45. Delgado Echeverría, *El descubrimiento*; M. J. Santesmases, 'Size and the Centromere: Translocations and Visual Cultures of Human Genetics', in L. Campos and A. von Schwerin (eds), *Making Mutations: Objects, Practices, Contexts* (Berlin: Max Planck Institute for the History of Science, 2010), pp. 189–204.
46. N. Jouve de la Barreda, 'Don Enrique Sánchez-Monge y Parellada, impulso de la mejora genética de plantas', in M. Candela (ed.), *Los orígenes de la genética en España* (Madrid: Sociedad Estatal de Conmemoraciones Culturales, 2003), pp. 397–422. On the power of the slides, see M. J. Santesmases, 'Samples, Cultures and Plates: Early Human Chromosomes', in I. Löwy (ed.), *Microscope Slides: Reassessing a Neglected Historical Resource* (Berlin: Max Planck Institute for the History of Science, 2011), pp. 25–34.
47. Delgado Echeverría, *El descubrimiento*, pp. 542–53; Pinar, 'The Emergence of Modern Genetics in Spain', pp. 136–40.
48. A chair at the Conde de Cartagena Foundation of the Real Academia de Ciencias, Exactas, Físicas y Naturales was created for Zulueta in 1931 as an academic honour, while at the university there were no chairs. See Pinar, 'The Emergence of Modern Genetics in Spain', p. 123.
49. Jouve de la Barreda, 'Don Enrique Sánchez-Monge'.
50. Tjio CV, NIH Archives. The Joseph P. Kennedy Jr Foundation was created by the Kennedys in 1946 to support people with mental retardation. It was headed by Eunice Kennedy until her death in 2009.
51. See M. J. Santesmases, 'Hacia descendencias saludables: algunos orígenes del diagnóstico prenatal en España', *Asclepio*, 59 (2007), pp. 129–50.
52. Interview with Enrique Sánchez-Monge, Madrid, 4 December 2007.
53. The contributions were published in 1976: see E. Sánchez-Monge, 'Genética y sociedad', in J. Botella and L. Izquierdo (eds), *Problemas actuales de genética humana* (Madrid: Instituto de España, 1976).
54. P. Nowell, J. Rowley and A. Knudson, 'Cancer Genetics, Cytogenetics: Defining the Enemy Within', *Nature Medicine*, 4 (1998), pp. 1107–8; P. Nowell, 'Phytohemagglutinin: An Initiator of Mitosis in Normal Human Leucocytes', *Cancer Research*, 20 (1960), pp. 462–8.
55. Levan and Tjio, 'Induction of Chromosome Fragmentation by Phenols'; J. H. Tjio and A. Levan, 'The Use of Oxyquinoline in Chromosome Analysis', *Anales de la Estación Experimental Aula Dei* (1950), pp. 21–62.

10 de Chadarevian, 'Putting Human Genetics on a Solid Basis: Human Chromosome Research, 1950s–1970s'

1. Exceptions are Daniel Kevles, who in his pioneering study on the history of human genetics dedicated a chapter to human cytogenetics, as does Susan Lindee in her recent history of medical genetics: see D. J. Kevles, *In the Name of Eugenics: Genetics and the Uses of Human Heredity. With a New Preface by the Author* (New York: Harvard University Press, 1995), and M. S. Lindee, *Moments of Truth in Genetics and Medicine* (Baltimore,

MD: Johns Hopkins University, 2005). Other recent studies include Aryn Martin's fresh look at the recounting of the number of human chromosomes in 1956 and Sarah Richardson's forthcoming book on the history of sex chromosomes: see A. Martin, 'Can't Anybody Count? Counting as an Epistemic Theme in the History of Human Chromosomes', *Social Studies of Science*, 34 (2004), pp. 923–4, and S. Richardson, *Sex Itself: Male and Female in the Human Genome* (Chicago, IL: Chicago University Press, forthcoming). For most valuable histories of the field by cytogeneticists, see, among others, J. L. Hamerton, 'Human Population Cytogenetics: Dilemmas and Problems', *American Journal of Human Genetics*, 28 (1976), pp. 107–22; T.-C. Hsu, *Human and Mammalian Cytogenetics: An Historical Perspective* (New York: Springer, 1979); and, most recently, P. S. Harper, *First Years of Human Chromosomes: The Beginning of Human Cytogenetics* (Bloxham: Scion Publishing, 2006). Many of the aspects discussed in this essay will be further developed in a book that is in preparation.

2. On the more general link between the nuclear age and postwar genetics, see J. Beatty, 'Genetics in the Atomic Age: The Atomic Bomb Casualty Commission, 1947–1956', in B. Benson, J. Maienschein and R. Rainger (eds), *The Expansion of American Biology* (New Brunswick, NJ: Rutgers University Press, 1991), pp. 284–324; M. S. Lindee, *Suffering Made Real: American Science and the Survivors at Hiroshima* (Chicago, IL: Chicago University Press, 1994); and S. de Chadarevian, 'Mice and the Reactor: The "Genetic Experiment" in 1950s Britain', *Journal of the History of Biology*, 39 (2006), pp. 707–35.
3. J. H. Tjio and A. Levan, 'The Chromosome Number of Man', *Hereditas*, 42 (1956), pp. 1–6; C. E. Ford and J. L. Hamerton, 'The Chromosomes of Man', *Nature*, 178 (1956), pp. 1010–23. Challenges to the new chromosome count persisted for a few years, but by the late 1950s it was generally accepted that the normal number of human chromosomes was 46.
4. For details on Ford's career, see M. F. Lyon, 'Charles Edmund Ford, 24 October 1912–7 January 1999', *Biographical Memoirs of Fellows of the Royal Society*, 47 (2001), pp. 189–201.
5. Medical Research Council, *Hazards to Man of Nuclear and Allied Radiations* (London: HMSO, 1956), Cmd 9780; *The Biological Effects of Atomic Radiation: A Report to the Public* (Washington, DC: National Academy of Sciences-National Research Council, 1956).
6. In 1961 the *Lancet* published a letter signed by a group of geneticists calling for the abandonment of the term 'mongolism' from the medical vocabulary. With time the term Down (or Down's) syndrome prevailed in both medical and lay discourse; see A. Gordon et al., 'Mongolism (Correspondence)', *Lancet*, 277 (1961), p. 775; M. L. Rodríguez-Hernández and E. Montoya, 'Fifty Years of Evolution of the Term Down's Syndrome', *Lancet*, 378 (2011), p. 402.
7. D. G. Harnden, 'Early Studies on Human Chromosomes', *Bioessays*, 18 (1996), pp. 162–8, on p. 165.
8. C. E. Ford, K. W. Jones, P. E. Polani, J. C. Cabral de Almeida and J. H. Briggs, 'A Sex-Chromosome Anomaly in a Case of Gonadal Dysgenesis (Turner's Syndrome)', *Lancet*, 273 (1959), pp. 711–13.
9. On Polani's role in establishing the new field of clinical cytogenetics in Britain, see D. T. Zallen, 'Medical Genetics in Britain: Laying the Foundation (1940s–1960s)', in *Encyclopedia of Life Sciences* (Chichester: John Wiley and Sons, 2009), at http://www.els.net/WileyCDA/ElsArticle/refId-a0005603.html [accessed 25 May 2013].
10. P. A. Jacobs and J. A. Strong. 'A Case of Human Intersexuality Having a Possible XXY Sex-Determining Mechanism', *Nature*, 183 (1959), pp. 302–3. In 1959 Strong was appointed as an honorary physician at the same unit.
11. On the contested role of Marthe Gautier, including the misspelling of her name in the key publication, see M. Gautier and P. Harper, 'Fiftieth Anniversary of Trisonomy 21:

Returning to a Discovery', *Human Genetics*, 126 (2009), pp. 317–24. Before Lejeune became widely known for his work on trisonomy 21, he published various papers with Turpin on the mutational effect of radiation used for diagnostic effects in the clinic. The research was funded by the French Atomic Energy Commission and the French National Institute of Health. Their studies showed that women exposed to diagnostic X-ray produced less male offspring, which led the two researchers to warn of the risk of radiation. The research was ongoing when Lejeune, together with laboratory intern Gautier, who had some previous experience with cell culturing techniques, started the cytogenetic study of Down patients that set him on a new path. On the broader 'natalist' context of the work of the French group and the following tensions between geneticists and paediatricians in the diagnosis of childhood diseases in French hospitals, see J.-P. Gaudillière, 'Le Syndrome Nataliste: Étude de l'Hérédité, Pédiatrie et Eugénisme en France (1920–1960)', *Histoire de la Médecine et Des Sciences*, 13 (1997), pp. 1165–71; J.-P. Gaudillière, 'Whose Work Shall We Trust? Geneticists, Pediatrics, and Hereditary Diseases in Postwar France', in P. Sloan (ed.), *Controlling Our Destinies: Historical, Philosophical, Ethical, and Theological Perspectives on the Human Genome Project* (Notre Dame, IN: University of Notre Dame Press, 2000), pp. 17–46. In the 1970s Lejeune, then the director of the cytogenetics laboratory at the Hôpital Necker Enfants-Malades, would take a vocal anti-abortionist stance, distancing himself from many geneticists.

12. L. Penrose, 'Human Chromosomes', [marked up typescript for a lecture], 22 October 1959, p. 11; file 88/1, Penrose Papers, University College London Special Collections. Penrose is here most likely referring to the chromosome image of the Klinefelter Down patient that Ford produced on his suggestion. I thank Robert Bud for pointing out the historical connection to the Soviet moon mission to me.
13. L. Penrose to C. E. Ford, 25 July 1960; file 132/5, Penrose Papers, UCL Special Collections.
14. Penrose, 'Human Chromosomes', p. 5. In another lecture just a year later, Penrose included the new findings on the structure of DNA in his considerations on the future of human genetics, yet the decisive turning point was still marked by the fact that 'now we can see our own chromosomes ... and can sometimes make an exact diagnosis from them'. In the same lecture Penrose also noted that 'a chromosome contains many strands of DNA, possibly 64 or 128'. All quotes from 'Molecular Basis of Heredity', typescript for lecture at Medical Society of London, 11 January 1960; file 88/2, Penrose Papers, UCL Special Collections.
15. L. S. Penrose, 'Mongolism', talk presented at the 'Discussion on Human Chromosomes in Relation to Disease in Childhood' at the R.S.M.-Paediatrics Section, 27 May 1960 [typescript] p. 1; file 62/5, Penrose Papers, UCL Special Collections.
16. Penrose, 'Human Chromosomes', p. 11.
17. T. Puck, Why Low-Level Human Radiation Damage is Difficult to Assess, but Dangerous to Ignore, n.d.; uncatalogued file box, Theodore T. Puck Collection, University of Denver, Penrose Library Special Collections, Denver, CO. I thank Daniella Perry for pointing me to this document.
18. The observation of forty-six chromosomes in some cases of Down syndrome was explained with the translocation of the additional chromosomal material to another chromosome. On the first of a series of standardization conferences that convened in Denver in 1960, see Lindee, *Moments of Truth*, pp. 90–119. The agreement on a standard nomenclature for the human karyotype was a crucial step for the use of cytogenetics in the clinic and beyond.

19. P. A. Jacobs, A. G. Baikie, W. M. Court Brown, T. N. MacGregor and D. G. Harnden, 'Evidence for the Existence of the Human "Super Female"', *Lancet*, 274 (1959), pp. 423–5.
20. A. A. Sandberg, G. F. Koepf, T. Ishihara and T. S. Hauschka, 'An XYY Human Male', *Lancet*, 278 (1961), pp. 488–9.
21. Following the suggestion of the inactivation of the second X chromosome in female cells in 1961, the Barr bodies were interpreted as representing the inactivated and therefore condensed X chromosomes in cells. The hypothesis about the inactivation of the second X chromosome, also known as Lyon hypothesis (now Lyon law), was formulated by Mary Lyon while working on the genetics of radiation-induced mutations in mice at the MRC Radiobiological Research Unit at Harwell. Lyon headed the genetic section at Harwell from 1962 to 1987.
22. F. Miller, '"Your True and Proper Gender": The Barr Body as a *Good Enough* Science of Sex', *Studies in History and Philosophy of Science, Part C*, 37 (2006), pp. 459–83. See also N. Q. Ha, 'Marking Bodies: A History of Genetic Sex in the Twentieth Century' (PhD dissertation, Princeton University, 2011), ch. 4.
23. Note that an XYY chromosome set does not show up as unusual in the Barr body test. The first XYY case was unexpectedly found when the father of a Down syndrome child was karyotyped to establish a possible genetic link; see Sandberg et al., 'An XYY Human Male'. For the controversy that erupted around the XYY karyotype in the mid-1960s, see below.
24. J. Hood-Williams, 'Sexing the Athletes', *Sociology of Sports Journal*, 12 (1995), pp. 290–305, on p. 300.
25. P. A. Jacobs, M. Brunton, M. M. Melville, R. P. Brittain and W. F. McClemont, 'Aggressive Behavior, Mental Sub-Normality and the XYY Male', *Nature*, 208 (1965), pp. 1351–2.
26. Interview of the author with Patricia Jacobs, Salisbury, UK, 2 June 2010. Jacobs later expressed regret about the title, but she was far from the only researcher making the connection between Y chromosome and aggressive behaviour; see P. A. Jacobs, 'The William Allan Memorial Award Address: Human Population Cytogenetics: The First Twenty-Five Years', *American Journal of Human Genetics*, 34 (1982), pp. 689–98, on p. 695. For a critical analysis of the role of gender stereotypes in the interpretation of the function of sex chromosomes, including the 'super female' and the XYY male, see Richardson, *Sex Itself*. As Richardson points out, the interpretation of the sex chromosome anomalies ran against the usual interpretation that an additional chromosome produced instability of chromosome function rather than overperformance.
27. P. A. Jacobs, W. H. Price, S. Richmond and R. A. W. Ratcliff, 'Chromosome Surveys in Penal Institutions and Approved Schools', *Journal of Medical Genetics*, 8 (1971), pp. 49–58.
28. W. M. Court Brown, 'Males with an XYY Sex Chromosome Complement', *Journal of Medical Genetics*, 5 (1968), pp. 341–59.
29. See, for instance, R. D. Lyons, 'Genetic Abnormality is Linked to Crime; Genetics Linked to Violent Crimes', *New York Times*, 21 April 1968, p. 1. The front-page article in the *New York Times* was followed by two further articles in the following two days. For an analysis of the role of the media in the controversy, see J. Green, 'Media Sensationalisation and Science: The Case of the Criminal Chromosome', in T. Shinn and R. Whitley (eds), *Expository Science: Forms and Functions of Popularisation* (Dordrecht: Reidel Publishing Company, 1985), pp. 139–61.
30. See L. Miller, 'What Becomes of the XYY Men?', *Lancet*, 305 (1975), pp. 221–2. The consent protocols varied in each prospective study. For instance, in the Edinburgh study parents whose children were enrolled into the study were, at least initially, not informed

about the karyotype of their children, as this was seen to introduce a bias. However, researchers did inform the respective family doctors of the test results. Controls were included into the study. In contrast, in the prospective study set up at the Harvard Medical School in Boston, parents were informed about the test results, which in the eyes of critics rendered the studies not only damaging but useless. For a detailed response to the accusations by a geneticist involved in the prospective studies, see Hamerton, 'Human Population Cytogenetics'. For a review of the XYY debate, especially as it developed in the USA, see the Hastings Center, 'Special Supplement: The XYY Controversy: Researching Violence and Genetics', *Hastings Center Report*, 10:4 (1980), pp. 1–31.

31. Arthur Jensen's article that controversially defended a hereditarian standpoint in respect to race and IQ appeared in 1969: see A. Jensen, 'How Much Can We Boost IQ and School Achievement?', *Harvard Educational Review*, 39 (1969), pp. 1–123.
32. W. M. Court Brown, 'Sex Chromosomes and the Law', *Lancet*, 280 (1962), pp. 508–9.
33. K. Royce, *The XYY Man* (London: Hodder and Stoughton, 1970). The subsequent volumes of the series carried different titles, although they featured the same hero. The series was later adapted into a thirteen-part television show with the same title.
34. W. M. Court Brown, 'Contributions of Human Cytogenetics to Clinical Medicine', MRC 67/357 – CR 67/26, 16 March 1967, p. 2; FD 9/1281, National Archives, Kew, UK.
35. J. S. Weiner and J. A. Lourie, *Human Biology: A Guide to Field Methods. IBP Handbook No. 9*, 131–9 (Oxford and Edinburgh: Blackwell Scientific Publications, 1969); J. S. Weiner, *International Biological Programme: Guide to the Human Adaptability Proposals* (ICSU: Special Committee for the International Biological Programme, 1965), p. 12.
36. G. Glover, 'Chromosomal Stripy Socks' artwork, see http://ginaglover.com/html/work/gallery2002/gallery06/pages/01.html [accessed 12 February 2012]. The artwork is currently hanging in Guy's Hospital in London.

11 Friedman, 'The Disappearance of the Concept of Anticipation in the Post-War World'

1. L. Penrose, *Outline of Human Genetics* (London: Heinemann, 1959), p. 44.
2. C. Darwin, *The Origin of Species by Means of Natural Selection*, ed. and intro. J. W. Burrow (1859; London: Penguin Books, 1985), p. 76; F. Galton, *Hereditary Genius: An Inquiry into its Laws and Consequences*, 2nd edn repr. (London: Macmillan and Co. Ltd, 1914), pp. 320–1.
3. P. S. Harper, H. G. Harley, W. Reardon and D. J. Shaw, 'Anticipation in Myotonic Dystrophy: New Light on an Old Problem', *American Journal of Human Genetics*, 51:1 (1992), pp. 10–16; P. Harper, *A Short History of Medical Genetics* (Oxford: Oxford University Press, 2008), pp. 428–53.
4. C. J. Höweler, 'A Clinical and Genetic Study in Myotonic Dystrophy' (MD thesis, Erasmus University of Rotterdam, 1986), pp. 9–10.
5. G. R. Sutherland, E. A. Hann, E. Kremer, M. Lynch, M. Pritchard, S. Yu and R. I. Richards, 'Hereditary Unstable DNA: A New Explanation for Some Old Genetic Questions?', *Lancet*, 338:8762 (1991), pp. 289–92.
6. For a brief overview of the history of anticipation, see J. Friedman, 'Anticipation in Hereditary Disease: The History of a Biomedical Concept', *Human Genetics*, 130:6 (2011), pp. 705–14. A monograph on this topic is currently under preparation.

7. E. Nettleship, 'On Some Hereditary diseases of the Eye. Being the Bowman Lecture Delivered on Thursday, June 10th, 1909', *Transactions of the Royal Ophthalmological Society of the United Kingdom*, 29 (1909), pp. 52–198; F. W. Mott, 'A Lecture on Heredity and Insanity', *Lancet*, 117:4576 (1911), pp. 1251–9; E. Rüdin, *Studien über Vererbung und Entstehung geistiger Störungen, I: Zur Vererbung und Neuentstehung der Dementia praecox* (Berlin: Julius Springer, 1916), pp. 129–30; A. Gaule, 'Das Auftreten der Chorea Huntington in einer Familie der Nordostschweiz', *Schweizer Archiv für Neurologie und Psychiatrie*, 29 (1932), pp. 90–112; W. J. Adie and J. G. Greenfield, 'Dystrophia Myotonica (Myotonia Atrophica)', *Brain*, 46:1 (May 1923), pp. 73–127.
8. On theoretical arguments against anticipation, see, for example, K. Pearson, 'On an Apparent Fallacy in the Statistical Treatment of 'Antedating' in the Inheritance of Pathological Conditions', *Nature*, 90:2247 (1912), pp. 334–5; A. S. Paterson, '"Anticipation" in Mental Disease', *Eugenics Review*, 24:3 (1932), pp. 191–3; L. S. Penrose, *The Influence of Heredity in Disease: Buckston Browne Prize Essay, 1933* (London: H. K. Lewis and Co. Ltd, 1934), p. 17.
9. J. Bell, *The Treasury of Human Inheritance. Vol. 4, Nervous Diseases and Muscular Dystrophies, Part 4: On Pseudohypertrophic and Allied Types of Progressive Muscular Dystrophy*, ed. R. A. Fisher (Cambridge: Cambridge University Press, 1943), pp. 289–95; J. Bell, *The Treasury of Human Inheritance. Vol. 4, Nervous Diseases and Muscular Dystrophies, Part 5: Dystrophia Myotonica and Allied Diseases*, with clinical notes by J. Purdon Martin, ed. L. S. Penrose (Cambridge: Cambridge University Press, 1947), pp. 352–3.
10. Penrose, *Influence of Heredity*, pp. 6–7, 15–18.
11. Thomas F. Gieryn, 'Boundary Work and the Demarcation of Science from Non-Science: Strains and Interests in Professional Ideologies of Scientists', *American Sociological Review*, 48:6 (December 1983), pp. 781–95.
12. L. Penrose, 'The Problem of Anticipation in Pedigrees of Dystrophia Myotonica', *Annals of Eugenics*, 14 (1948), pp. 125–32.
13. Ibid., p. 128
14. Ibid.
15. In 1938 the German-born American developmental biologist Richard Goldschmidt had found a lone example of what seemed to be anticipation in a strain of fruit flies, which had a mutation in one locus that, dependent upon modification from other genetic factors, resulted in a range of damage to the wings from slight to severe; R. Goldschmidt, '"Progressive Heredity" and "Anticipation": The Possibility of a Genetic Explanation of Certain Odd Hereditary Phenomena Observed in Man', *Journal of Heredity*, 29:4 (April 1938), pp. 140–2. Penrose referred to Goldschmidt's treatment of the problem as 'obscure'; Penrose, 'Problem', p. 130.
16. Penrose, 'Problem', p. 129.
17. Ibid., p. 130.
18. Ibid., pp. 130–1.
19. Ibid., p. 131.
20. Höweler, 'Clinical and Genetic Study', pp. 14–23.
21. Chris Höweler, correspondence with Judith Friedman, 18 March 2004.
22. See N. Comfort, *The Science of Human Perfection: How Genes Became the Heart of American Medicine* (New Haven, CT: Yale University Press, 2012), p. xi; also D. Paul, *The Politics of Heredity: Essays on Eugenics, Biomedicine, and the Nature-Nurture Debate* (Albany, NY: State University of New York Press, 1998), pp. 133–56.
23. See J.-P. Gaudillière, 'Making Heredity in Mice and Men: The Production and Uses of Animal Models in Postwar Human Genetics', in J.-P. Gaudillière and I. Löwy (eds), *Heredity and Infection: The History of Disease Transmission* (London: Routledge, 2001), pp. 181–202, on p. 182; V. McKusick, 'The Growth and Development of Human Genetics as a Clinical Discipline', *American Journal of Human Genetics*, 27 (1975), pp. 264–9.

24. H. J. Muller, 'Progress and Prospects in Human Genetics', *American Journal of Human Genetics*, 1:1 (September 1949), pp. 1–2.
25. Muller, 'Progress and Prospects', pp. 2–3. Trofim Lysenko's genetic theories were based upon the inheritance of acquired characteristics. The controversy between Mendelian genetics (supported by the West) and Lysenkoism (supported in the Communist Bloc) became embroiled in the Cold War. See, for example, R. Selya, 'Defending Scientific Freedom and Democracy: The Genetics Society of America's Response to Lysenko', *Journal of the History of Biology*, 45:3 (August 2012), pp. 418–22.
26. Muller, 'Progress and Prospects', pp. 7–10, 12–14.
27. O. T. Avery, C. M. Macleod and M. McCarty, 'Studies on the Chemical Transformation of Pneumococcal Types', *Journal of Experimental Medicine*, 79 (1944), pp. 137–58; A. D. Hershey and M. Chase, 'Independent Functions of Viral Proteins and Nucleic Acid in Growth of Bacteriophage', *Journal of General Physiology*, 36 (1952), pp. 39–56; J. D. Watson and F. H. C. Crick, 'Molecular Structure of Nucleic Acids. A Structure for Deoxyribose Nucleic Acid', *Nature*, 171 (25 April 1953), pp. 737–8; J. D. Watson and F. H. C. Crick, 'Genetical Implications of the Structure of Deoxyribonucleic Acid', *Nature*, 171 (30 May 1953), pp. 964–7; F. H. C. Crick, 'On Protein Synthesis', *Symposia for the Society of Experimental Biology*, 12 (1958), pp. 138–63.
28. P. Abir-Am, 'The Rockefeller Foundation and the Rise of Molecular Biology', *Nature Reviews Molecular Cell Biology*, 3 (January 2002), pp. 65–70; S. de Chadarevian, *Designs for Life: Molecular Biology after World War II* (Cambridge: Cambridge University Press, 2002), pp. 33–43, 300–24; L. Kay, *The Molecular Vision of Life: Caltech, the Rockefeller Foundation, and the Rise of the New Biology* (New York: Oxford University, 1993), pp. 225–39, 269–77; D. Kevles, *In the Name of Eugenics: Genetics and the Uses of Human Heredity*, with a new preface (Cambridge, MA: Harvard University Press, 1995), pp. 212–50.
29. J. Sapp, *Beyond the Gene: Cytoplasmic Inheritance and the Struggle for Authority in Genetics* (New York: Oxford University Press, 1987), pp. 115–22.
30. Ibid., pp. 163–180; N. Krementsov, *Stalinist Science* (Princeton, NJ: Princeton University Press, 1997), pp. 169–83; W. deJong-Lambert and N. Krementsov, 'On Labels and Issues: The Lysenko Controversy and the Cold War', *Journal of the History of Biology*, 45:3 (August 2012), pp. 374–8.
31. J. Krige, *American Hegemony and the Postwar Reconstruction of Science in Europe* (Cambridge, MA: MIT Press, 2006), pp. 115–51.
32. Sapp, *Beyond the Gene*, pp. 121–2, 202–3, 231–3.
33. Penrose to Morison, 3 May 1946, folder 233, box 16, series 401a, RG 1.1, Rockefeller Foundation Archives, Rockefeller Archive Center, Sleepy Hollow, New York, USA (hereafter RAC).
34. H. Harris, 'Lionel Sharples Penrose 1898–1972 Elected F.R.S. 1953', *Biographical Memoirs of Fellows of the Royal Society*, 19 (1973), pp. 537–8.
35. Muller, 'Progress and Prospects', p. 7.
36. J. B. S Haldane to the Provost University College London, 9 August 1944, Penrose Papers, 49/1, University College London Library Special Collections, University College London, London, England (hereafter UCL Special Collections); quotation from J. B. S. Haldane to the Principal, Ruskin College, Oxford, 12 March 1953, Haldane Papers, 5/1/4/115, UCL Special Collections.
37. Funding Motion RF 46085, 21 June 1946, folder 222, box 16, series 401a, RG 1.1, Rockefeller Foundation Archives, RAC; Funding Motion RF 50315, 22 September 1950,

folder 222, box 16, series 401a, RG 1.1, Rockefeller Foundation Archives, RAC; Funding Motion RF 55078, 20 May 1955, folder 222, box 16, series 401a, RG 1.1, Rockefeller Foundation Archives, RAC; Funding Motion RF 60160, 23 September 1960, folder 222, box 16, series 401a, RG 1.1, Rockefeller Foundation Archives, RAC.

38. Book with the names and addresses of Voluntary Workers at the Galton Laboratory, 1933–66; address book of visitors and workers in the Galton Laboratory, 1945–59; typed list of postgraduate workers in the Galton Laboratory, 1945–65, Penrose Papers, 49/2, UCL Special Collections.
39. T. Kuhn, *The Structure of Scientific Revolutions*, 2nd edn, enlarged (Chicago, IL: University of Chicago Press, 1970), p. 10.
40. For example, the English translation of the influential German textbook by E. Baur, E. Fisher and F. Lenz discussed anticipation as an 'illusion' while noting that it had been seen in a variety of diseases. R. R. Gates likewise noted that anticipation was often seen by physicians and that while many believed these findings to be false, he did not entirely dismiss them. E. Baur, E. Fisher, F. Lenz, *Human Heredity*, trans. E. Paul and C. Paul (London: George Allen and Unwin Ltd, 1931), pp. 243–4, 354–6, 418–21; R. R. Gates, *Human Genetics*, Vol. 1 (New York: The Macmillan Company, 1946), pp. 32–3, 202, 224, 265–6, 546–50.
41. J. Neel, 'Curt Stern 1902–1981', *Annual Review of Genetics*, 17:1 (December 1983), pp. 1–4.
42. C. Stern, *Principles of Human Genetics* (San Francisco, CA: Freeman and Co., 1949), p. viii.
43. Lionel Penrose, London, ON to Curt Stern, Rochester, NY, 16 January 1941, Curt Stern Papers, American Philosophical Society, Philadelphia, Pennsylvania, USA.
44. Curt Stern to Margaret Penrose, Radlett, England, 30 June 1972, Curt Stern Papers, American Philosophical Society, Philadelphia, Pennsylvania, USA.
45. Stern, *Principles*, p. 297.
46. Ibid., pp. 298–9.
47. E. Passarge, *Color Atlas of Genetics*, 2nd edn, rev. and enlarged (New York: Thieme, 2001), p. 8.
48. Neel, 'Curt Stern', p. 7.
49. Oral History Interview with Victor McKusick, 10–11 December 2001 (Ms. Coll. No. 316), Oral History of Human Genetics Collection, History and Special Collections Division, Louise M. Darling Biomedical Library, University of California, Los Angeles.
50. See, for example, A. G. Steinberg and R. M. Wilder, 'A Reconsideration of the Phenomenon of Anticipation in Diabetes Mellitus', *Proceedings of the Staff Meetings of the Mayo Clinic*, 25:23 (8 November 1950), pp. 625–30.
51. The two researchers were the German-born Swiss physician and medical geneticist David Klein and the New Zealand neurologist J. E. Caughey. Caughey's assertion that women with myotonic dystrophy were likely to have children with early onset of disease significantly precedes the 1972 paper by Harper and Dyken, which is usually seen as the one that established the maternal transmission of the congenital form of myotonic dystrophy. J. E. Caughey and J. Barclay, 'Dystrophia Myotonica and the Occurrence of Congenital Physical Defect in Affected Families', *Australasian Annals of Medicine*, 3:3 (August 1954), pp. 165–70; P. S. Harper and Paul R. Dyken, 'Early Onset Dystrophia Myotonica – Evidence Supporting a Maternal Environmental Factor', *Lancet*, 300:7767 (8 July 1972), pp. 53–5.
52. F. Clifford Rose, 'Lord Walton of Detchant', *Postgraduate Medical Journal*, 68:801 (July 1992), p. 497.

53. J. Walton, *The Spice of Life: From Northumbria to World Neurology* (London: Royal Society of Medicine Services Ltd, 1993), p. 176.
54. Ibid.
55. J. Walton, 'On the Inheritance of Muscular Dystrophy', *Annals of Human Genetics*, 20:1 (September 1955), pp. 1–13.
56. John Walton, correspondence with Judith Friedman, 18 February 2011.
57. Walton, 'On the Inheritance'; J. Walton, 'The Inheritance of Muscular Dystrophy: Further Observations', *Annals of Human Genetics*, 21:1 (September 1956), pp. 40–58.

12 Pemberton, '"The Most Hereditary of All Diseases": Haemophilia and the Utility of Genetics for Haematology, 1930–70'

1. N. Comfort, *The Science of Human Perfection: How Genes Became the Heart of American Medicine* (New Haven, CT: Yale University Press, 2012), p. 198.
2. Ibid., pp. x and 244. An instructive counterpoint to Comfort's interpretation can be found in R. S. Cowan, *Heredity and Hope: The Case for Genetic Screening* (Cambridge, MA: Harvard University Press, 2008).
3. P. S. Harper, *A Short History of Medical Genetics* (Oxford: Oxford University Press, 2008), p. 4. See also S. Lindee, *Moments in Truth in Genetic Medicine* (Baltimore, MD: Johns Hopkins University Press, 2005), and C. López-Beltrán, 'The Medical Origins of Heredity', in S. Müller-Wille and H. J. Rheinberger (eds), *Heredity Produced: At the Crossroads of Biology, Politics, and Culture, 1500–1870* (Cambridge, MA: MIT Press, 2007), pp. 105–32.
4. Harper, *Short History of Medical Genetics*, p. 4.
5. Ludwig Grandidier (1810–78), a spa doctor in Nenndorf, first labelled haemophilia 'the most hereditary of all diseases' in *Die Haemophilie oder die Bluterkrankheit, nach eigenen und fremden Beobachtungen monographisch bearbeitet* (Leipzig: Otto Wigand, 1855).
6. The word 'haematologist' is utilized throughout this essay to describe physicians from various specialties (especially, pathology and internal medicine) who took a concerted interest in understanding blood's role in health and illness and/or in treating blood-related disorders. Such usage might seem anachronistic because specialty examinations in haematology only emerged in North America in the early 1970s. However, as shown by Keith Wailoo, enthusiasm for haematology took root within organized medicine in the early 1900s and played a major role in shaping hospital practice as well as the identities of various specialties and diseases over the course of the century. See K. Wailoo, *Drawing Blood: Technology and Disease Identity in Twentieth-Century America* (Baltimore, MD: Johns Hopkins University Press, 1997), pp. 1–16, 188–200.
7. See S. Pemberton, *The Bleeding Disease: Hemophilia and the Unintended Consequences of Medical Progress* (Baltimore, MD: Johns Hopkins University Press, 2011), pp. 20–5.
8. J. C. Otto, 'An Account of an Hemorrhagic Disposition Existing in Certain Families', *Medical Repository*, 6 (1803), p. 1.
9. Aside from Otto, John Hay, an American physician, is widely credited in the Anglophone literature with the first accurate description of the sex-linked inheritance in haemophilia in 1813; see J. Hay, 'Account of a Remarkable Hemorrhagic Disposition Existing in Many Individuals of the Same Family', *New England Journal of Medicine and Surgery*, 2 (1813), pp. 221–5, and V. McKusick, 'Hemophilia in Early New England: A

Follow-Up of Four Kindreds in which Hemophilia Occurred in the Pre-Revolutionary Period', *Journal of the History of Medicine and Allied Sciences*, 17 (1962), pp. 342–65.

10. J. W. Legg, *Treatise on Haemophilia, Sometimes Called the Hereditary Haemorrhagic Diathesis* (London: H. K. Lewis, 1872), p. 30.
11. See Pemberton, *The Bleeding Disease*, pp. 25–31.
12. Christian Friedrich Nasse's seminal work on haemophilia is 'Von einer erblichen Neigung zu tödtlichen Blutungen', *Archiv für medizinische Erfahrung im Gebiete der praktischen Medizin und Staatsarzneikunde, hrsg. von Horn, Nasse und Henke* (Berlin: Mai-Juni, 1820), pp. 385–434, on p. 385. See O. Ratnoff, 'Why Do People Bleed?' in M. Wintrobe (ed.), *Blood, Pure and Eloquent* (New York: McGraw-Hill, 1980), pp. 600–57, on p. 626, and A. Rushton, *Genetics and Medicine in the United States, 1800–1922* (Baltimore, MD: Johns Hopkins University Press, 1994), p. 7.
13. Pemberton, *The Bleeding Disease*, pp. 54–5.
14. The medical literature was quite mixed on the question of whether haemophilic males could be 'transmitters' before the rise of Mendelism; see, for example, W. Bulloch and P. Fildes, 'Haemophilia', in K. Pearson (ed.), *Treasury of Human Inheritance*, Vol. 1 (London: Cambridge University Press, 1912), pp. 169–354, on pp. 185, 267–71; R. R. Gates, *Heredity in Man* (London: Constable, 1929), p. 205; and C. B. Kerr, 'The Fortunes of Haemophiliacs in the Nineteenth Century', *Medical History*, 7 (1963), pp. 359–70.
15. Bulloch and Fildes, 'Haemophilia', pp. 169, 174–6; occasionally referenced as *Eugenics Laboratory Memoirs XII, Francis Galton Laboratory for National Eugenics, University of London* (London: Dulau, 1911), pts V and VI, sec. XIVa.
16. Bulloch and Fildes, 'Haemophilia', pp. 177–81, esp. 179.
17. Ibid., pp. 184–6.
18. The author thanks Peter Harper for identifying Karl Pearson's directive to Bulloch and Fildes to refrain from engaging Mendelism in their contribution to *The Treasury of Human Inheritance*.
19. V. McKusick, *Human Genetics, Second Edition* (Englewood Cliffs, NJ: Prentice-Hall, 1969), pp. 55–7.
20. Pemberton, *The Bleeding Disease*, pp. 37–47, 84–6.
21. W. H. Howell, 'The Condition of the Blood in Hemophilia, Thrombosis, and Purpura', *Archives of Internal Medicine*, 13 (January 1914), pp. 76–95, on p. 89.
22. C. A. Mills, 'The Transmission of Hemophilia', *Journal of the American Medical Association*, 94 (17 May 1930), pp. 1571–2.
23. See, for example, P. Clough, 'Hemophilia', in *Diseases of the Blood* (New York: Harper and Brothers Publishers, 1929), p. 236, and Pemberton, *The Bleeding Disease*, pp. 81–3 and 86.
24. The diagnostic criteria can be found in H. Joules and R. G. Macfarlane, 'Pseudo-Haemophilia in a Woman', *Lancet*, 1 (26 March 1938), pp. 715–18.
25. See J. B. S. Haldane, 'The Rate of Spontaneous Mutation of a Human Gene', *Journal of Genetics*, 31 (1935), pp. 317–26, and D. Kevles, *In the Name of Eugenics: Genetics and the Uses of Human Heredity* (Cambridge, MA: Harvard University Press, 1995), pp. 204–5.
26. C. Birch, 'Hemophilia', *Proceedings of the Society for Experimental Biology and Medicine*, 28 (April 1931), pp. 752–3.
27. R. G. Macfarlane, 'Russell's Viper Venom, 1934–64', *British Journal of Haematology*, 13 (1967), pp. 437–51, quote on p. 439.
28. Birch, 'Hemophilia', *Proceedings*, pp. 752–3.

29. 'Successfully Treats Two for Hemophilia: Chicago Woman Doctor Arrests Inherent Bleeding by Use of Ovarian Extract', *New York Times*, 15 March 1931, p. A15. See also 'Ovaries for Bleeders', *Time*, 18 (13 July 1931), p. 45.
30. C. Birch, 'Hemophilia and the Female Sex Hormone', *JAMA*, 97 (31 July 1931), p. 244.
31. C. Birch, 'Hemophilia', *JAMA*, 99 (5 November 1932), pp. 1566–72, quote on p. 1571.
32. See R. Brown and F. Albright, 'Estrin Therapy in a Case of Hemophilia', *New England Journal of Medicine*, 209 (28 September 1933), pp. 630–2; J. Brem and J. Leopold, 'Ovarian Therapy: Relationship of the Female Sex Hormone to Hemophilia', *JAMA*, 102 (20 January 1934), pp. 200–2; and R. Stetson, C. Forkner, W. Chew and M. Rich, 'Negative Effect of Prolonged Administration of Ovarian Substances in Hemophilia', *JAMA*, 102 (7 April 1934), pp. 1122–6.
33. See C. Birch, *Hemophilia: Clinical and Genetic Aspects* (Urbana, IL: University of Illinois Press, 1937), p. 38.
34. The biological phenomenon that Birch was trying to account for in clinical terms would be given a satisfying genetic explanation in the 1960s following the work of England's Mary Lyon and others. According to the Lyon hypothesis, all X chromosomes in excess of one are deactivated at an early stage of embryogenesis, and this hypothesis allowed haemophilia researchers to account for the fact that female carriers of haemophilia (X^hX) typically have normal clotting times. See McKusick, *Human Genetics, Second Edition*, pp. 6, 20, 103–5, 204.
35. S. Resnik, *Blood Saga: Hemophilia, AIDS, and the Survival of a Community* (Berkeley, CA: University of California Press, 1999), and Pemberton, *The Bleeding Disease.*
36. See Birch, *Hemophilia: Clinical and Genetic Aspects*, p. 40; M. Warde, 'Haemophilia in the Female', *British Medical Journal*, 2 (6 October 1923), p. 599–600; M. T. Macklin, 'Heredity in Hemophilia', *American Journal of the Medical Sciences*, 175 (February 1928), pp. 218–223, on p. 222; and Gates, *Heredity in Man*, pp. 207–8.
37. K. M. Brinkhous and J. B. Graham, 'Occurrence of Hemophilia in Females', *Journal of Laboratory and Clinical Medicine*, 34 (1949), pp. 1587–8, and K. M. Brinkhous and J. B. Graham, 'Hemophilia in the Female Dog', *Science*, 111 (30 June 1950), pp. 723–4.
38. M. C. Isreales, H. Lempert, and E. Gilbertson, 'Haemophilia in the Female', *Lancet*, 1 (1951), p. 1375, and C. Merskey, 'The Occurrence of Haemophilia in the Human Female', *Quarterly Journal of Medicine*, 20 (1951), pp. 299–312, on p. 299. There was also a debate as to whether female 'carriers' manifested detectable symptoms of a bleeding disorder. See C. Merskey and R. G. Macfarlane, 'The Female Carrier of Haemophilia', *Lancet*, 1 (1951), pp. 487–90, on p. 487, and A. Margolius and O. Ratnoff, 'A Laboratory Study of the Carrier State in Classic Hemophilia', *Journal of Clinical Investigation*, 35 (1956), pp. 1316–23.
39. S. Pemberton, 'Canine Technologies, Model Patients: The Historical Production of Hemophiliac Dogs in American Biomedicine', in S. Schrepfer and P. Scranton (eds), *Industrializing Organisms: Introducing Evolutionary History* (New York: Routledge, 2004), pp. 191–214.
40. Ibid.
41. See J. N. Lozier and K. M. Brinkhous, 'Gene Therapy and the Hemophilias', *JAMA*, 271 (1994), pp. 47–51.
42. J. B. Graham, *How It Was: Pathology at UNC 1896–1973* (Chapel Hill, NC: University of North Carolina Press, 1996), p. 163
43. See, for example, J. B. Graham, 'Biochemical Genetics of Blood Coagulation', *American Journal of Human Genetics*, 8 (June 1956), pp. 63–79; J. B. Graham, 'Genetic Problems:

Hemophilia and Allied Diseases', in K. Brinkhous (ed.), *Hemophilia and Hemophiliod Diseases: International Symposium* (Chapel Hill, NC: University of North Carolina, 1957), pp. 137–62; and J. B. Graham, 'The Inheritance of "Vascular Hemophilia": A New and Interesting Problem in Human Genetics', *Journal of Human Genetics*, 11 (1959), pp. 385–96.

44. P. M. Aggeler, S. G. White, M. B. Glendenning et al., 'Plasma Thromboplastin Component (P.T.C.) Deficiency: A New Disease Resembling Hemophilia', *Proceedings of the Society of Experimental Biology and Medicine*, 79 (1952), pp. 692–4; I. Schulman and C. H. Smith, 'Hemorrhagic Disease in an Infant Due to Deficiency of a Previously Undescribed Clotting Factor', *Blood*, 7 (1952), pp. 794–807; and R. Biggs, A. S. Douglas, R. G. Macfarlane et al., 'Christmas Disease: A Condition Previously Mistaken for Haemophilia', *British Medical Journal*, 2 (1952), pp. 1378–82.
45. W. Dameshek, 'Introduction to Symposium: What is Hemophilia?', *Blood*, 9 (March 1954), pp. 244–5.
46. See R. Biggs and R. G. Macfarlane, *Human Blood Coagulation and its Disorders* (Springfield, IL: Charles C. Thomas, 1953, 1st edn; 1957, 2nd edn). Nearly four hundred articles on blood coagulation appeared in the 1949–50 academic year (1st edn, p. 3), and over six hundred appeared in the 1953–4 academic year (2nd edn, p. 3). Citations on blood clotting and related subjects from the *Index Medicus* for 1945–5 corroborate this claim.
47. Compare M. Stefanini's 'Hemophilia: Specific Entity or Syndrome?', *Blood*, 9 (1954), pp. 273–80, L. Tocantins's 'Hemophilic Syndromes and Hemophilia', *Blood*, 9 (1954), pp. 281–5, and F. Koller's 'Is Hemophilia a Nosologic Entity?', *Blood*, 9 (1954), pp. 286–90, to R. G. Macfarlane's 'Hemophilia, Christmas Disease, and Matters of Terminology', *Blood*, 9 (1954), pp. 258–64, and K. Brinkhous and J. B. Graham, 'Hemophilia and the Hemophiliod States', *Blood*, 9 (1954), pp. 254–64, 273–80, 281–90.
48. See Pemberton, *The Bleeding Disease*, pp. 89–90 and 104–5.
49. Resnik, *Blood Saga*, pp. 20–5, and Pemberton, *The Bleeding Disease*, pp. 91–2.
50. See S. Dietrich, *Hemophilia: A Total Approach to Treatment and Rehabilitation* (Los Angeles, CA: Orthopaedic Hospital, 1968).

13 Paul, 'How PKU Became a Genetic Disease'

1. J.-P. Gaudillière, 'Bettering Babies: Down's Syndrome, Heredity and Public Health in Post-War France and Britain', in I. Löwy and J. Krige (eds), *Images of Disease: Science, Public Policy and Health in Post-War Europe* (Luxembourg: European Community, 2001), pp. 89–108.
2. K. Wailoo and S. Pemberton, *The Troubled Dream of Genetic Medicine: Ethnicity and Innovation in Tay-Sachs, Cystic Fibrosis, and Sickle Cell Disease* (Baltimore, MD: Johns Hopkins University Press, 2006), p. 74.
3. This history is told in greater detail in D. B. Paul and J. P. Brosco, *The PKU Paradox: A Short History of a Genetic Disease* (Baltimore, MD: Johns Hopkins University Press, 2013).
4. V. E. Schuett, *Low Protein Food List for PKU*, 3rd edn (CreateSpace, 2010). The section 'Fruits and Vegetables' is on pp. 45–65, and 'Grain Products' on pp. 147–61.
5. A. MacDonald, H. Gokmen-Ozel, M. van Rijn and P. Burgard, 'The Reality of Dietary Compliance in the Management of Phenylketonuria', *Journal of Inherited Metabolic Disorders*, 33 (2010), pp. 665–70.

6. On average, children treated early and continuously have IQ scores in the normal range but below those of the general population or their siblings. Adults often experience social and emotional difficulties, generalized anxiety, phobias and social isolation. See G. M. Enns, R. Koch, V. Brumm, E. Blakely, R. Suter and E. Jurecki, 'Suboptimal Outcomes in Patients with PKU Treated Early with Diet Alone: Revisiting the Evidence', *Molecular Genetics and Metabolism*, 101 (2010), pp. 99–109; S. E. Waisbren, 'Phenylketonuria', in S. Goldstein and C. R. Reynolds (eds), *Handbook of Neurodevelopmental and Genetic Disorders in Children*, 2nd edn (New York: Guildford Press, 2011), pp. 398–424, on pp. 404–9.
7. J. S. Alper and M. R. Natowicz, 'On Establishing the Genetic Basis of Mental Disease', *Trends in Neurosciences*, 16 (1993), pp. 387–9.
8. C. R. Scriver, 'The PAH Gene, Phenylketonuria, and a Paradigm Shift', *Human Mutation*, 28:9 (2007), pp. 831–45.
9. A. J. Clarke, 'Newborn Screening', in P. S. Harper and A. J. Clarke (eds), *Genetics, Society, and Clinical Practice* (Oxford: Bios Scientific Publishers, 1997), pp. 107–17, on p. 107.
10. Committee for the Study of Inborn Errors of Metabolism, National Research Council, *Genetic Screening: Programs, Principles, and Research* (Washington, DC: National Academy of Sciences, 1975), pp. 51, 92, quotation on p. 92.
11. Ibid., p. 44.
12. On the rDNA controversy, see: S. Wright, *Molecular Politics: Developing American and British Regulatory Policy for Genetic Engineering, 1972–1982* (Chicago, IL: University of Chicago Press, 1994); H. Gottweis, *Governing Molecules: The Discursive Politics of Genetic Engineering in Europe and the United States* (Cambridge, MA: MIT Press, 1998); D. S. Frederickson, *The Recombinant DNA Controversy: A Memoir* (Herndon, VA: ASM Press, 2001); M. J. Peterson, 'Asilomar Conference on Laboratory Precautions', *International Dimensions of Ethics Education in Science and Engineering* (2010), at www.umass.edu/sts/ethics/asilomar.html [accessed 5 July 2013].
13. The comment is from Richard Nixon's statement on signing the bill, at http://www.presidency.ucsb.edu/ws/index.php?pid=3413#axzz1UYYbiwS8 [accessed 5 July 2013]. See R. S. Cowan, *Heredity and Hope: The Case for Genetic Screening* (Cambridge, MA: Harvard University Press, 2008), pp. 175–8.
14. Committee for the Study of Inborn Errors, *Genetic Screening*, p. 195.
15. For an expanded version of this argument, see D. B. Paul, 'What Is a Genetic Test and Why Does It Matter?' *Endeavour*, 23 (1999), pp. 159–61.
16. N. A. Holtzman, 'Anatomy of a Trial', *Pediatrics*, 60 (1977), pp. 932–4.
17. A. Jensen, 'How Much Can We Boost IQ and Scholastic Achievement?', *Harvard Educational Review*, 39 (1969), pp. 1–123.
18. R. J. Herrnstein, 'I.Q.', *Atlantic*, 228 (1971), pp. 63–4; R. J. Herrnstein, *I.Q. in the Meritocracy* (Boston, MA: Little Brown, 1973).
19. L. Kamin, *The Science and Politics of IQ* (Potomac, MD: Lawrence Erlbaum, 1974), p. 1.
20. N. J. Block and G. Dworkin, 'IQ, Heritability, and Inequality', in N. J. Block and G. Dworkin (eds), *The IQ Controversy* (New York: Pantheon, 1976), pp. 410–542, on p. 489; see also S. Rose, 'Environmental Effects on Brain and Behaviour', in K. Richardson, D. Spears and M. Richards (eds), *Race, Culture and Intelligence* (Baltimore, MD: Penguin, 1972), pp. 128–44, on p. 135.
21. P. Kitcher, *Vaulting Ambition: Sociobiology and the Quest for Human Nature* (Cambridge, MA: MIT Press, 1985), p. 128.
22. R. Wright, 'Dumb Bell', *New Republic*, 2 January 1995, p. 6.

23. L. Hood, The Book of Life', Commencement Address, Whitman College, 19 May 2002, at http://www.systemsbiology.org/download/whitman.pdf [accessed 4 September 2011].
24. W. Gilbert, 'A Vision of the Grail', in D. J. Kevles and L. Hood (eds), *The Code of Codes: Scientific and Social Issues in the Human Genome Project* (Cambridge, MA: Harvard University Press, 1992), pp. 83–97, on p. 94.
25. L. Hood, 'Biology and Medicine in the Twenty-First Century', D. J. Kevles and L. Hood (eds), *The Code of Codes: Scientific and Social Issues in the Human Genome Project* (Cambridge, MA: Harvard University Press, 1992), pp. 112–63, on p. 138.
26. J. D. Watson, 'A Personal View of the Project', D. J. Kevles and L. Hood (eds), *The Code of Codes: Scientific and Social Issues in the Human Genome Project* (Cambridge, MA: Harvard University Press, 1992), pp. 164–73, on p. 167.
27. C. DiLisi, 'Meetings that Changed the World: Santa Fe 1986: Human Genome Baby-Steps', *Nature*, 455 (16 October 2008), pp. 876–7. See also R. Cook-Deegan, *The Gene Wars: Science, Politics, and the Human Genome* (New York: W. W. Norton, 1994), V. K. McElheny, *Drawing the Map of Life: Inside the Human Genome Project* (New York: Basic Books, 2010).
28. R. C. Lewontin, 'The Dream of the Human Genome', *New York Review of Books*, 39:10 (1992), pp. 31–40.
29. H. N. Kirkman, 'Projections of a Rebound in Frequency of Mental Retardation from Phenylketonuria', *Applied Research in Mental Retardation*, 3 (1982), pp. 319–28, on p. 326.
30. Transcript, 'Talk of the Nation' programme, NPR, 15 November 1996. Host: Ira Flatow.
31. Transcript, Noah Adams interview with Francis Collins, 'All Things Considered', NPR, 2 December 1999.
32. D. L. Hartl and E. W. Jones, *Genetics: Analysis of Genes and Genomes*, 7th edn (Sudbury, MA: Jones and Bartlett, 2008), p. 2.
33. J. J. Mitchell, 'Phenylalanine Hydroxylase Deficiency', *Gene Reviews* , at www.ncbi.nlm.nih.gov/books/NBK1504 [last updated 31 January 2013; accessed 5 July 2013].
34. On numbers of types of mutations at the PAH locus, see M. Phommarnih and C. R. Scriver, 'Phenylalanine Hydroxylase Mutation Map (revised Jan. 8, 2007)', PAH db Phenylalanine Hydroxylase Locus Knowledgebase, at http://www.pahdb.mcgill.ca/Information/MutationMap/mutationmap.pdf [accessed 20 June 2012].
35. S. Kaufman, *Overcoming a Bad Gene* (Bloomington, IN: AuthorHouse, 2004), pp. 77–9.
36. D. Nelkin and L. Tancredi, *Dangerous Diagnostics: The Social Power of Biological Information* (Chicago, IL: University of Chicago Press, 1994), pp. 41–2.
37. J. Phelan, *What Is Life? A Guide to Biology with Physiology* (New York: W. H. Freeman, 2011), p. 273.

14 Cottebrune, 'The Emergence of Genetic Counselling in the Federal Republic of Germany: Continuity and Change in the Narratives of Human Geneticists, *c.* 1968–80'

1. For example, S. Kühl, *The Nazi Connection: Eugenics, American Racism, and German National Socialism* (New York: Oxford University Press, 1994); H. P. Kröner, *Von der Rassenhygiene zur Humangenetik: Das Kaiser-Wilhelm-Institut für Anthropologie, menschliche Erblehre und Eugenik nach dem Zweiten Weltkrieg* (Paderborn: G. Fischer,

1998); D. Hahn, *Modernisierung und Biopolitik: Sterilisation und Schwangerschaftsabbruch in Deutschland nach 1945* (Frankfurt: Campus, 2000); R. v. Bruch and B. Kaderas (eds), *Wissenschaften und Wissenschaftspolitik: Bestandsaufnahmen zu Formationen, Brüchen und Kontinuitäten im Deutschland des 20. Jahrhunderts* (Stuttgart: Steiner, 2002); R. Mackensen and J. Reulecke (eds), *Das Konstrukt 'Bevölkerung' vor, im und nach dem 'Dritten Reich'* (Wiesbaden: VS Verlag für Sozialwissenschafte, 2005); J. Ehmer, U. Ferdinand and J. Reulecke (eds), *Herausforderung Bevölkerung: Zu Entwicklungen des modernen Denkens über die Bevölkerung vor, im und nach dem "Dritten Reich"* (Wiesbaden: VS Verlag für Sozialwissenschafte, 2007); R. Wecker, S. Braunschweig and G. Imboden (eds), *Wie nationalsozialistisch ist die Eugenik? Internationale Debatten zur Geschichte der Eugenik im 20. Jahrhundert* (Wien: Böhlau, 2009); R. Argast and P.-A. Rosenthal (eds), *Eugenics after 1945*, *Journal of Modern European History*, 10:4 (2012).

2. P. Weingart, J. Kroll and K. Bayertz, *Rasse, Blut und Gene: Geschichte der Eugenik und Rassenhygiene in Deutschland* (Frankfurt: Suhrkamp, 1992), p. 664; J. Habermas, *Die Zukunft der menschlichen Natur: Auf dem Weg zu einer liberalen Eugenik?* (Frankfurt: Suhrkamp, 2005); T. Lemke, 'Zurück in die Zukunft? – Genetische Diagnostik und das Risiko der Eugenik', in S. Graumann (ed.), *Die Gen-Kontroverse* (Freiburg: Herder, 2001), pp. 37–44; T. Lemke, *Gouvernementalität und Biopolitik* (Wiesbaden: VS Verlag für Sozialwissenschafte, 2008); K. Lange, *Was ist neu an der neuen Eugenik: Eine kritische Analyse am Beispiel der Pränataldiagnostik und der Präimplantationsdiagnostik* (Erfurt: GRIN Verlag, 2005).
3. A. Waldschmidt, *Das Subjekt in der Humangenetik* (Münster: Westfälisches Dampfboot, 1996); A. Bogner, *Grenzpolitik der Experten. Vom Umgang mit Ungewissenheit und Nichtwissen in pränataler Diagnostik und Beratung* (Birkach: Velbrück Verlag, 2005); Hahn, *Modernisierung*; S. Samerski, *Die verrechnete Hoffnung. Von der selbstbestimmten Entscheidung durch genetische Beratung* (Münster: Westfälisches Dampfboot, 2002).
4. M. Reif and H. Baitsch, *Genetische Beratung. Hilfestellung für eine selbstverantwortliche Entscheidung?* (Berlin: Springer, 1986).
5. Waldschmidt, *Subjekt*; Bogner, *Grenzpolitik*; Hahn, *Modernisierung*; E. Beck-Gernsheim, 'Gesundheit und Verantwortung im Zeitalter der Gentechnologie', in E. Beck-Gernsheim and U. Beck (eds), *Riskante Freiheiten: Individualisierung in modernen Gesellschaften* (Frankfurt: Suhrkamp, 1994), pp. 316–35; A. Lösch, *Tod des Menschen – Macht zum Leben. Von der Rassenhygiene zur Humangenetik* (Pfaffenweiler: Centaurus, 1998); C. Althaus and C. Knobloch, 'Zur Debatte über die Selbstoptimierung des Menschen', *Sozialwissenschaftliche Informationen*, 31 (2002), pp. 4–11; J. Reyer, 'Ellen Key und die eugenische "Verbesserung" des Kindes im 20. Jahrhundert: Von der autoritären zur liberalen Eugenik?', in W. Bergsdorf et al. (eds), *Herausforderungen der Bildungsgesellschaft: 15 Vorlesungen* (Weimar: Rhino-Verlag, 2002), pp. 59–88; M. Wolf, *Eugenische Vernunft. Eingriffe in die in die reproduktive Kultur durch die Medizin 1900–2000* (Wien: Böhlau, 2008).
6. S. C. Reed, 'A Short History of Genetic Counselling', *Social Biology*, 21 (1974), pp. 332–9, on p. 335.
7. Ibid. In 1951 there were already ten genetic counselling centres in the United States.
8. G. Terrenoire, 'L'évolution du conseil génétique aux Etats-Unis de 1940 à 1980: Pratique et légitimation', *Sciences sociales et santé*, 4:3–4 (1986), pp. 51–79, particularly on p. 68.
9. In 1974 the International Directory of Genetic Services already listed 387 centres in the United States; ibid., p. 69.
10. Reed, *Short History*, p. 337.

11. In 1955 there were four centres of genetic counselling in the UK, one in Leeds, the other three in London. See O. Lahmann, 'Genetische Beratung und pränatale genetische Diagnostik in der Bundesrepublik Deutschland, in Großbritannien und in den Vereinigten Staaten. Eine vergleichende Studie' (MD dissertation, Marburg University, 1982).
12. WHO, 'Genetic Counselling. Third Report of the WHO Expert Committee on Human Genetics', Technical Report Series, 416 (1969), p. 13, at http://apps.who.int/iris/handle/10665/40725 [accessed 18 July 2013].
13. Ibid.
14. T. Schlich and U. Tröhler (eds), *The Risks of Medical Innovation: Risk Perception and Assessment in Historical Context* (London: Routledge, 2006), pp. 5–6.
15. The name of the conference was 'Human Genetics in the Biological Revolution'.
16. The Forum opened in Spa Hotel Ortenberg.
17. Bundesarchiv Koblenz, Bundesministerium für Jugend, Familie und Gesundheit, gesundheitliche Modellaktion, B189/34001.
18. Bundesministerium für Jugend, Familie und Gesundheit, *Genetische Beratung, ein Modellversuch der Bundesregierung in Frankfurt und Marburg* (Bonn: Bundesministerium für Jugend, Familie und Gesundheit, 1979), p. 7.
19. D. Drohm, C. Lohrengel and K. Merz, 'Risikoermittlung und ärztliche Ratgebung in der genetischen Beratung', in Bundesministerium für Jugend, Familie und Gesundheit, *Genetische Beratung*, pp. 46–53.
20. Ibid., pp. 48–9.
21. E. Passarge and F. Vogel, 'The Delivery of Genetic Counseling Services in Europe', *Human Genetics*, 56 (1980), pp. 1–5.
22. Contergan, a non-prescription sleeping and tranquillizing agent sold by the German company Grünenthal, caused one of the biggest pharmaceutical scandals in German post-war history. At the turn of 1961–2, it was revealed that a large number of stillbirths and deformities of thousands of children were due to ingestion of Contergan. Despite public outrage, the company stubbornly refused to take contergan off the market. In November 1961 Hamburg geneticist Widukind Lenz, who had discovered a link between the deformities and thalidomide use, personally intervened at Grünenthal to urge a halt to the drug's production. Sales were stopped only after health officials threatened to ban the drug a few days later. In result of a lawsuit conducted between 1968 and 1970, the company was sentenced to pay approximately 100 million marks as compensation for the victims. See P. Osten, 'Spätes Erwachen. Vor 50 Jahren begann der Verkauf des Schlafmittels Contergan', *Berliner Zeitung*, 29 September 2007, at http://www.berliner-zeitung.de/archiv/vor-50-jahren-begann-der-verkauf-des-schlafmittels-contergan---und-eine-katastrophe-nahm-ihren-lauf-spaetes-erwachen,10810590,10508248.html [accessed 22 July 2013]; B. Kirk, *Der Contergan-Fall: eine unvermeidbare Arzneimittelkatastrophe? Zur Geschichte des Arzneistoffs Thalidomid* (Stuttgart: WVG, 1999).
23. Nachtsheim was the only senior researcher of the Kaiser Wilhelm Institute for Anthropology, Human Heredity and Eugenics (Kaiser-Wilhelm- Institut für Anthropologie, menschliche Erblehre und Eugenik) able to maintain his previous research department after the war. See H. P. Kröner, *Von der Rassenhygiene zur Humangenetik: Das Kaiser-Wilhelm-Institut für Anthropologie, menschliche Erblehre und Eugenik nach dem Krieg* (Münster: G. Fischer, 1994).
24. Only few human geneticists who had already working in the field during the Weimar Republic were able to continue university careers after World War II. By contrast, almost all the young human geneticists trained during the Third Reich had to reorient themselves outside of academic human genetics due to their earlier political involvement. However, this did not mean they had no relations to the university or had to give up their genetic research completely. See E. Klee, *Das Personenlexikon zum Dritten Reich: Wer war*

was vor und nach 1945 (Frankfurt: G. Fischer, 2003). On the post-war career of former human geneticists and anthropologists, see B. Massin, 'Anthropologie und Humangenetik im Nationalsozialismus oder: Wie schreiben deutsche Wissenschaftler ihre eigene Wissenschaftsgeschichte?', in H. Kaupen-Haas and C. Saller (eds), *Wissenschaftlicher Rassismus: Analysen einer Kontinuität in den Human- und Naturwissenschaften* (Frankfurt: Campus, 1999), pp. 12–64.

25. G. Wendt (ed.), *Genetik und Gesellschaft: Marburger Forum Philippinum* (Stuttgart: Wissenschaftliche Verlagsgesellschaft, 1970), pp. 1–2.
26. See the contributions of Lionel S. Penrose and of Helmut Baitsch, who made clear that 'it was too simple a model to view a characteristic either as an advantage or a disadvantage'; L. S. Penrose, 'Genetik und Gesellschaft', in Wendt (ed.), *Genetik und Gesellschaft*, pp. 3–9, on p. 4; H. Baitsch, 'Das eugenische Konzept – einst und jetzt', in Wendt (ed.), *Genetik und Gesellschaft*, pp. 59–71, on p. 64.
27. 'Based on a careful estimate, every human being is likely to have several harmful mutations in their gene makeup. With this wakeup call, all hopes for completely eliminating all harmful genes collapse'; Baitsch, 'Das eugenische Konzept', p. 64.
28. For example, the human geneticist Peter Emil Becker argued that the controlled breeding of human beings with valuable genetic potential was not desirable because variability is needed in a society that requires specialization and division of labour. See Wendt (ed.), *Genetik und Gesellschaft*, pp. 141–2.
29. U. Theile, *Genetische Beratung: Motivationsanalyse* (Munich: Urban und Schwarzenberg, 1977), p. 64.
30. Wendt (ed.), *Genetik und Gesellschaft*, pp. 135–6.
31. F. Vogel, 'Ist mit einer Manipulierbarkeit auf dem Gebiet der Humangenetik zu rechnen?', *Medizin und Kultur*, 16 (1967), pp. 648–50.
32. F. Lenz, 'Über die Grenzen praktischer Eugenik', *Acta Genetica et Statistica Medica*, 6 (1956–7), pp. 13–24, on p. 14.
33. Baitsch, 'Das eugenische Konzept', p. 66.
34. W. Fuhrmann, 'Genetische Beratung als ärztliche Aufgabe', *Diagnostik*, 5 (1972), pp. 500–2.
35. H. Ritter, 'Populationsgenetik und Zukunft des Menschen', in Wendt (ed.), *Genetik und Gesellschaft*, pp. 102–8, on p. 108.
36. F. Vogel, 'Genetische Beratung', in Wendt (ed.), *Genetik und Gesellschaft*, pp. 95–101, on p. 100.
37. Ibid.
38. Wendt (ed.), *Genetik und Gesellschaft*, p. 156.
39. W. Fuhrmann, 'Die Tätigkeit des Arztes und die biologische Zukunft des Menschen', Materia Medica Nordmark, 22:11–12 (1970), pp. 512–24, on p. 518.
40. See, for example, F. Vogel, 'Die eugenische Beratung beim Retinoblastom (Glioma retinae)', *Acta Genetica et Statistica Medica*, 7 (1957), pp. 565–72; F. Vogel, 'Formale Genetik und eugenische Beratung bei Retinoblastom', *Acta faculta medica Universita brunen*, 25 (1965), pp. 238–45, on p. 241; F. Vogel, *Lehrbuch der allgemeinen Humangenetik* (Berlin: Springer, 1961).
41. Fuhrmann, 'Genetische Beratung', p. 500.
42. W. Fuhrmann and F. Vogel, *Genetische Familienberatung. Ein Leitfaden für Studenten und Ärzte* (Berlin: Springer, 1982), p. 176.
43. K.-H. Degenhardt, *Humangenetik. Ein Leitfaden für Studium, Praxis und Klinik* (Köln: Deutscher Ärzte-Verlag, 1973).

44. G. Broberg and N. Roll-Hansen, *Eugenics and the Welfare State: Sterilization Policy in Denmark, Sweden, Norway, and Finland* (East Lansing, MI: Michigan State University Press, 1996); L. Koch, 'The Meaning of Eugenics: Reflections on the Government of Genetic Knowledge in the Past and the Present', *Science in Context*, 17:3 (2004), pp. 315–31.
45. The Cornelius Helferich Foundation supports social facilities that provide assistance and care for people with mental and physical disabilities and for elderly and sick individuals.
46. G. Wendt, *Die Zahl der Behinderten nimmt zu: Analyse der Situation und Darstellung der notwendigen Konsequenzen* (Frankfurt: Stiftung für das behinderte Kind, 1978), p. 6.
47. E. Bösl, *Politiken der Normalisierung: Zur Geschichte der Behindertenpolitik in der Bundesrepublik Deutschland* (Bielefeld: Transcript Verlag, 2009); H.-W. Schmuhl, *Exklusion und Inklusion durch Sprache: Zur Geschichte des Begriffs Behinderung* (Berlin: IMEW, 2010).

15 Lindee, 'Performing Anger: H. J. Muller, James V. Neel and Radiation Risk'

1. The quote is in fn. 12 of J. Beatty, D. B. Paul and R. Lewontin, 'Weighing the Risks: Stalemate in the Classical/Balance Controversy', *Journal of the History of Biology*, 20 (1987), pp. 289–319.
2. M. S. Lindee, 'Experimental Wounds: Science and Violence in Mid-Century America', in S. Smith (ed.), 'Health Legacies: Militarization, Health, and Society', *Journal of Law, Medicine and Ethics*, 39 (2011), pp. 8–20; D. Slaney, 'Eugene Rabinowitch, the *Bulletin of the Atomic Scientists* and the Nature of Scientific Internationalism in the Early Cold War', *Historical Studies in the Natural Sciences*, 42 (2012), pp. 114–42.
3. K. Bird and M. J. Sherwin, *American Prometheus: The Triumph and Tragedy of J. Robert Oppenheimer* (New York: A. A. Knopf, 2005); K. Moore, *Disrupting Science: Social Movements, American Scientists, and the Politics of the Military, 1945–1975* (Princeton, NJ: Princeton University Press, 2008); J. Wang, *American Science in an Age of Anxiety: Scientists, Anticommunism, and the Cold War* (Chapel Hill, NC: University of North Carolina Press, 1998).
4. J. Rohde, 'Gray Matters: Social Scientists, Military Patronage, and Democracy in the Cold War', *Journal of American History*, 96 (2009), pp. 99–122.
5. P. Galison and B. Bernstein, 'In Any Light: Scientists and the Decision to Build the Superbomb, 1952–1954', *Historical Studies in the Physical and Biological Sciences*, 19 (1989), pp. 267–347.
6. J. C. Jolly, 'Linus Pauling and the Scientific Debate over Fallout Hazards', *Endeavour*, 26 (2002), pp. 149–153; J. C. Jolly, *Thresholds of Uncertainty: Radiation and Responsibility in the Fallout Controversy. Dissertation Abstracts International, A 64* (2004), 4600.
7. Rohde, 'Gray Matters'.
8. A. Hochschild, *The Managed Heart: Commercialization of Human Feeling*, 20th anniversary edn, with a new afterword (Berkeley, CA: University of California Press, 2003).
9. K. H. Ng and J. L. Kidder, 'Toward a Theory of Emotive Performance: With Lessons from How Politicians Do Anger', *Sociological Theory*, 28 (2010), pp. 193–214; see also J. Bourke, 'Fear and Anxiety: Writing about Emotion in Modern History', *History Workshop Journal*, 55 (2003), pp. 111–22.

10. W. Laemmli, 'Alpha Males: Science, Conflict, and Masculinity, 1960–1980' (unpublished seminar paper, University of Pennsylvania, 2010).
11. J. Samuel Walker, in his 1994 *Isis* article, proposed that the Atomic Energy Commission had been successful in addressing the scientific aspects of the issue but somewhat less so in addressing the political ones; J. S. Walker, 'The Atomic Energy Commission and the Politics of Radiation Protection, 1967–1971', *Isis*, 85 (1994), pp. 57–78, on p. 57.
12. E. A. Carlson, *Genes, Radiation, and Society: The Life and Work of H. J. Muller* (Ithaca, NY: Cornell University Press, 1981).
13. J. V. Neel, *Physician to the Gene Pool* (New York: John Wiley, 1994).
14. See exchanges in the fall of 1950 over a demand that Neel appear at the AEC to explain problems with the genetics programme, detailed in Neel to Thomas M. Rivers, 2 November 1950, in ABCC Program Components, Alphabetical File, A–G, Genetics, 1949–1955 3B, National Academy of Sciences. See also various discussions in my book, S. Lindee, *Suffering Made Real: American Science and the Survivors at Hiroshima* (Chicago, IL: University of Chicago Press, 1994).
15. The entire relevant copy of *Saga: The Magazine for Men*, April 1962, is in Series II, Professional Atomic Energy Commission, Papers of Bentley Glass, American Philosophical Society, Philadelphia, Pennsylvania (hereafter Glass, APS).
16. The figures are from the 1963 Atomic Energy Commission budget, in Series II, Professional Atomic Energy Commission, Glass, APS.
17. S. Kirsch, 'Harold Knapp and the Geography of Normal Controversy: Radioiodine in the Historical Environment', *Osiris*, 2nd ser., 19: 'Landscapes of Exposure: Knowledge and Illness in Modern Environments' (2004), pp. 167–81; I. Semendeferi, 'Legitimating a Nuclear Critic: John Gofman, Radiation Safety, and Cancer Risks', *Historical Studies in the Natural Sciences*, 38 (2008), pp. 259–301.
18. R. Borofsky, *Yanomami: The Fierce Controversy and What We Can Learn from It* (Berkeley, CA: University of California Press, 2005).
19. The reports of UNSCEAR are now readily available and downloadable from their website. The 1958 report in its entirety is at http://www.unscear.org/unscear/en/publications/1958.htm [accessed 25 March 2012].
20. WHO, *Effect of Radiation on Human Heredity, Report of a Study Group Convened by WHO Together with Papers Presented by Various Members of the Group* (Geneva: World Health Organization, 1957), p. 11 (hereafter WHO, 1957).
21. E. A. Carlson recounts a moment when the meeting recorder noted, after Muller left the room, that 'now that Muller is away we should be able to get something done', Carlson, *Genes, Radiation, and Society*, pp. 409–10. Beatty cites meeting minutes around this time in which Neel called himself the 'bête noir' in these debates; J. Beatty, 'Scientific Collaboration, Internationalism, and Diplomacy: The Case of the Atomic Bomb Casualty Commission', *Journal of the History of Biology*, 26 (1993), pp. 205–23.
22. WHO, 1957, p. 139. The prepared summaries of the informal discussions provoked so many more discussions by mail that they were abandoned and not published. I ran across multiple discussions of the summary for genetics in the Papers of Alexander Hollaender, American Philosophical Society, Philadelphia, Pennsylvania (hereafter Hollaender, APS). A. C. Stevenson had prepared these, and Muller became extremely upset about them, which led Stevenson to complain to Hollaender. Also complaining was Sterling Emerson, then geneticist in the Biology Branch of the AEC's Division of Biology and Medicine. See also Emerson to Hollander, 10 October 1956, Hollaender, APS.

23. Neel, 'Estimation of Mutation Rates in Animal and Man', in WHO, 1957, pp. 139–50, on p. 140.
24. Muller to Stevenson, 5 October 1956, Hollaender, APS.
25. Muller to Neel, Joe to Jim, 24 October 1956, Neel Folder 6, Curt Stern Papers, APS (hereafter Stern, APS). See also Neel to Muller, 18 October 1956, Neel Folder 6, Stern, APS.
26. A. P. Davis and M. J. Justice, 'An Oak Ridge Legacy: The Specific Locus Test and its Role in Mouse Mutagenesis', *Genetics*, 148 (1998), pp. 7–12.
27. Muller to Neel, 3 November 1956, Hollaender, APS.
28. Neel to Muller, 18 October, Muller, Hollaender, APS.
29. Muller to Neel, 7 December 1956, Neel Folder 6, Stern, APS.
30. Ibid.
31. Ibid.
32. Neel to Hollaender, 11 December 1956, Neel, Hollaender, APS.
33. Neel to Stern, 11 December 1956, Neel Folder 6, Stern, APS.
34. K. A. Rader, 'Alexander Hollaender's Postwar Vision for Biology: Oak Ridge and Beyond', *Journal of the History of Biology*, 39 (2006), pp. 685–706.
35. E. Novitski, *Sturtevant and Dobzhanksy: Two Scientists at Odds* (Philadelphia, PA: XLibris, 2005); J. F. Crow, D. Lindsley and J. Lucchesi, 'Edward Novitski: Drosophila Virtuoso', *Genetics*, 174 (2006), pp. 549–53.
36. Novitski to Neel, 15 December 1956, Hollaender, APS.
37. Hollander was also the referee for Muller and Stevenson (Stevenson was angered by Muller's criticisms of his draft summary of the discussion); see his letter to Hollaender, 11 October 1956, in A. C. Stevenson folder, Hollaender, APS.
38. Muller, 'Damage from Point Mutations', in WHO, 1957, pp. 25–47, on p. 41.
39. Neel, 'Estimation of Mutation Rates in Animal and Man', in WHO, 1957, pp. 139–50, on p. 143.
40. Neel to Stern, 9 January 1957, Neel Folder 6, Stern, APS.
41. Neel to Muller, 15 January 1957, Neel Folder 6, Stern, APS.
42. Ibid.
43. 5 April 1957. Copy of a letter sent by Muller to Raymond K. Appleyard at the UN, which was sent to Hollaender at Oak Ridge with a note to Alex from Joe – bringing up the extrapolation problem as he saw it. Muller refers to his own paper with Morton and Crow, 'refuting the now popular (and AEC promoted) claim that a random increase in heterozygosity is likely to be advantageous'; Muller to Appleyard, 5 April 1957, in Hollaender, APS.
44. Semendeferi, 'Legitimating a Nuclear Critic', p. 261.
45. A copy of the transcript of the interview is in Hollaender, APS. It was at UCLA on 8 April 1971, and was part of Carlson's efforts to follow up a rumour he had heard – that it was not Strauss but Libby who had blocked Muller's participation in the 1955 conference at Geneva (though Strauss took public responsibility).
46. Quoted in Philip M. Boffey's blow-by-blow account of the fight between Gofman and his colleague and co-author Arthur Tamplin on one side, and the AEC and Lawrence Livermore on the other. P. M. Boffey, 'Gofman and Tamplin: Harassment Charges against AEC, Livermore', *Science*, 169 (1970), pp. 838–43, on p. 840.
47. There were certainly other cases where scientists found themselves at odds with the AEC over questions of scientific importance. See, for example, the effort by Earl Cook, later a dean at Texas A&M, who served on the National Academy of Sciences Committee

on the Geological Aspects of Radioactive Waste Disposal, to publish on waste disposal practices of the AEC. Earl Cook to John W. Gofman, 24 February 1970, Gofman Folder, Stern, APS.

48. Kirsch, 'Harold Knapp', p. 180.
49. J. Beatty and A. Moore, 'Should we Aim for Consensus?' *Episteme*, 7 (2010), pp. 198–214.
50. Report is filed in 'Federation of American Scientists', Hollaender, APS.
51. R. Proctor, *Golden Holocaust: Origins of the Cigarette Catastrophe and the Case for Abolition* (Berkeley, CA: University of California Press, 2012).
52. S. Lindee, *Moments of Truth in Genetic Medicine* (Baltimore, MD: Johns Hopkins University Press, 2005).
53. J. Radin, 'Life on Ice' (PhD dissertation, University of Pennsylvania, 2012).
54. S. S. West, 'Ideology of Academic Scientists', *IRE Transactions on Engineering Management*, 7 (1960), pp. 54–62.

16 Cassata, 'The Struggle for Authority over Italian Genetics: The Ninth International Congress of Genetics in Bellagio, 1948–53'

1. G. Montalenti and A. Chiarugi (eds), *Atti del IX Congresso internazionale di genetica. Bellagio (Como), 24–31 agosto 1953*, 2 vols (Florence: Florentiae, 1954), vol. 1, p. 16.
2. N. Krementsov, *International Science between the World Wars: The Case Of Genetics* (Abingdon and New York: Routledge, 2005), p. 5.
3. On Buzzati–Traverso and Montalenti, see in particular: F. Cassata, *L'Italia intelligente. Adriano Buzzati-Traverso e il Laboratorio internazionale di genetica e biofisica (1962–69)* (Rome: Donzelli, 2013); M. Capocci and G. Corbellini, 'Adriano Buzzati-Traverso and the Foundation of the International Laboratory of Genetics and Biophysics in Naples (1962–1969)', *Studies in History and Philosophy of Science Part C: Biological and Biomedical Sciences*, 33:3 (2002), pp. 489–513; F. De Sio and M. Capocci, 'Southern Genes. Genetics and its Institutions in the Italian South, 1930s–1970s', *Medicina nei Secoli*, 20:3 (2008), pp. 791–826.
4. R. S. Morison officer's diary, Rome, Italy, 23–5 September 1953, p. 109, in Record Group (RG), 12.1, Rockefeller Foundation Archives, Rockefeller Archive Center, Sleepy Hollow, New York.
5. For a comprehensive history of Italian eugenics, with a specific focus on Gini's role, see in particular F. Cassata, *Building the New Man: Eugenics, Racial Science and Genetics in Twentieth-Century Italy* (New York and Budapest: Central European University Press, 2011).
6. On Gini's role as statistician and demographer, see in particular J.-G. Prévost, *A Total Science: Statistics in Liberal and Fascist Italy* (Montreal: McGill-Queen's University Press, 2009); F. Cassata, *Il fascismo razionale. Corrado Gini fra scienza e politica* (Rome: Carocci, 2006).
7. C. Barigozzi, 'I nuovi orizzonti della citogenetica', *Genus*, 3:3–4 (June 1939), pp. 35–72.
8. A. Buzzati-Traverso, 'I nuovi orizzonti della radiogenetica', *Genus*, 3:3–4 (June 1939), pp. 73–130.
9. G. Montalenti, 'I recenti studi sul problema della determinazione del sesso e dei caratteri sessuali secondari negli animali', *Genus*, 3:3–4 (June 1939), pp. 193–214.
10. G. Montalenti, 'L'VIII Congresso internazionale di Genetica (Stoccolma, 7–14 luglio 1948)', *La Ricerca Scientifica*, 19 (1949), pp. 130–1.

11. Buzzati-Traverso and Barigozzi to Montalenti, 1 January 1949, Carte Giuseppe Montalenti, Università di Roma 'La Sapienza', Sezione di Storia della Medicina (hereafter AM), b. 24, f. 2, sf. 8. The letter was sent to Montalenti for comments.
12. Buzzati-Traverso and Barigozzi to Montalenti, 1 January 1949, AM, b. 24, f. 2, sf. 8.
13. Minutes of the meeting of the Provisory Committee for the Ninth International Congress of Genetics, 3 November 1951, AM, b. 28, f. 9. The other permanent members – Carlo Jucci, professor of zoology in Pavia; and Silvio Ranzi, professor of zoology, and Sergio Tonzig, professor of botany, both at the University of Milan – were connected with both Buzzati and Barigozzi.
14. For more details, see Cassata, *Building the New Man*, pp. 295–308.
15. C. Gini, 'The Physical Assimilation of the Foreign Settlements in Italy', in Montalenti and Chiarugi (eds), *Atti del IX Congresso internazionale di genetica*, vol. 1, pp. 246–53, on p. 252.
16. See F. Boas, *Changes in the Bodily Form of Descendants of Immigrants* (Washington, DC: Senate Document 208, 1911).
17. Gini explicitly adopted the term 'sub-Lamarckian': see C. Gini, 'Cause e carattere adattativo dell'evoluzione delle forme viventi', *Genus*, 17:1–4 (1961), pp. 1–42.
18. See Cassata, *Building the New Man*, pp. 147–91.
19. On Gini's post-war scientific racism and his collaboration with the *Mankind Quarterly*, see Cassata, *Building the New Man*, pp. 362–77. On IAAEE and the *Mankind Quarterly*, see in particular W. H. Tucker, *The Science and Politics of Racial Research* (Urbana, IL: University of Illinois Press, 1994), and J. P. Jackson, Jr, *Science for Segregation: Race, Law and the Case against Brown v. Board of Education* (New York: New York University Press, 2005).
20. Gini presented the same paper at a workshop held at the Milan Serotherapeutic Institute in 1949 and in 1956 at the First International Congress of Human Genetics, in Copenaghen. In both circumstances, he was criticized respectively by Haldane and by Montalenti.
21. A. Buzzati-Traverso, 'Nonsenso biologico del razzismo', *La Rassegna d'Italia*, 1:1 (January 1946), pp. 1–8 (offprint).
22. A. Buzzati-Traverso, 'Genetica, medicina e uomo', *Recenti progressi in medicina*, 8:1 (January 1950), pp. 1–26 (offprint).
23. L. Gianferrari, 'Il contributo dell'Università al Centro di studi di genetica umana', *Gli Annali della Università d'Italia*, 3:1 (29 October 1941), pp. 24–8.
24. L. Gianferrari, 'Sull'organizzazione e sull'attività svolta dal Centro di studi di genetica umana nel primo quadriennio dalla sua fondazione', *Natura*, 35 (1944), pp. 112–16, on p. 114.
25. Ibid., p. 113.
26. Ibid., p. 115.
27. Ibid., p. 116.
28. L. Gianferrari, 'Importanza, urgenza di ricerche genetiche in popolazioni endogame', *Atti e memorie della Società Lombarda di Medicina*, 5:8 (1937), pp. 581–4.
29. L. Gianferrari, 'Il Centro di Studi di Genetica umana dell'Università di Milano ed i Consultori di genetica umana dell'Università e del Comune di Milano', *Natura*, 41 (1950), pp. 75–81, on p. 76.
30. L. Gianferrari, 'Introduzione alla profilassi delle malattie ereditarie', *Acta Geneticae Medicae et Gemellologiae*, 2 (May 1952), pp. 113–17, on p. 117.
31. L. Gianferrari, 'Genetica umana', in *Atti del IV Congresso internazionale dei medici cattolici (Roma, 24 settembre–2 ottobre 1949)* (Rome: Orizzonte Medico, 1950), p. 129.

32. L. Gianferrari, 'Il problema genetico delle leucemie', in Montalenti and Chiarugi (eds), *Atti del IX Congresso internazionale di genetica*, pp. 390–434.
33. Ministerial decree by Antonio Segni, 15 June 1953, Archivio Centrale dello Stato, Ministero della Pubblica Istruzione, Direzione Generale Istruzione Superiore (hereafter ACS, MPI, DGIS), Divisione I, Commissione libere docenze 1938–1953, b. 74, f. 1052.
34. Barigozzi and Buzzati-Traverso appeal to the State Council, 27 August 1953, ACS, MPI, DGIS, Divisione I, Commissione libere docenze 1938–1953, b. 74, f. 1052.
35. Appeal by Montalenti to the Head of State, 14 December 1953, in ACS, MPI, DGIS, Divisione I, Commissione libere docenze 1938–1953, b. 74, f. 1052.
36. L. Gedda, 'Genetica, medicina e costituzione', *Acta geneticae medicae et gemellologiae*, 1 (January 1952), pp. 1–6, on p. 5.
37. L. Gedda (ed.), *Genetica Medica. Primum Symposium Internationale Geneticae Medicae Roma 6–7 settembre 1953* (Rome: Edizioni dell'Istituto Gregorio Mendel, 1953).
38. Buzzati-Traverso to Montalenti, 2 February 1953, AM, b. 28, f. 9.
39. C. Foà, 'Discorso pronunciato nella cerimonia inaugurale dell'Istituto G. Mendel il 6 settembre 1953', in Gedda (ed.), *Genetica Medica*, pp. 447–8, on p. 447.
40. Ibid., pp. 447–8.
41. L. Gedda, 'Profilo scientifico della genetica medica', in Gedda (ed.), *Genetica Medica*, pp. 3–18, on pp. 13–14.
42. Ibid., p. 6.
43. Ibid.
44. 'Address of His Holiness Pope Pius XII to those attending the Primum symposium internationale geneticae medicae', in Gedda (ed.), *Genetica Medica*, p. 429.
45. Ibid.
46. T. Dobzhansky, 'Comment on the Discussion of Genetics by His Holiness, Pius XII', *Science*, 118:3071 (November 1953), pp. 561–3.
47. A. Buzzati-Traverso, 'Review of L. Gedda (ed.), *Genetica Medica. Primum Symposium Internationale Geneticae Medicae Roma 67 settembre 1953* (Rome: Edizioni dell'Istituto Gregorio Mendel, 1953)', *Science*, 122:3161 (July 1955), p. 206.
48. Ibid., p. 206.
49. Barigozzi to Montalenti, 4 March 1953, AM, b. 28, f. 9.
50. G. Montalenti, 'The Genetics of Microcythemia', in Montalenti and Chiarugi (eds), *Atti del IX Congresso internazionale di genetica*, vol. 1, pp. 554–88.

INDEX

abortion, 136, 183, 184, 189
Albanians, 221
Africa, 62, 67
  Africans, 222
Agricultural College (Berlin), 114–16
agricultural research, 6, 9, 73, 114–15, 127, 130–1, 134, 138
agronomy, 127, 129–31, 137–8
Aktion Sorgenkind (Germany), 197, 202
Albareda, José M., 132
alkaptonuria, 3, 6, 13
allele frequency, 63, 69, 75–6
allelic modification, 156, 161
Allison, Anthony, 48
Allmänna Svenska Utsädesaktiebolaget (Sweden), 130
Alps, 61, 87, 91, 96–8, 223
Alzheimer's disease, 188
American Eugenics Society, 29, 34
American Society of Human Genetics, 158
amniocentesis, 146, 184, 204
Anglo-American International Association for the Advancement of Ethnology and Eugenics (IAAEE) 222
anaemia, 53, 106, 108, 109, 184
animal genetics, 48, 59, 219
animal breeding, 114–15
anthropology
  biological, 55–6, 61
  cultural and social, 11, 66, 86, 101, 102, 104, 105
  physical, 43, 57, 66, 86, 99, 221
  racial, 90–1, 95, 98–9
anthropometry, 62, 86, 221
anticipation, 10, 153–63
antiserum production, 71–2, 74
Apache, 62
Army Blood Transfusion Service (UK), 79
Asilomar Conference, 121, 183
Atomic Bomb Casualty Commission, 209
Atomic Energy Commission 106, 207, 208
Atomic Energy Research Establishment (Harwell, UK), 117–18, 125, 142–4
atomic energy, 142, 209, 212
atomic weapons, 142, 143, 205, 206
Aula Dei Experimental Station (Spain), 127, 130, 132–137
Auschwitz, 23
Austen, Jane, 207
Australia, 62, 107, 159, 180
  Aborigines, 62
autarchy, 134
autism, 53
Avery, Amos, 132

bacteriology, 14, 24
Baden, 14
Baden-Württemberg, 197
Baitsch, Helmut, 199–200
Bakeslee, Albert F., 132
Balling, Rudi, 123–4
Bandung (Java), 130
Barber, Bernard, 215
Barigozzi, Claudio, 217–22, 224, 227
barley (*Hordeum*), 127, 130, 132–3
Barr body, 137, 146, 147
Barr, Murray L., 137
Basques, 61
Baur, Erwin, 115
Bavaria, 21
Beadle, George, 3
Beatty, John, 214
Bell, George Douglas Hutton, 135

Bell, Julia, 154–5, 157
Bellagio, 217–22, 224–5, 227
Bene Israel, 64–5
Berlin, 22–3, 34, 115, 117
Bern, 34
Bernard, Claude, 113
Bernstein, Felix, 3
Betancourt, Rafael Molina, 107
Bianco, Ida, 218
Biesele, John J., 135
Birmingham, 34
biochemistry, 12, 110
  biochemical markers, 12, 63, 103
biohistorical narrative, 65–7
biometry, 5, 18, 42–4
biopsy, 139
biotechnology, 1–2, 6, 165, 188
Birch, Carroll LaFleur, 171–3
birth control, 45, 50
Blacker, C. P., 50
blood
  coagulation, 176–7
  depots, 70–1, 73, 77
  disease, 109, 168, 170
  donation, 71, 73–5, 82
  groups, 3–4, 6, 10, 52, 57, 60, 62–5, 69–71, 75, 86–7, 90–9, 107–9, 111, 222, 224
    incompatibility, 80–3, 223
    testing, 71, 74, 78, 81, 86, 91, 107, 223
  sampling, 64–65, 69, 76, 80, 82, 105, 106–109, 111, 139
  transfusion, 8, 70, 78, 169–170, 172–174
Blood Transfusion Research Committee (UK), 71, 78
Boas, Franz, 43–5, 49, 102, 104, 221
Bogor (Indonesia), 129
Bologna, 219, 221
Botanical Institute (Bogor, Indonesia), 129
Bowditch, Henry Pickering, 41, 43
Boyd, William C., 60, 63
Boyer, Samuel H., 34
Brazil, 60–2, 102, 225
Bremen, 19
Brinkhous, Kenneth, 173–5
British Blood Group Survey, 76
British Medical Journal, 71, 74, 78
broad bean (*Vicia faba*), 133
Bucharest, 221
Buerger's disease, 36
Bulloch, William, 168–70
Burt, Cyril, 40, 43, 46, 50, 51, 186
Bush, Vannevar, 31
Bussey Institution, 114
Buzzati-Traverso, Adriano, 217–22, 224–7

Caja de Ahorros y Monte de Piedad de Aragón y Rioja, 132
Calabria, 221
Canada, 142, 159
Cancer Research Centre (Bombay, India), 60
cancer, 5, 26, 34, 90, 121–2, 132, 141–4, 150, 189, 215, 217
Cardiff, 34
Cárdenas, Lázaro, 104
Carlson, Elof Axel, 213, 207
Carnegie Institution, 4, 30–2
Carr-Saunders, Alexander M., 46
Carstairs (UK), 147
Cattell, Raymond B., 45, 51
Caso, Alfonso 104, 105, 107, 110
caste system (India), 61, 63–4, 77
cataract, 117, 122–3
Catholicism, 218–19, 228
Cavalli-Sforza, Luigi, 61, 207, 217, 221–2, 224, 227
census, 21, 25
central dogma of molecular biology, 158
cereal breeding, 128–30, 132, 134
Charité clinic, Berlin, 116
Chicago, 108, 110
child growth, 40–1, 43–5, 47
Childs, Barton, 159, 184
chromosome, 1, 9, 36, 128–9, 131–2
  aberration, 10, 12
  fragmentation, 131, 135
  human, 127, 129, 136–7, 141–51
Churchill Hospital (Oxford, UK), 144
CIBA Symposium, 199
citizenship, 94–5, 98
civil rights movement, 148
Clarke, Angus, 182
clerical work, 74–5
clinical medicine, 2, 6, 8, 78–80, 82, 127, 138–9, 153, 156, 161–2, 166, 169–71, 176–8

clinical observation, 23, 35
clinical psychiatry, 21
cloning, 1
colchicine, 128–9, 132–3, 135–6, 139
Cold Spring Harbour Symposium on Quantitative Genetics, 59
Cold War, 90, 147, 158, 206, 207, 215, 216
Collier, John, 102, 104
Collins, Francis, 189
Cologne, 34
colonialism, 59
colour blindness, 63
Columbia University, 47, 60, 104, 161
  Institute for the Study of Human Variation, 60, 63
Comfort, Nathaniel, 6, 165
computing, 73
concentration camp, 22, 129
Condon, E. U., 206
consanguinity, 58–61
Consejo Superior de Investigaciones Científicas (Spain), 132
constitution (medicine), 1, 10, 20, 22, 29, 34, 41, 219, 225–6
constitutional pathology, 20, 29, 219, 225, 226, 228
contagion, 19
Cornelius Helferich Foundation, 203
Contergan scandal, 197
Cornet, Georg, 14
coronary diseases, 35
coroner, 17
counselling (eugenic/ genetic), 11, 24, 32, 177, 193–204, 223
Court Brown, Michael, 144, 148, 150
cross-breeding, 61, 65
cystic fibrosis, 179
cytogenetics, 127, 129, 131–2, 134, 137–9, 141–6, 148–52, 165
cytology, 127, 131, 135
cytoplasmic inheritance, 158

D'Ancona, Umberto, 224
Dall'Aqua, Giovanni, 224
Dameshek, William, 176
D'Ancona, Umberto, 224
Darwin, Charles, 153
Darwinian evolution, 61, 97
Datura, 133
Davenport, Charles, 3, 4
degeneration, 153
Degenhardt, Karl-Heinz, 203
dementia praecox, 154
demography, 45, 57, 61, 66, 220–1
Denmark, 127
Department of Atomic Energy (Chalk River, Canada), 142
depression, 188
diabetes, 154
diagnosis, 18–19, 82, 127, 138, 165, 168, 170
diathesis, 14, 19, 226
Dice, Lee Raymond, 175
Diehl, Karl, 22–5
Dight Institute for Human Genetics, University of Minnesota, 32, 194
Di Guglielmo, Giovanni, 224
disability, 196–7, 202–4
DNA, 158, 165, 183, 188
Dobzhansky, Theodosius, 57–58, 60, 63, 97, 205, 208, 212, 222, 226
dog, 173–4
dominance, 75, 80
Donald, Malcolm, 29
Down syndrome, 137, 144–5
Draper, George, 29
Draper, Wickliffe P., 29
Drosophila, 120, 123, 136, 139, 142, 147, 157, 161, 169, 205, 211–13, 217
Drury, Alan, 78
Duncan, Otis Dudley, 47
Dunker community, 61–2
Dunn, Leslie Clarence, 2, 57–8, 60, 68, 97
Dunning, Gordon, 214
Dutch East Indies, 129
dynamic mutation, 162

East Prussia, 20
Ebro (Spain), 132
Eddy, James E., 30
Edinburgh, 144, 147–50, 221
Edinburgh University, 46
Ehling, Heidede, 118–20
Ehling, Udo, 117–23, 125
electrophoresis, 106, 111

Elvas Plant Breeding Experimental Station (Portugal), 130
embryonic tissue, 136–7
Emergency Blood Transfusion Service, 69–72, 76
Emergency Public Health Laboratory Service (UK), 72
endogamy, 58, 62, 65
  endogamous group, 56, 59–60, 65
England, 76
Environmental Mutagen Society, 120
epidemiology, 2, 14, 17, 90, 195
epilepsy, 116
Erythroblastosis fetalis, 79–80
Estaçao Agronomica Nacional (Sacavem, Portugal), 132
Estación de Biología Experimental de Cogullada (Zaragoza, Spain), 130
Esteruelas, Ramón, 130, 132
ethnography, 75
ethnology, 61, 66, 76–7
eugenics, 4–5, 10–11, 18–19, 21, 23–5, 42–3, 46–7, 50–1, 53, 57, 73, 143, 158, 165, 193, 201, 204, 222
Eugenics Record Office (Cold Spring Harbor, USA), 3, 27–30
Eugenics Society, 46, 47, 51
Eugster, Jakob, 90
Europe, 65
Eve, I. S., 212
evolutionary synthesis, 56
experiment, 58–9, 63–4, 80
Experimental Breeding Station (Swedish Seed Association, Svalöf), 127, 130–1, 134, 136
experimental design, 65, 154
Experimental and Education Centre for Radiation Protection, Munich, 119–20, 122, 124–5
experimental medicine, 166, 169, 173, 175–6

familial inheritance, 167
family history, 14, 80, 153–5, 157, 167, 169
fascism (Italian), 221–7
Favor, Jack, 122–3
Federal University of Paraná, 60
federalism, 93–6, 98
Federation of American Scientists, 214
feebleminded ('morons', 'imbeciles', 'idiots'), 36, 42–4, 48, 49, 52
Ferguson-Smith, Malcolm, 34
fertility, 39, 45, 46, 48–53
field biology, 58
field researcher (human genetics), 27, 30–1, 223
Fildes, Paul, 168–70
Fisher Box, Joan, 73
Fisher, Ronald A., 40, 42–3, 45, 48–50, 52, 60, 69, 72–83, 159
Fleck, Ludwick, 6
fly room, 161
Foà, Carlo, 225–6
Følling, Asbjørn, 179
Food and Drug Administration (USA), 174
Ford, Charles, 142–4, 147
Fox, Robin, 207
Framingham study, 225
France, 5, 153
Franco dictatorship, 127, 134
Frankfurt-on-Main, 196, 203
Fraser-Roberts, John A., 45, 50
Freire-Maia, Newton, 60
frog, 183
Fuhrmann, Walter, 196, 200–2

Gallástegui, Cruz, 137
Galton, Francis, 3, 5, 14–15, 41–3, 50, 153
Gamio, Manuel, 102, 104
Gannett, Lisa, 94
Gautier, Marthe, 145
Grajales, Francisco, 107
Garay, Alfonso León de, 107
Garrod, Archibald, 3, 6
Gaudilliére, Jean-Paul, 2, 179
Gedda, Luigi, 218–19, 222, 224–8
gene, 1, 165
  gene frequency, 60, 62, 66, 76, 95–6
  gene pool, 59, 200, 204
  gene transfer, 165
genealogy, 14–15, 25
generation, 17
genetic distance, 62
genetic drift, 59, 98
genetic engineering, 199
genetic hygiene, 194–5, 199

genetic load, 61, 199, 208, 211
genetic markers, 62–3, 67
genetic therapy, 175, 188, 190
genetic variation, 55–6
genetics, 2, 51, 134, 137–8, 158, 165–6, 174–5, 177–8, 179, 182, 183, 185, 187–90
  biochemical, 175
  comparative, 116, 119, 124
  correlation in, 22
  medical, 11–12, 55–6, 60, 67, 101, 103, 105, 107, 108, 110–12, 127, 153, 158–63, 165, 177–8, 183, 184, 226
  molecular, 183, 188, 190
Geneva, 34, 195
genomics, 125, 151, 165
genotype, 81, 173
Genus (journal), 219
German Mouse Clinic, 114, 125
German Research Foundation, 114–15
German Research Institution for Psychiatry, 21
German Society for Blood Group Research, 75, 91
German Society for Racial Hygiene, 18
German Tuberculosis Society, 25
Germany, 5, 14, 18, 114, 118, 125, 167, 193–204
germ-plasm poisoning, 154
Ghigi, Alessandro, 221
Gianferrari, Luisa, 218–19, 222–5, 227–8
Gilbert, Walter, 188
Gini, Corrado, 218–21
Giordano, Alfonso, 224
Glass, David V., 46, 47, 52
Glover, Gina, 151
Goddard, Henry H., 41–2, 44, 48
Gofman, John W., 208, 209, 213
Goldschmidt, Richard, 161
Gottstein, Adolf, 19
Graham, John, 173–6
grass (*Phleum echinatum*), 133
Greece, 93
Gregor Mendel Institute of Medical Genetics and Twin Research (Rome), 225–6, 228
Griesemer, James, 94
Gruening, Ernst, 102
guinea pig, 114
Guisan, Henry, 90
Gürich, Hellmuth, 116
Guthrie, Robert, 180, 185
Guy's Hospital, London, 144

Hadorn, Ernst, 90
Haecker, Valentin, 19
Hanhart, Ernst, 96
haematology, 70, 166–7, 172–3
haemophilia, 13, 166–78, 223
  carriers, 168
  female transmission, 168–9
Haldane, J. B. S., 39, 44, 52, 73, 82, 154, 159, 171
Halsey, A. H., 52
Hamburg, 19
Hamerton, John, 142
Hardy, George, 76
Hardy-Weinberg equilibrium, 42, 52, 75–7, 82
Harlan, John M., 29
Harvey, A. McGehee, 33
Harper, Peter, 165–6
Harris, Harry, 159
Heidelberg, 34, 197
hereditary disease, 14–15, 26, 165–8, 177–8
hereditary disposition, 167
hereditary talent, 223
heredity clinics, 27–37, 195
  Heredity Clinic (University of Michigan), 175
heredity, 5, 6, 9, 17, 19, 25–6, 129, 153, 166
Herrnstein, Richard, 185, 187
heritability, 10, 22
Herskovits, Melville J., 68
heterozygosity, 43, 48, 49, 183, 190
Hiernaux, Jean, 63, 67–8
Hiroshima, 207, 209, 210
Hobsbawm, Eric, 6
Hochschild, Arlie, 206, 207
Hogben, Lancelot, 39, 44, 47, 73, 154
Hollaender, Alexander, 119–20, 212
homosexuality, 53
homozygosity, 48, 49, 173
Hood, Leroy, 188
Hôpital Trousseau (Paris, France), 144

Hospital de Enfermedades de la Nutrición, 108
Hospital for Sick Children (London, UK), 195
hospital population, 16–18
hospital records, 8, 17–18, 222
Höweler, Chris, 157
Howell, William Henry, 169
Hrabé de Angelis, Martin, 123–4
Hsia, David, 159
Hsu, Tao-Chiuh, 136
Hug, Otto, 119
human diversity, 55, 67
human evolution, 55, 67
Human Genetics Committee (Medical Research Council), 73, 82
human genetics, 1, 6, 11, 55, 57, 67, 69, 74, 76, 82–3, 138, 153–4, 158–63, 165, 173, 175, 194, 197–8, 202, 204, 219–20
Human Genome Project, 122–4, 187, 189
human heredity, 6, 17, 21, 74, 153
Hungerford, David A., 143
Huntington's chorea, 13, 154
Hurler's syndrome, 36
Hutchinson, G. Evelyn, 52
hybrid vigour (heterosis), 48, 52, 53
hybridization, 135
hygiene, 14, 19, 23

Iceland, 76
Ikin, Elizabeth, 72
immigration, 76, 97, 221
immunity, 2, 19, 79, 172
in vitro fertilization, 1
inbreeding, 58, 60–1, 65
incest, 58
index cards, 75
India, 61, 63
Indiana University, Bloomington, 208, 209
indigenous populations (*Indigenismo, indigenista*), 101–12
infection, 2, 23
inheritance of acquired characteristics, 154, 158
Institute of Bacteriology (Lund, Sweden), 136
Institute of Forest Genetics (Placerville, California), 30
Institute of Genetics (University of Lund, Sweden), 131
Institute of Human Variation (University of Michigan), 175
insurance companies, 8, 15, 19, 20, 25, 226
intelligence (mental ability, IQ), 39–54, 148, 185–7, 190
interbreeding, 58
Inter-American Congress of Indigenous Affairs, 102, 104
Inter-American Institute for Indigenous Affairs, 104
interdisciplinarity, 67, 177
International Association of Athletics Federation, 147
International Biological Program, 151
International Congress of Catholic Physicians, 223
International Congress of Genetics, 217–20, 224–5
International Congress of Human Genetics, 59, 145
International Congress of the Latin Eugenics Societies, 221
International Programme for Human Biology, 66
International Wheat Genetics Symposium, 135
Iowa Child Welfare Station, 44
islanders, 61
isolate, 8, 56, 58, 60–1, 65, 95, 97, 221, 223
Istituto Sieroterapico Milanese, 60
Italian Committee for the Study of Population (CISP), 218–21
Italian Genetics Society 219, 227
Italian National Institute of Statistics, 218
Italian National Research Council, 219
Italian Society of Genetics and Eugenics (SIGE), 218–21, 227
Italian Society of Medical Genetics, 225, 227
Italian State Council, 224
Italy, 217–28

Jackson Laboratory, 114
Jacobs, Patricia, 144
Jaenisch, Rudolf, 183

jaundice, 154
Java, 127, 129, 130
Jennings, H. S., 42
Jensen, Arthur, 185, 187, 207
Jews, 94, 222
Johns Hopkins Hospital (Baltimore, Maryland), 31–4
Johns Hopkins Medical School (Baltimore, Maryland), 169
Jørgensen, C. A., 133
Joseph P. Kennedy, Jr Foundation, 137
Journal of Pathology and Bacteriology, 78
Julius Klaus Foundation, 91–2
Junta de Relaciones Culturales (Spain), 130

Kahn test (syphilis), 74
Kaiser Wilhelm Institute for Biology (Berlin), 161
Kaiser-Wilhelm Institute for Anthropology, Human Heredity and Eugenics, 22, 116–17
Kälin, Joseph, 94
Kamin, Leon, 186
Karl, Adolfo, 108
karyotyping, 9, 141–4, 145–51
Kemp, Tage, 194, 199
Kevles, Daniel, 5, 47
Khanolkar, V. R., 56, 60, 64–5
King's College (Newcastle upon Tyne), 162
Kirkman, Neil, 175
Kirsch, Scott, 214
Klinefelter syndrome, 144, 146, 147
Knapp, Harold, 208, 214
Knut and Alice Wallenberg Foundation (Sweden), 131
Koumaris, Ioannis, 93
Krementsov, Nikolai, 217
Kretschmer, Ernst, 20
Kroeber, Alfred 104
Krokowski, Ernst, 117–18
Kühn, Alfred, 116
Kuhn, Thomas S., 6, 159

Laboratory for Studies in Human Variation (Bombay, India), 60, 63
Laboratory of Human Genetics (Federal University of Paraná), 60
Laemmli, Whitney, 207
Lajtha, Lazlo G., 144
Lakatos, Imre, 40
Lamarckism, 158
Landsteiner, Karl, 79
Lange, Bruno, 23
Laughlin, Harry H., 27–32, 35, 37
Laurence, William L., 117
Lawrence Livermore National Laboratory, 213
Leber's hereditary optic neuropathy, 154
Leicester, 45
Léjeune, Jérôme, 137, 145, 179
Lenz, Fritz, 198–9
leukaemia, 139, 143, 144, 224
Levan, Albert, 127, 131, 139, 142
Libby, Willard F., 213
Lilienfeld, Abraham, 221
linguistics, 67, 93–4
linkage, 80, 162
Lisker, Rubén, 103, 107–12
Lister Institute for Preventive Medicine (UK), 60, 83
Liverpool, 16
Livingstone, Frank B., 66
Logan, Cheryl, 113
Lombardy, 223–4
London, 34, 107, 110
London County Council (LCC), 43
Löwy, Ilana, 2
Ludmerer, Kenneth, 4
Lund (Sweden), 132, 136, 142
Luxenburger, Hans, 21–2
Lysenkoism, 158

Macfarlane, Robert Gwyn, 172, 176
Mackenzie, Donald, 4
MacKey, James, 131
Madrid School of Agronomy, 130
Magni, Giovanni, 218
malaria, 106, 109–11
Malling, Heinrich, 122
manic depression, 21, 188, 223
Mankind Quarterly (journal), 222
Manuila, Alexander, 93
mapping, 73, 87–9, 92, 94, 96
Marburg, 196, 198–200
Marfan's syndrome, 35–6

marriage
  laws, 64, 226
  registers, 66
mathematization, 62, 75
Mather, Kenneth, 50
Mayr, Ernst, 205
Max Planck Society, 117, 119
Max Planck Institute for Comparative and Medical Genetics, 117, 197
Mazumdar, Pauline, 4, 53
McKusick, Victor, 27, 33–7, 161
meadow saffron (*Colchicum autumnale*), 128
medical records, 23, 25, 34, 37
Medical Research Council (UK), 70–1, 73, 77–8, 83, 106, 143, 144, 148, 149
medical statistics, 17
Mendel, Gregor, 3, 61
Mendelism, 3, 6, 28, 113, 158, 169–71
  Mendelian inheritance, 3, 9, 13, 18–19, 21–2, 26, 42–4, 49, 156, 169, 176
mental disease, 20, 26
mental retardation, 182, 189, 190
Merriam, John C., 30–1
Mexico, 101–12
Microcythaemia, 218
microscope, 78, 131, 136
migration, 57, 59, 63, 68
Milan, 34, 217–18, 222, 225
military medicine, 90–2, 226
Miller, Fiona, 146
minorities (ethnic), 93, 97
Ministry for Atomic Affairs (West Germany), 118
Ministry of Health (Mexico), 105, 106, 109
Ministry of Health (UK), 71
Ministry of Health (US), 106
Ministry of Health (West Germany), 196
Ministry of Public Education (Italy) 224
Ministry of Public Education (Mexico) 105
Ministry for Scientific Research (West Germany), 120
miscegenation, 68
Misión Biológica de Galicia (Spain), 137
mitosis, 128–9, 133, 136, 139
Mittwoch, Ursula, 159
model organism, 2, 9, 24, 113, 125, 156, 173–4
model population, 21
Mohr, Jan, 159
molecular biology, 178
molecular medicine, 165
molecularization, 158, 178
Mollison, Patrick, 80
'mongols', 36
  see also Down syndrome; feebleminded
monogenic disease, 13, 22
Montalenti, Giuseppe, 217–22, 224–5, 227
Moore, Joseph E., 33
morbidity, 14
Morgan, Thomas Hunt, 161, 169, 208
Morison, Robert S., 218
Morris, Desmond, 207
mortality, 16–18, 25
Moscow Treaty, 119
mother-daughter pairs, 36
Motulsky, Arno, 3, 108, 159
Mourant, Arthur, 60, 92, 107, 110
mouse, 114, 118–22, 132, 183, 210, 211
Muller, Herman J., 158–9, 205, 207–13, 215
Müller-Wille, Staffan, 85
multi-allelic loci, 157
Munich, 34
Munich crisis, 70
Münster, 34, 197
Müntzing, Arne, 131
Murray, Charles, 187
Museum of Natural Sciences (Madrid), 137
mutagenesis tests, 118, 120–4
mutagens, chemical, 120–4
mutation, 57, 59, 62, 116, 156, 171, 190, 199–201, 208, 210–12
myotonic dystrophy, 154–5, 157
myth, 64, 66, 68

Nachtsheim, Hans, 114–20, 124–5, 197–8, 203
Nagasaki, 207, 209, 210
Naples, 218, 224
Nasse, Christian Friedrich, 167
National Academy of Sciences, 184, 214
National Council of Mental Hygiene, 44
National Institute for Genomic Medicine (Mexico), 112
National Institute of Cardiology (Mexico), 106
National Institute of Nutrition (Mexico), 106

National Institutes of Health (Bethesda, Maryland), 106, 137–8, 174
National Nuclear Energy Commission (Mexico), 107
National Polytechnic Institute (Mexico), 108
Native Americans, 61
native place, 94
National University of Mexico, 104
Nattras, F. J., 162
Nazi regime, 4–5, 10, 23–4, 57, 85, 158, 161, 193, 198, 204
Nebel, B. R., 132
Neel, James V., 61, 161, 175, 205, 207–13, 215
Neue Zürcher Zeitung, 92
Neuhäuser-Klaus, Angelika, 123
neurology, 115–16, 153, 162
New York State Agronomic Experimental Station, 132
New York City, 29, 106, 110, 135–6, 167
New Zealand, 159, 180
Newcastle Medical School, 162
Nixon, Richard, 184
nomenclature, 79–80, 82
non-Mendelian inheritance, 154
North America, 158
Novitski, Ed, 212
Nowell, Peter, 139
nuclear research, 9, 61
numerical taxonomy, 68
Nüsslein-Volhard, Christiane, 123
nutrition, 19, 40, 45, 47, 51

Oak Ridge National Laboratories (Tennessee, USA), 118–21, 205, 212
occupational groups, 17, 19
Office for Indian Affairs of the United States, 102
Ohio, 32
Oklahoma, 32
Oldenburg, 116
Olympics, 147, 151
Oppenheimer, J. Robert, 206
orcein, 131, 135
Osborn, Frederick, 29, 32, 50
Ostertag, Bernhard, 115
Otto, John Conrad, 167
Oxford, 34
oxyquinoline, 132

Panton, Philip Noël, 81
Parkinson's disease, 116
Passarge, Eberhard, 161, 196
Pathology Society (UK), 76
pathology, 175
Paul, Diane, 53
Pauling, Linus, 206
Pauly, Philip, 4
Pavia, 217–18, 224
Pearl Harbor, 211
Pearson, Karl, 15–16, 18, 43, 49, 154, 168–9
pedigree, 14–15, 19, 28, 31, 34–5, 42, 156, 169, 175, 222, 223, 224
Pemberton, Stephen, 179
penicillin, 33, 132
Penrose, Lionel, 39–40, 44–5, 47–53, 73, 144, 145, 153–63, 179, 180, 199
peripheral blood (human), 137, 139
peroneal atrophy, 154
phenogenetics, 116–17
phenol, 131–2, 135
phenylalanine, 179–2, 185, 187, 190–1
phenylketonuria, 12, 53, 179–91
phenylthiocarbamide (PTC) taste sensitivity, 62–3
Philip, Ursula, 162
physician, 26, 153–4, 162, 165–6, 168–9, 175
physiology, 169
Pius XII (Pope), 225–6
PKU *see* phenylketonuria
plant breeding, 130–1, 134, 142
plant genetics, 48
plant pathology, 73
plasma fractionation, 173
Polani, Paul, 144
polyploidy, 128–9, 133–4, 137–8
population, 57–8, 63, 66
  paradigm, 66
  records, 17
population genetics, 11, 18, 55, 57, 60–2, 67, 87, 96–7, 103, 106, 110, 149–51, 222
Population Genetics Research Unit (Oxford), 150
Population Investigation Committee, 46, 47
Post, Richard H., 95–6
Porter, Theodore, 4
Porter, William Townsend, 41–5
Portugal, 130

potato blight, 129
pregnancy, 81–2
prenatal diagnostics, 203–4
Presbyterian Hospital, New York City, 29
primitive groups, 66
Prinzing, Friedrich, 17
Prior, Eileen, 72
prophylaxis, 172, 200
psychiatry, 21, 153
Puck, Theodore T., 137, 145
Punnett, R. C., 42, 52
pure line, 61
pure race, 61
pyrogallol, 133

rabbit, 24, 114–17, 119
race, 4, 10–11, 56–7, 61, 64–5, 66, 85–7, 91–2, 95–9, 104, 185
Race, Robert, 72, 80, 83
racial hygiene, 4, 107, 193, 196, 198
radiation, 4, 9, 61, 139, 142–5, 150, 151, 205–15
  radiation genetics, 9, 120, 209, 219
  risk, 117, 205, 209, 213–15
radiographs, 23, 26
radioisotopes, 117
Ramey, James T., 213
random mating, 42, 60, 77
rat, 114, 121, 132
Real Academia de Ciencias Exactas, Físicas y Naturales (Spain), 137
Reardon, Jenny, 85
recombination, 80
Red (Soviet) Army, 117
Red Cross, 92
Reed, Sheldon C., 32, 194, 195
Regional Blood Transfusion Service (UK), 75
Reiche, Franz, 18
Renwick, Chris, 5
Renwick, James, 159
representativeness, 16, 19
reproductive barrier, 58
reproductive community, 58
reproductive isolation, 66–7
Revolution (Mexico), 101–6, 110
Rhesus blood groups, 79–81
Riffel, Alexander, 14, 19
Río, Pablo Martínez del, 104, 105, 107, 110
risk determination, 15, 20, 118, 121, 123, 171, 196, 198
risk group, 12, 190, 195, 200
Ritter, Horst, 199–200
Robert Koch Institute, 23
Rockefeller Foundation, 29, 60, 70, 83, 158–9, 161, 218
Roelcke, Volker, 86
Romansh, 62
Rome, 34, 220, 225
Rosal, Corona del, 107
Rosenberg, Charles, 5
Rosewood State Training School, 36
Rosin, Siegfried, 87, 90–2, 94–9
Rothamsted Experimental Station (UK), 69, 73, 76, 82
Royal Agricultural and Veterinary College (Copenhagen, Denmark), 133
Royal Eastern Counties Institution for Mental Defectives (Colchester, UK), 44
Royal Veterinary and Agricultural College (Copenhagen, Denmark), 130
Royal Commission on Population, 46
Royce, Kenneth, 149
Rüdin, Edith, 159
Rüdin, Ernst, 21
Russell, Liane, 118, 120
Russell, William, 118, 120–3
rye (*Secale*), 129, 133–4

Salazar-Mallén, Manuel, 103, 106, 107, 108
sampling, 18
sanatorium, 16
Sánchez-Monge, Enrique, 127–35
Sanger, R., 107
Sanghvi, L. D., 56, 60, 62, 63–5
Sapir, Edward, 104
Sardinia, 221
Scandinavia, 203
Schinz, Hans R., 90
schizophrenia, 21–2, 53
Schlaginhaufen, Otto, 86, 90–1, 95, 99
School of Agronomy (Bogor, Indonesia), 129
Schull, William J., 208
Schütz, Alfred, 91, 95
Scossiroli, Renzo, 218
Scotland, 76
Scottish Mental Survey, 40, 45–7, 49

Scottish Council for Research in Education, 46
screening, 24, 146–50, 152, 180–5, 189
Scriver, Charles, 182
Saénz, Moisés, 102, 104
Segni, Antonio, 224
selection bias, 20, 21, 154–5, 157, 161
selection (natural), 97, 201
Semendeferi, Ionna, 213
serology, 8, 56–7, 60, 71, 76–7
sex hormones, 171–2
sex-linked inheritance, 169–1, 173, 176
Shebeski, Leonard H., 135
sickle cell anaemia, 48, 53, 184
Siemens, Hermann W., 20
Silvestri, Luigi, 217
Silvestroni, Ezio, 218
Simpson, Barbara, 73, 75, 77
Singer, Karl, 108
Slavs, 93
slide (microscopy), 131, 136
Sloan-Kettering Institute (New York), 135
Smith, Cedric, 162
Snyder, Laurence, 51
social medicine, 5, 13
sociobiology, 187, 190
sociology, 66–7
Solanum, 129
Spain, 132, 134, 137
Spanish Civil War, 70, 134
Spearman, Charles, 43
spouse method, 17
St Thomas's Hospital (London), 78
Staimer, Georg, 120
staining (microscopy), 131, 135
statistics, 6–7, 14, 18, 20, 21, 23–4, 25, 74, 77, 83, 95, 154, 158, 161–2, 218
  correlation, 16, 41, 43, 45, 48, 52, 54, 155–7
stature (height), 40–5, 47, 49, 51–4
Stein, Zena, 47
sterilization, 24, 49, 50, 53, 198, 203, 226
Stern, Curt, 159, 161, 212
Stevenson, Alan, 150
Stiftung für das behinderte Kind (German Foundation), 197
Stiftung Rehabilitation (German Foundation), 197
stigma, 20
Stockholm, 220, 221
Strandskov, Herluf H., 58
Strong, John A. 144
Stuttgart, 16
Sturtevant, Alfred, 212
surveillance, 16, 24
survey, 17, 23, 39, 40, 44, 45–7, 75
Susi, Ada, 180, 185
Susser, Mervyn, 47
Svalöf (Sweden), 127, 130
Swadesh, Morris, 109
Sweden, 127, 130–1
Swedish Association for Seed Improvement, 130
Swiss National Science Foundation, 92, 94
Switzerland, 61–2, 86–7, 90–9
syphilis, 33, 74
syringomyelia, 115

Tay-Sachs disease, 184
Taylor, George, 69, 71, 74, 76, 78–80, 83
Teller, Edward, 206
testing, 9, 12, 22
Texas, 32
textbook, 82, 159–60
therapeutics, 170, 178
Tierney, Patrick, 209
Tiger, Lionel, 207
Tipper, George, 72
tissue
  culture, 136
  human, 136–7
Tjio, Joe Hin, 127–35, 142, 144
Thomson, Godfrey, 46
toxicity, 139
toxicogenetics, 120–3
transfusion medicine, 169, 177
transnational research, 59, 66, 127, 134
Triticale, 129, 133–5
tuberculosis, 13–26
  care stations, 16, 20, 22–5
  sanatorium, 16, 20, 22–3
  susceptibility to, 22, 24–5
Turner syndrome, 144, 146, 147
Turpin, Raymond, 144
twin studies, 22–5
typology, 20

unit character, 9
United Nations Educational, Scientific and Cultural Organization (UNESCO), 57, 85–6, 222, 227
United Nations Scientific Committee on the Effects of Atomic Radiation (UNSCEAR), 121, 210
US Environmental Protection Agency (EPA), 121
University College London, 42, 43, 47, 60, 69–70, 73, 77, 144
  Galton Chair of Eugenics, 42, 153–4, 159
  Galton Laboratory for National Eugenics, 154–5, 159, 162, 168
  Galton Serological Laboratory, 72, 73, 83
University of Bonn (Germany), 167
University of California, Berkeley, 212
University of Cambridge (UK), 70
  Department of Pathology, 72
  Galton Serum Unit, 69–70, 73–4, 76–8, 80, 82
University of Colorado Medical Center, 137
University of Copenhagen, 210
University of Illinois, 171
University of Madrid
  Faculty of Science, 137
  Medical School, 137
  School of Agronomy, 137
University of Manitoba, Winnipeg
  Faculty of Agriculture, 135
University of Pennsylvania, 207
  Department of Pathology, 139
University of North Carolina, 32, 173–4
University of Rochester (New York), 161
Utah, 32

Vatican, 219, 228
Vaughan, Janet, 70–3, 75–6, 78–9, 81
Vega, Jimena Fernández de la, 137
Verschuer, Otmar von, 22–5, 197
Viking conquest, 76
Virginia, 35
Visconti di Modrone, Niccolò, 217
visualization, 129, 136, 139, 155–6
Vogel, Friedrich, 3, 120, 196, 199, 201–2

Wailoo, Keith, 179
Wales, 76
Waller, John, 5
Walser (Swiss ethnic minority), 62, 91, 97
Walton, John (Baron Walton of Detchant), 162
Washington, DC, 30, 35, 137
Washington University, 189
Waterston, Robert, 189
Watson, James D., 188, 207
Weinberg, Alvin, 118
Weinberg, Wilhelm, 15–18, 21, 76
Weindling, Paul, 5
Weber, Max, 205
Wendt, Gerhardt, 196–8, 201, 203
Werner syndrome, 35
West, Samuel Stewart, 215
Western General Hospital (UK), 144
wheat (*Triticum*), 129, 131–4
Whitby, Lionel, 79
Wiener, Alexander, 79–80, 107
Wilson, E. O., 207
Die Woche (Swiss newspaper), 92
Worcester (Massachusetts), 43
working class, 16
World Health Organization (WHO), 12, 66, 67, 120, 150–1, 195, 210–12, 215
World War I, 2, 93, 95, 168–9
World War II, 4, 6, 13, 27, 32, 36, 66, 70, 83, 90, 102, 103, 105, 106, 108, 110, 111, 134, 141, 142, 153, 166, 177, 193
Wragge, Bernhard, 116
Württemberg, 17

X-rays, 132–3

Young, Hugh, 33

Zapata, Emiliano, 103
Zaragoza, 127, 130
Zeitschrift für induktive Abstammungs- und Vererbungslehre, 116
Zeitschrift für Rassenphysiologie, 75
Zepeda, J. Preciado, 107
Zulueta, Antonio de, 137
Zurich Society for Blood Group Research, 90–1

Milton Keynes UK
Ingram Content Group UK Ltd.
UKHW031144141024
449569UK00024B/1096

9 781138 662292